FOUNDATIONS OF MODERN BIOCHEMISTRY SERIES

Lowell Hager and Finn Wold, editors

ORGANIC CHEMISTRY OF BIOLOGICAL COMPOUNDS*
Robert Barker

INTERMEDIARY METABOLISM AND ITS REGULATION
Joseph Larner

PHYSICAL BIOCHEMISTRY
Kensal Edward Van Holde

MACROMOLECULES: STRUCTURE AND FUNCTION
Finn Wold

SPECIAL TOPICS:

BIOCHEMICAL ENDOCRINOLOGY OF THE VERTEBRATES
Earl Frieden and Harry Lipner

* Published jointly in Prentice-Hall's *Foundations of Modern Organic Chemistry Series.*

PRENTICE-HALL INTERNATIONAL, INC., *London*
PRENTICE-HALL OF AUSTRALIA, PTY. LTD., *Sydney*
PRENTICE-HALL OF CANADA, LTD., *Toronto*
PRENTICE-HALL OF INDIA PRIVATE LIMITED, *New Delhi*
PRENTICE-HALL OF JAPAN, INC., *Tokyo*

INTERMEDIARY METABOLISM AND ITS REGULATION

JOSEPH LARNER

Professor of Pharmacology
University of Virginia

Prentice-Hall, Inc., Englewood Cliffs, New Jersey

To FRAN, ANDY, JIMMY, and PAUL

and to WELLFLEET, MASSACHUSETTS
where most of the writing was done

Current printing (last digit)

10 9 8 7 6 5 4 3 2 1

Library of Congress
Catalog Card No. 70-172888

13-470658-7 (C)

13-470641-2 (P)

Printed in the United States of America

FOREWORD

Biochemistry has been and still is the major meeting place for biological and physical sciences, and most introductory courses in biochemistry have a rather unique and heterogeneous population of advanced students from all branches of the natural sciences. Such courses, therefore, have equally unique and heterogeneous requirements for background material and textbooks. The content of a first-year course in biochemistry based on two years of chemistry and biology would probably not be too difficult to define, but to write a single text which contains the needed material for all students becomes a much more controversial issue. As a solution to this dilemma, presenting the material in several packages offers some interesting possibilities. Without in any way compromising the basic content, such a multivolume text should above all allow for a great deal of flexibility: flexibility for the student to supplement previous experience with only the parts which represent new and unique features; flexibility for the instructor to offer a course covering an area of modern biochemistry with something less than the comprehensive text; and the flexibility to keep a text current by rewriting any outdated part without having to reject the whole text.

These thoughts were fundamental in formulating the Foundations of Modern Biochemistry series. So was the philosophy that a major purpose of a textbook is perhaps not so much to be encyclopedic as to select for the student the important principles and to illustrate and explain these in some depth. With this basic plan in mind, the next step was to divide the whole into logical subdivisions or parts. The science of biochemistry seeks the answer to three basic questions:

1. What is the nature of the molecules and structures found in living cells?
2. What is the biological function of these molecules and structures?
3. How are they synthesized (and broken down) in the cell?

These questions were adopted as the basis for the division of this text. The first question, related to the qualitative and quantitative characterization of the biochemical world and to the methods available for structural analysis, is covered in two books: *Organic Chemistry of Biological Compounds* and *Physical Biochemistry*. The second question, concerning the elucidation of the biological function of these molecules, is discussed in *Macromolecules: Structure and Function*. The third question, covering all aspects of intermediate metabolism and metabolic regulation, is considered in *Intermediary Metabolism and Its Regulation*. As the work on the individual books progressed, it became apparent that this subdivision had one unexpected advantage; namely that the physical presentation of material as diversified as the mathematical derivations in physical chemistry, the many structures of organic chemistry, and the long and complicated road maps of intermediate metabolism can be handled much more rationally in the individual format of separate books than in a single volume.

Thus, the Foundations of Modern Biochemistry series came into being consisting of four *individual* books. The books can hopefully be used either separately or in any combination to meet the requirements of the individual student according to his particular background and goals. The absence of a numbered sequence represents a deliberate effort to emphasize that the books can be used in any order. The integration of the four parts into the total program is done by extensive cross-references between the individual books. Trying to retain the individuality and utility of the separate books and at the same time aiming for an integrated program required some compromises in the selection and distribution of the material to be covered. Quite expectedly, the main price paid for this dual purpose has turned out to be some duplication, which hopefully is not extensive enough to become a serious flaw.

In arriving at the definition of the Foundations of Modern Biochemistry content and at the philosophy represented by this set of books, the thinking of the "editorial board" (the four authors and Dr. Lowell P. Hager) underwent an extensive evolution. The evolutionary pressures were graciously, patiently, and sometimes even enthusiastically provided by colleagues, by the publishers, and most importantly by students, too many to mention individually. To all of these good people we express our sincere thanks.

FINN WOLD

CONTENTS

|| # INTRODUCTION

Our starting point may be considered to be the cell. The *cell* is the unit of life and by definition successfully solves all the problems that must be solved for life to exist. What are the problems? What are the solutions?

The problems are twofold: *maintenance* of the living state and *reproduction*, providing a faithful copy for the next generation. Reproduction leads directly into *growth and development*, the transformation of the young into the adult.

The cell meets both types of challenges with solutions which are extraordinary in their utter and beautiful precision. Nothing has been left unconsidered.

Reproduction, growth, and development require that the information stored in the adult cell be copied accurately. The copied information serves then as a set of instructions faithfully followed to construct all of the cellular components. The new young cell grows and develops into its final distinctive state. The energy considerations are shown in Figure 1.1. In this situation, a constantly increasing energy input is required to maintain controlled growth and development until the maintenance state is achieved.

Maintenance of the living state in terms of energy is something like walking on the edge of an energy precipice (Figure 1.1). On the one side is the chasm represented by increased entropy (increased randomness), the exergonic state which occurs at cell death. On the other side is the hill representing increased energy input, leading to controlled or uncontrolled growth and

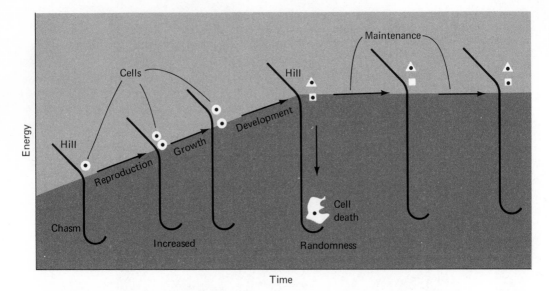

Figure 1.1   Energy pathway of cell reproduction and maintenance. The hill represents
the energy imput required for reproduction, growth, and development leading to the maintenance state. The chasm represents the exergonic state with
increased entropy and cell death.

development. The problem is to maintain motion along the defined ener-
getic pathway at the edge without deviating.

The *energy balance* in the maintenance state is required for life; and all
life is involved in, and dependent on, an *energy flow*. The energy flow has
the sun as its source and light from the sun is captured by green plants and
certain microorganisms by means of pigments which absorb the energy and
channel it into the synthesis of cellular constituents. This process is termed
photosynthesis, and the captured solar energy is stored as chemical energy
principally in the form of carbohydrate. During photosynthesis, part of the
light energy is converted directly into another form of chemical energy,
namely, adenosine triphosphate, ATP

This form of energy can be used to drive a large number of energy-requiring processes in the cell and is used for that purpose by most cells. The majority of biological systems, that is, those which cannot carry out photosynthesis, depend upon a supply of degradable materials from which they can obtain energy in the form of ATP. There is a flow of material through the cell from which energy is derived and utilized for growth or maintenance (Figure 1.2). These processes require that gases such as oxygen, nitrogen, and carbon dioxide and *required* nutrients such as minerals and vitamins be taken into the cell through the cell membrane, and pass from one subcellular site to another to be *converted to products,* or to *serve a catalytic role* in the conversion reactions. Products are either stored, utilized in cellular processes, or passed out of the cell through the cell membrane in the reverse direction. Passage through the membrane may be either *passive,* that is, diffusion-controlled, or *active,* that is, uphill against a concentration gradient. Usually, even with diffusion-controlled processes, there is some selectivity with regard to the chemical nature of the materials which pass across the membrane.

Before continuing with a general discussion of the energy flow that is required for life, a brief consideration of the kinds of chemical compounds that are the constituents of living cells and the precursor materials that can be used for their synthesis is in order. The five main classes of materials are listed in Table 1.1 and include proteins, carbohydrates, lipids, nucleic acids and inorganic materials. An indication is given of the precursors for their syn-

TABLE 1.1 THE MAJOR CONSTITUENTS OF LIVING SYSTEMS, FUNCTION, AND PRECURSORS

Class	Function	Precursors	
		In Higher Forms	In Simple Forms
Proteins	Catalysts in all chemical reactions; structural integrity of all cell organelles	Some twenty amino acids, carbohydrates, lipids	Carbon dioxide, nitrogen or nitrates
Carbohydrates (polysaccharides)	As polymers, structural components; storage of energy; recognition function	Monosaccharides, amino acids	Carbon dioxide, water
Lipids	As components of membranes; storage of energy	Fatty acids, monosaccharides, amino acids	Carbon dioxide
Nucleic acids	Genetic information storage; regulation of growth and development	Monosaccharides, amino acids	Carbon dioxide, water, nitrogen or nitrate, carbohydrate, amino acids
Inorganic materials	Many cell functions, movement, catalysis, structural role; as ions Ca^{2+}, HPO_4^{2-}	As ions and organic derivatives	

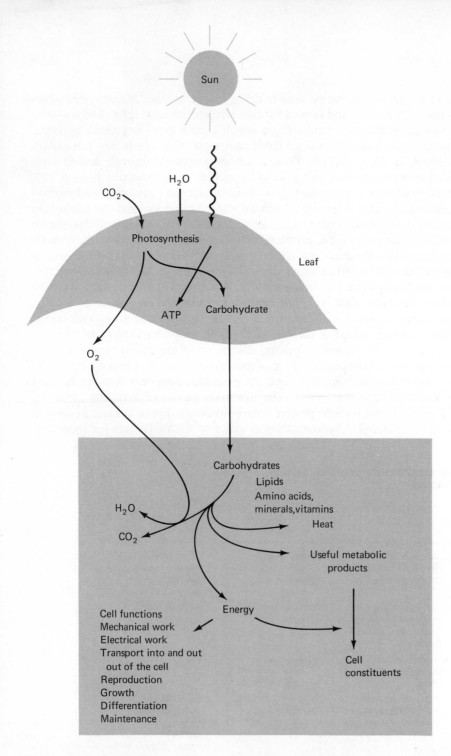

Figure 1.2 The cellular energy flow. Energy from the sun is converted to carbohydrate and ATP by photosynthesis. Carbohydrates and other cellularly synthesized constituents such as lipids and amino acids are combusted by the cell to provide energy as heat or to drive cellular processes as listed.

4

thesis in cells of higher life forms, such as the mammals, and in simpler forms, such as the bacteria. The five classes, with the exception of the inorganic ions, exist in cells in very complex forms, many of which are very large molecules with molecular weights ranging to the millions. Since most cell membranes, under ordinary circumstances, are permeable to molecules having molecular weights below a few hundred daltons (the *dalton* is the unit of atomic and molecular weight) and having relatively few charged groups, the synthesis of large, charged polymers within the cell depends upon the availability of low-molecular-weight precursors, their transport into the cell, their conversion to a suitable form for polymerization, and finally their condensation into the polymer. Table 1.2 lists the nutritional requirements of the human. In addition to the vitamins, a number of organic compounds including amino acids, polyunsaturated fatty acids, as well as inorganic materials are essential or probably essential for life.

TABLE 1.2   HUMAN NUTRITIONAL REQUIREMENTS[e]

Amino Acids	Elements	Vitamins
Established as Essential		
Isoleucine	Calcium	Ascorbic acid
Leucine	Chlorine	Choline[b]
Lysine	Copper	Folic acid
Methionine	Iodine	Niacine[c]
Phenylalanine	Iron	Pyridoxine
Threonine	Magnesium	Riboflavin
Tryptophan	Manganese	Thiamine
Valine	Phosphorus	Vitamine B_{12}
	Potassium	Vitamins A, D[d], E, K
	Sodium	
Probably Essential		
Arginine[a]	Fluorine	Biotin
Histidine[a]	Molybdenum	Panthothenic acid
	Selenium	Polyunsaturated fatty acids
	Zinc	

[a] Probably required for growth of children.
[b] Met by adequate dietary methionine.
[c] Met by synthesis from adequate dietary tryptophan.
[d] Met by exposure to sunlight in children. No evidence for a requirement in adults.
[e] From White, A., Handler, P., and Smith, E. W., *Principles of Biochemistry*, 4th edition, New York: McGraw-Hill Book Company, 1968, with permission.

Metabolism consists of the sum of all of the reactions concerned with the biosynthesis or *anabolism* and degradation or *catabolism* of cell constituents.

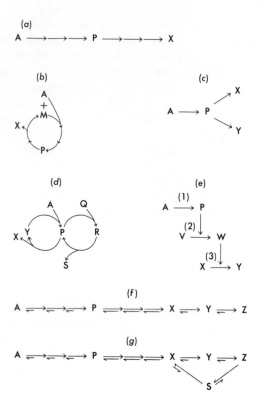

Figure 1.3

The forms of metabolic pathways. (a) linear; (b) cyclic; (c) branched; (d) two interlocking cycles; (e) tiered or layered; (f) directly reversible; and (g) indirectly reversible (the size of the arrows indicates roughly the extent of reversibility at each separate step).

Essentially all of the thousand or so separate reactions that occur in a metabolizing living cell are catalyzed by enzymes—even those associated with the *entry and exit* processes (see F. Wold's book in this series, Chapters 9 and 10 for a discussion of these processes). Since metabolism is chiefly intracellular in location, the movement of metabolites through various membranes within the cell itself as well as into and out of the cell is of great importance in maintaining its energy balance.

The pathways of biosynthesis and of degradation are varied in their arrangements. Some are linear [Figure 1.3(a)], with each enzyme-catalyzed reaction producing a product which serves as the substrate for the next reaction. Cyclic pathways [Figure 1.3(b)] require that the starting material A be carried through the cycle by a substance M and that each turn of the cycle regenerates M, which serves a "catalytic" role in the overall sequence. There are also more complex patterns, which include branching points [Figure 1.3(c)], and two (or more) interlocking cycles [Figure 1.3(d)] in which precursors A and Q form products X and S, respectively; here P is the common intermediate and is formed from either Y or R. There are tiered or layered hierarchical arrangements [Figure 1.3(e)] in which P, produced in the first reaction (1) serves to stimulate the conversion of V to W in the second reaction (2), and so on. This type of arrangement is commonly found when a rapid build-up of the end product Y is needed. Since P is a catalyst for formation of W, which in turn catalyzes the formation of Y, the overall process can also serve to *amplify* an event which stimulates the initial reaction. Reversibility of pathways may be direct [Figure 1.3(f)] or may not be direct [Figure 1.3(g)]. The presence of starting material A and a set of catalysts for its conversion to Z provides the cell with a useful product, but it also presents the cell with the problem of controlling the process. The demands of the cell for any product vary with time and its survival depends upon the *regulation* of all of the processes of which it is capable to produce the balance of events that constitute life.

It is extraordinary to consider how closely defined are the limits of life in terms of temperature, pH, degree of hydration, pressure, etc. Controls are exerted at several levels and by several mechanisms, all of which are related to the control of the activity of various catalytic and transport systems, including enzymes. Controls may be intrinsic and represent responses to the changes in the levels of *metabolites* (intermediates or products) in the metabolic process itself. This regulation is termed *nonhormonal control.* Other controls are imposed on metabolism by means of glandular secretions (hormones) and are extrinsic or *hormonal* controls; they are characteristic of multicellular and multiorgan life forms. Indeed, only by a wide variety of control mechanisms can a truly "fine" or graded control be achieved.

These general processes are used to solve the problems of the mature cell. In another volume of this series (Wold) the transfer of information in reproduction, growth, and development through the biosynthesis of informational polymers is discussed.

The fact that an organism must maintain an energy balance to continue living, even though it has reached maturation, leads directly to the conclusion that the organism must simultaneously maintain a *material balance.* It is taking in foodstuffs for energy, repair and maintenance and excreting wastes. It must therefore excrete as many of each kind of atom as it takes in or it will fall out of balance. It will become fatter or thinner depending upon which way its material balance is upset. The concept of the existence of a material balance leads directly into a consideration of nutrition and nutritional requirements. What are the minimum requirements for the material balance present during the maintenance phase? What are the minimum requirements for the altered balance of reproduction, growth, and development? In a similar vein, what are the minimum lethal tolerances for various toxic materials which are polluting land, sea, and air?

Metabolism presents interesting questions and problems to many disciplines. Questions concerning the chemistry of the intermediates in the reactions, the mechanisms of the transformations, are of great interest to the organic chemist. These questions are discussed in another volume of this series by R. Barker. To the physical chemist, the questions of the energetics, the considerations of the kinetics, the processes of transport and diffusion through cell membranes as model systems are of great interest. Also the physical chemistry of the macromolecules of biology are of great importance. These topics are discussed in another volume of this series by K. E. Van Holde. For the chemical engineer, there are similar interests, as well as interests concerned with the systems analysis of control mechanisms. Using available data coupled with computer techniques, the chemical engineer is also interested in providing integrated models of living systems.

For the physician and medical scientist, the questions concerned with the alterations in metabolism brought on by disease states are of primary concern. It is perhaps pertinent to point out that for each enzyme-catalyzed reaction, there is theoretically one or more genetically controlled disease states in which the enzyme is deficient or absent. In addition to all of the above aspects, the biochemist is concerned with metabolism and its control from the point of view of the relationship between the simplified systems studied in the test tube (in vitro) (literally in glass) and events in the living cell (in vivo) (literally in life). What is the *quantitative* significance of an in vitro reaction to the in vivo process? What is the directionality of a reaction in vivo which is reversible in vitro? When there are more than one set of pathways known in vitro, how is the metabolic flow apportioned through these pathways in vivo? By what approaches and techniques may these questions be answered? We may now define the study of metabolism in terms of an ultimate goal. This would be the complete understanding of all *reactions* of living cells from all points of view including their interactions and interdependence with *control* systems in normal and diseased states, so that a complete understanding of the higher ordered in vivo relationships at the physiologic level can be attained.

The present volume deals with metabolism and its control or regulation from a biochemical point of view. The methods and systems used to work out the ordering of the reactions of metabolic pathways are described first; the energy balance is considered and the "burning" of the metabolic fuels, the carbohydrates and the lipids, is presented as flow diagrams and discussed in terms of reaction types, thermodynamics, reaction (enzyme) location within the cell, organ distribution, and physiologic significance. The metabolism of the N-containing components follows next, with presentation and discussion along similar lines.

The control of metabolism is introduced by a consideration of the problem of translating results obtained in vitro to the in vivo system. A general discussion of control mechanisms together with a discussion of approaches and techniques used to establish these mechanisms follows and the control of the metabolism of the metabolic fuels, the N-containing compounds, and the energy cycle is next. Finally the control of the energy cycle by metabolites and the control of metabolism by components of the energy cycle unify the regulation of all of metabolism.

APPROACHES USED TO DELINEATE METABOLIC PATHWAYS

TWO

Let us begin our discussion of metabolism by asking the following questions: How were the thousand or so reactions which make up the total metabolism identified? How were they ordered into the sequences, cycles, and interlocking networks which constitute the metabolic "roadmaps" of today? This was accomplished by a variety of experimental approaches. In this chapter we will examine several specific techniques, and the in vivo-in vitro "chain" of approaches developed to answer these questions.

In general, the larger metabolic sequences were first established by studies of the conversion of *precursor* to *product,* according to the rules of a *material balance.* These were in turn broken down to smaller component parts, and finally into individual reactions. Inherent in these studies was the idea of the catalytic nature of the reactions. A complete chain of biochemical systems was developed starting with the whole animal or plant on the one end capable of carrying out a complete conversion and ending with the homogeneous enzyme at the other, capable of catalyzing a single step in the sequence. The organ, slice, single cell, homogenate and extract each occupy intermediate positions in the experimental development.

The historical roots of our understanding of metabolism can be traced to studies of digestion, putrefaction, and fermentation. *Digestion*, originally defined as the breaking down of organic material by organic juices, was the subject of elegant experimentation by Reaumur (1752) and Spallanzani (1783). Reaumur trained a pet kite to swallow sponges, which were indigestible and soon regurgitated. The gastric juice squeezed from the sponges was shown to dissolve meat. Spallanzani himself swallowed bits of bread and meat sewn in linen bags. After passing through the intestine, the bags were recovered intact, but the bread and meat were dissolved. It came to be appreciated that stomach secretions played a very important role in this process.

2.1 PRECURSOR-PRODUCT, AND MATERIAL BALANCE RELATIONSHIPS

The conversion of precursor to product by the action of a catalyst was demonstrated by Kirchhoff (1815), who showed that when starch was heated with acid it dissolved and was converted to sugar. In the process, there was *no loss* of acid. Dubrunfaut (1830) soon showed that an extract of malt could catalyze the same reaction. Just three years later, Payen and Persoz successfully accomplished the first enzyme isolation when they precipitated the active amylase enzyme from the malt extract with alcohol, obtaining the enzyme as a dry powder, a truly great achievement. The digestion of starch by the juices of saliva was also soon demonstrated by Leuchs (1831). Shortly thereafter, the two meat-liquifying enzymes were identified, pepsin by Schwann (1836) and trypsin by Corvisart (1856). By these studies, it became appreciated that similar chemical reactions took place in the test tube or under milder conditions in the gastrointestinal tract. Complex insoluble materials were transformed into soluble products. Catalysts, either acid or enzymes which themselves were not destroyed, accelerated these reactions.

Studies of *putrefaction* (formation of foul-smelling substances from organic materials) and especially of *fermentation* (formation of gases from organic materials) laid the foundations of the material balance approach, and emphasized the importance of catalysis. It was demonstrated, for example, that in fermentation of sugar by yeast, all of the carbon could be accounted for by the products CO_2 and alcohol.

$$C_6H_{12}O_6 \longrightarrow 2CO_2 + 2C_2H_5OH \tag{1}$$

Carbon was thus neither formed nor lost in the process, *but was changed from one form to another*. The problem was thus chemically defined, and the question, "By what process is precursor totally converted to product(s)?", could be asked.

The studies of Claude Bernard (1848) deserve mention because he pioneered some important techniques for the study of metabolism. Knowing that sugar, the product, was formed by the liver and secreted into the blood stream, he asked, "What is the nature of the sugar-forming substance in the liver?" Having shown, with a sound analytical method, that sugar is present in the livers of animals, Bernard began to examine the amount of sugar in the liver under a variety of conditions. Large variations were found, clearly *not* analytical in origin. *The results could not be averaged.* Carefully examining all of the experimental conditions, he found the answer in the element of time. If the liver were analyzed immediately after death, there was little sugar. If the liver were analyzed 24 hours after death, large amounts were present. Bernard, with great experimental elegance, injected a current of cold water forcibly through the hepatic vessels of an animal immediately after death to wash the liver completely free of sugar. If the liver were kept warm for a few hours and the experiment repeated, sugar reappeared in the wash water. This was in essence a liver perfusion (see Section 2.6). It demonstrated that the liver produced sugar after death, as it did in the living animal. Armed with this discovery, Bernard proceeded to isolate the polymeric material, glycogen, from the liver and to show that an enzyme system in liver converted it to sugar, similar to the conversion of starch to sugar by plant extracts and by salivary juices.

From these early experiments, the concepts of the transformations of precursors to products, material balance, and the fundamental role of catalysts in these transformations of organic matter came to be appreciated.

2.2 THE USE OF MARKERS AND TRACERS

The concept of using a marker which is fixed chemically to the precursor to trace its conversion to product is an extremely important technique. In spite of its early origin, it has been increasingly refined over the years and is still widely used. Knoop's studies (1904) with ω-phenyl-substituted fatty acids provide a classic example of the early approach. When ω-phenyl fatty acids are fed to dogs, their metabolism could be studied by following the urinary excretion of marked products. For example, when ω-phenyl-marked *even* carbon chain fatty acids are given, phenylacetic acid

$$\phi-\overset{\displaystyle H}{\underset{\displaystyle H}{C}}-\overset{\displaystyle H}{\underset{\displaystyle H}{C}}-\overset{\displaystyle H}{\underset{\displaystyle H}{C}}-COOH \longrightarrow \phi-\overset{\displaystyle H}{\underset{\displaystyle H}{C}}-COOH \qquad (2)$$

phenylacetic acid

is the oxidation product. It is converted in the liver to its glycine conjugate, phenylaceturic acid,

$$\phi-\underset{\underset{H}{|}}{\overset{\overset{H}{|}}{C}}-COOH + H_2N-\underset{\underset{H}{|}}{\overset{\overset{H}{|}}{C}}-COOH \longrightarrow \phi-\underset{\underset{H}{|}}{\overset{\overset{H}{|}}{C}}-\overset{\overset{O}{\|}}{C}-N-\underset{\underset{H}{|}}{\overset{\overset{H}{|}}{C}}-COOH \qquad (3)$$

phenylaceturic acid

which is excreted by the kidney and can be isolated from the urine. When ω-phenyl-marked *odd* carbon chain fatty acids are given,

$$\phi-\underset{\underset{H}{|}}{\overset{\overset{H}{|}}{C}}-\underset{\underset{H}{|}}{\overset{\overset{H}{|}}{C}}-COOH \longrightarrow \phi-COOH \qquad (4)$$

benzoic acid

benzoic acid is formed in the liver, similarly converted to hippuric acid

$$\phi-COOH + H_2N-\underset{\underset{H}{|}}{\overset{\overset{H}{|}}{C}}-COOH \longrightarrow \phi-\overset{\overset{O}{\|}}{C}-\overset{H}{N}-\underset{\underset{H}{|}}{\overset{\overset{H}{|}}{C}}-COOH \qquad (5)$$

hippuric acid

and excreted by the kidney, and it can be isolated from the urine. Knoop, from these experiments, correctly deduced that fatty acids were oxidized into two-carbon fragments.

The use of radioactive or stable heavy isotopic tracers whose distribution can be followed by *physical* (*not chemical*) methods represents a more sophisticated application of the labeling technique. In principle, labeled molecules (in contrast to marked molecules) are metabolically indistinguishable from nonlabeled ones. Hevesy and his coworkers pioneered in this work. Their experiments demonstrated that an isotopic tracer such as radioactive phosphate was very rapidly distributed into all parts of the body. Schoenheimer further developed the approach and used deuterium (^2H) and heavy nitrogen (^{15}N). He and his coworkers traced these heavy atoms into a wide variety of hydrogen- and nitrogen-containing compounds in cells and organs. It was concluded that macromolecules such as proteins and nucleic acids, as well as lipids, cholesterol, and a number of nitrogen-containing compounds, are constantly involved in chemical reactions in which they are broken down to and resynthesized from smaller fragments. The concept of the turnover of the body constituents" arose. This meant that the molecules of living matter were constantly being broken down and regenerated without an increase in mass.

For example, when a diet of bread and water (enriched in D_2O), was fed to mice, deuterium became incorporated into the newly synthesized fatty acids. When the time course of the synthesis was studied, a *half-time* (time to achieve half maximal synthesis) of several days was demonstrated. To study the reverse process (the degradation of fatty acids), mice were prefed a diet containing deuterated fat, which was then replaced with bread and water (H_2O). The deuterium isotope in the fatty acids decreased with time at a rate almost identical to that observed for synthesis. Based on the concept of the living cell as a combustion engine, the idea had arisen over the years of two *separate* types of metabolism, one exogenous and degradative (catabolism), the combustion of fuel to waste products, and the other endogenous and synthetic (anabolism), the maintenance of the engine. Since there was in fact a rapid and complete mixing of dietary constituents and metabolic breakdown products into a common mixed "pool" with no *de facto* segregation, this idea was no longer tenable. In Appendix Table A.1 some of the important heavy atom and radioactive tracers used in metabolic studies are listed.

The early experiments with tracers allowed the dissection of metabolism in broad categories. Recent refinements have allowed an even finer dissection. Several examples will be described.

In the conversion of precursor A to product X, for example, the question of whether P is an intermediate arises. To test this possibility, labeled A* is administered and, after a suitable reaction time, unlabeled P is added in large amount

$$A^* \longrightarrow P^* \longrightarrow X^* \atop {\uparrow \atop P}$$

(6)

It acts as a carrier for labeled P* formed in the reaction. Added P is then isolated, rigorously purified, and its radioactivity or heavy isotope content determined. The presence of label demonstrates that P* is indeed an intermediate. This technique is termed *isotopic trapping*.

Reverse isotopic trapping can be used to test for the presence of more than one pathway leading to a specific product. Labeled A* is administered over a time period rather than as a single dose. The extent of synthesis of product X from *unlabeled* precursors which may be A or some other material can be followed by measuring the proportion of label in the product X* (its specific activity) and comparing it to the A* administered. The term *specific activity* is an important one; it refers to the amount of activity per unit mass of material. For radioactive materials it is expressed as the number of nuclear disintegrations occurring per minute per mole of compound. Consider that X is synthesized from A in two different sites in the body, site 1 and site 2. One may ask, is the X formed from A in these two sites from a common A pool

$$
\begin{array}{lll}
A^* \longrightarrow X^* & \quad\text{Site 1} \\
\big\Updownarrow & & \quad\quad\quad\quad\quad\quad (7) \\
A \longrightarrow X^* & \quad\text{Site 2}
\end{array}
$$

or from two pools not in equilibrium with each other

$$
\begin{array}{lll}
A^* \longrightarrow X^* & \quad\text{Site 1} \\
A \longrightarrow X & \quad\text{Site 2} & \quad (8)
\end{array}
$$

In the former case, the increase of label in X^* will occur at the same rate in sites 1 and 2; in the latter case, it will increase at two different rates in the two sites, infinitely faster at site 1 than at site 2.

Overloading techniques have proved of great importance in defining metabolic pathways. For example, in the question posed above, "Is P an intermediate in the $A \to P \to X$ pathway?", the following experiment can be performed: Labeled A^{**} is administered in one experiment alone.

$$
A^{**} \longrightarrow P^{**} \longrightarrow X^{**} \qquad\qquad\qquad (9)
$$

and in a second experiment,

$$
\begin{array}{l}
A^{**} \longrightarrow P^{**} \longrightarrow X^* \\
\qquad\quad \uparrow \quad\Big\}P^* \qquad\qquad\qquad\qquad (10) \\
\qquad\quad P
\end{array}
$$

together with a large amount of unlabeled P (contrast this with the isotopic-trapping experiment). If P is an intermediate, two results are observed. First, the label in X^* is decreased in the second experiment as compared with the first because of the dilution of the label of P^{**} by unlabeled P. Second, as mentioned above, P^*, when isolated, will be labeled. Furthermore, if labeled P^* is itself now administered, it will be converted to X^*.

If we use labeled small molecules, we could readily study their conversion to large molecules. Thus began the classic studies of the biosynthesis of fatty acids and cholesterol from labeled acetate (Figure 2.1), and of heme, the purine bases, and a wide variety of N-compounds from labeled glycine. The study of cholesterol biosynthesis is a particularly elegant example and is shown in Figure 2.2. Using double-labeled acetate $^{14}CH_3{}^{13}COOH$, Bloch and others demonstrated that both carbon atoms were incorporated into the cholesterol molecule. It was next shown that the six-carbon (C-6) acid meva-

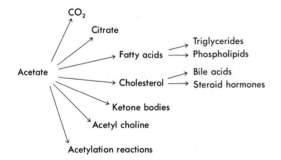

Figure 2.1

Pathways of acetate metabolism. The wide variety of products synthesized from acetate became appreciated from tracer techniques.

lonate was formed from three moles of acetate and was readily converted to cholesterol. Mevalonate was therefore an intermediate. This led next to the

$$\underset{\text{mevalonic acid}}{HOOC-CH_2-\overset{\overset{\displaystyle CH_3}{|}}{\underset{\underset{\displaystyle OH}{|}}{C}}-CH_2-COOH}$$

suggestion that the C-30 compound squalene, formed from six moles of mevalonate (mevalonate being itself first decarboxylated to a C-5 isopentenyl unit) might be an intermediate. Unlabeled squalene was given to rats synthesizing cholesterol from labeled acetate. When the squalene was reisolated, it

squalene

was found to be radioactive, proving that it was an intermediate. Thus the acetate ⟶ cholesterol pathway was further defined into the acetate ⟶ mevalonate ⟶ squalene ⟶ cholesterol pathway (Figure 2.2).

By similar approaches, studies of the biosynthesis of the macromolecules, proteins and nucleic acids, also were initiated. On the other hand, the biosynthesis of polysaccharides was worked out initially by isolating the enzymes responsible for the individual steps.

Some of the most elegant and sophisticated tracer methodologies have been devised and used in studies of biopolymer synthesis. Consider the question of the *polarity* of biopolymer formation. If a short pulse of a labeled monomer is fed to a system synthesizing a linear polymer of known structure, followed by unlabeled monomer, radioactivity will be introduced at the initiating end of the chain. As it is replaced by unlabeled monomer, the radioactivity will move down the chain *away* from the initiation point. If,

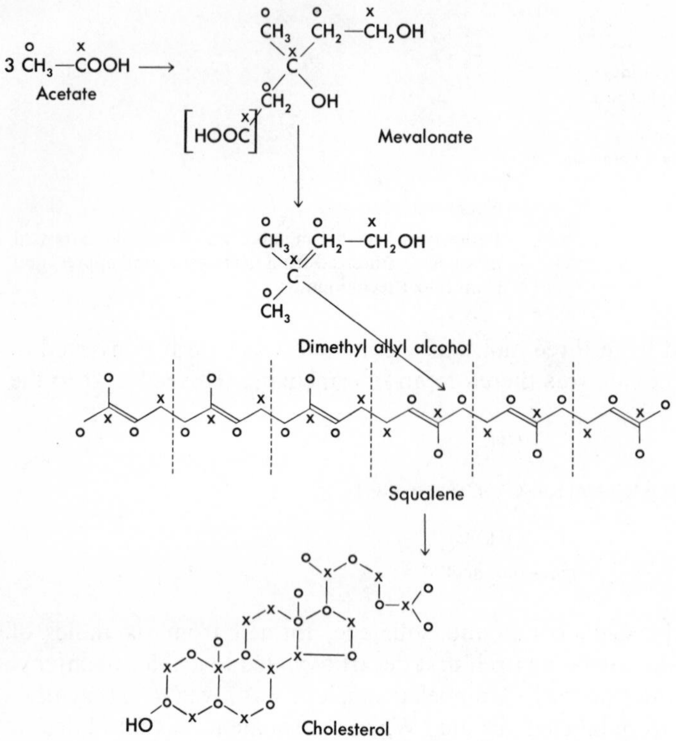

$$3 \; \overset{o}{C}H_3\overset{x}{-}COOH \longrightarrow$$

Acetate

Mevalonate

Dimethyl allyl alcohol

Squalene

HO   Cholesterol

Figure 2.2

The pathway of conversion of acetate to cholesterol via mevalonate and squalene using double labelled acetate. The metabolic origin of each carbon atom in cholesterol was thus established. Adapted from the work of Bloch, Gurin, Lynen, Popjak, Rudney, Tavormina and others. See also Figure 4.16 for the detailed pathway.

at the end of the reaction, the position of the radioactivity in the polymer can be determined, the polarity of the synthesis may be deduced. In Figure 2.3, labeled A* is fed into the system at times 1 through 3, followed by unlabeled A at times 4 through 5. The label moves down the chain from the Δ end to the ◀ end. If the labeled chain is broken down into three fragments of known structure, fragment 3 will be more highly labeled than fragment 2, and fragment 2, in turn, more labeled than fragment 1. The synthesis will thus have proceeded from its initiating end Δ to the opposite end ◀ in

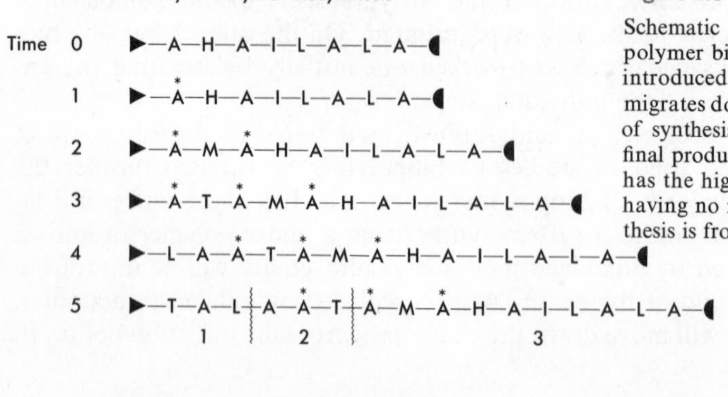

Directionality of Polymer Biosynthesis

Time 0   ▶—A—H—A—I—L—A—L—A—◀

1   ▶—Å—H—A—I—L—A—L—A—◀

2   ▶—Å—M—Å—H—A—I—L—A—L—A—◀

3   ▶—Å—T—Å—M—Å—H—A—I—L—A—L—A—◀

4   ▶—L—A—Å—T—Å—M—Å—H—A—I—L—A—L—A—◀

5   ▶—T—A—L⫲A—Å—T⫲Å—M—Å—H—A—I—L—A—L—A—◀
        1   2   3

Figure 2.3

Schematic representation of the directionality of polymer biosynthesis. At times 1–3 labelled A* is introduced into the system. At times 4–5 the label migrates down the chain away from the initial point of synthesis ▶ toward ◀. On degradation of the final product into fragments 1, 2 and 3, fragment 3 has the highest radioactivity followed by 2 with 1 having no radioactivity. Thus the polarity of synthesis is from ▶ ⟶ ◀.

the direction $\Delta \longrightarrow \blacktriangleleft$. Had the polarity of synthesis been opposite, the labeling pattern in the fragments would have been opposite. Such an elegant experiment was first done (in a more sophisticated form) with the synthesis of the protein hemoglobin and established the polarity of protein biosynthesis from the amino toward the carboxyl end of the chain.

Another ingenious use of labeling to elucidate the polarity of deoxyribonucleic acid is described in a volume in this series by Barker.

In another application heavy isotopes have been used for *separation* of nucleic acid molecules rather than for *detection* purposes. Systems can produce nucleic acids using precursors containing the heavy atoms ^{15}N or ^{13}C. When solutions of ribonucleic acid (RNA) or deoxyribonucleic acid (DNA) are centrifuged at high speed in the ultracentrifuge (100,000 × gravity) for prolonged time periods in cesium chloride solutions, the cesium chloride is distributed in a gradient of increasing density and concentration in the direction of the centrifugal field, and the nucleic acids form bands in the region of the gradient having the same density. Using this technique, it was possible to demonstrate that DNA is replicated during cell division, so that one half of the parent DNA is present in each new DNA molecule. This is a most important verification of the proposal that the system of information transfer of which DNA is the core uses the parent DNA molecule as a template for the formation of the daughter molecules.

Finally, a labeling technique has been used to show that the development of a new competence by a biological system is the result of the synthesis of a specific enzyme. For example, in bacterial systems the synthesis of enzymes in response to the presence of a new energy source in the bacterial environment can be demonstrated; in animals, hormonally-induced enzyme biosynthesis can be shown. A single-labeled amino acid is fed into the system together with a full complement of the other unlabeled amino acids, and biosynthesis is allowed to proceed. After its completion, the enzyme studied is extracted from the cells, partially purified, and then selectively precipitated with a specific antibody previously prepared for this purpose. From the radioactivity incorporated, and from the mass of the enzyme precipitated by the antibody, the separate rates of biosynthesis and of degradation of the enzyme can be calculated (see Chapter 9 for an example).

As may be appreciated from this discussion, the influence of this methodology, especially when used with another technique has been enormous.

2.3 THE ENZYMOLOGICAL APPROACH

Probably as important as isotopes in elucidating metabolic pathways has been the study of isolated enzymes. The power of the enzymological approach was demonstrated in the study of fermentation, which is described briefly here.

The biochemical studies of fermentation (Eq. 1) began when the brothers Büchner together with Hähn (1903) reported the (then) astonishing discovery that fermentation could be carried out by cell-free extracts of yeast, just as it occurred in intact cells. Following this discovery, efforts were made to subject the complex process to successive steps of *simplification*. The requirement for inorganic phosphate was a key early discovery. It was shown that the rate of fermentation rapidly fell off and that inorganic phosphate restored the rate but was consumed in the process. A study of the reason for this led to the isolation by Harden, Young, and Robison of several sugar phosphates which were themselves fermentable. Thus, in fermentation, inorganic phosphate was converted to organic forms and the sugar phosphates were intermediates in the process.

$$\text{glucose} + P_i \longrightarrow \quad \begin{array}{c} \text{sugar} \\ \text{phosphates} \end{array} \quad \longrightarrow \text{ethanol} + CO_2 \tag{11}$$

The ordering of the reactions involving the various sugar phosphates such as fructose-1,6-diphosphate, fructose-6-phosphate and glucose-6-phosphate proceeded over a period of years.

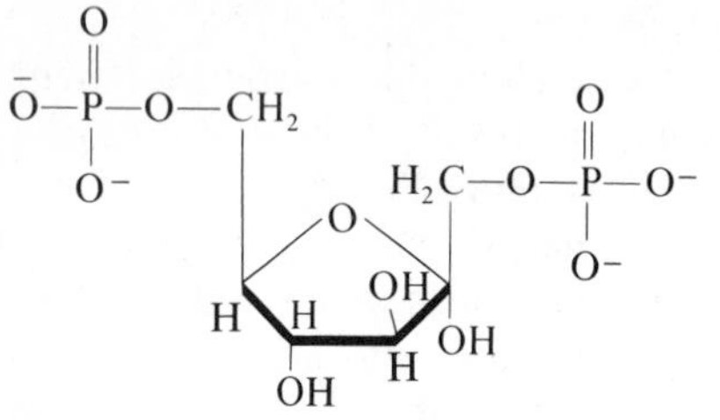

fructose-1,6-diphosphate

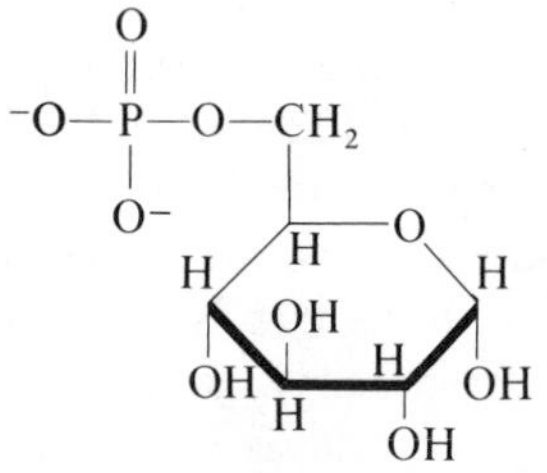

glucose-6-phosphate

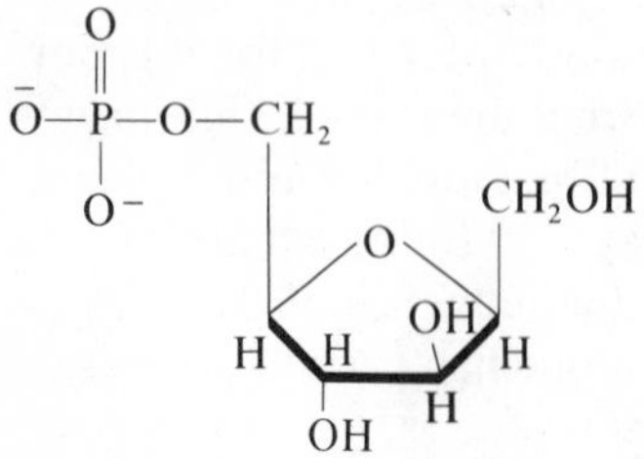

fructose-6-phosphate

Dialysis of the cell-free fermentative systems yielded further unexpected rewards in the form of low-molecular-weight materials which acted as cofactors in the enzymatic conversions of the sugars. Diphosphopyridine nucleotide or DPN (also termed NAD) was discovered in yeast and shown to

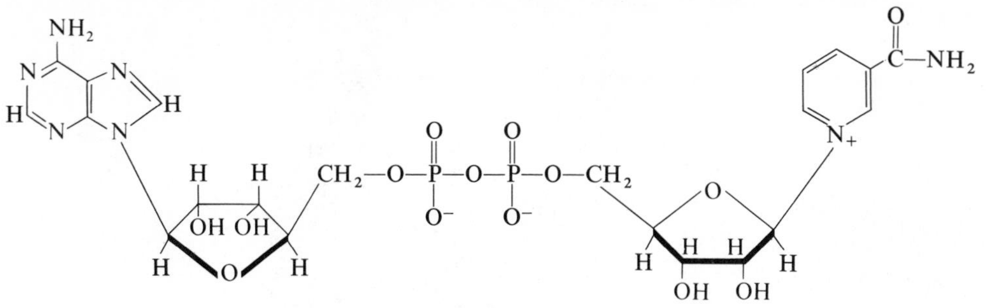

DPN (diphosphopyridine nucleotide) or
NAD (nicotinamide adenine dinucleotide)

be essential in several steps in the fermentation process. Similarly, triphosphopyridine nucleotide (TPN), (also termed NADP) was discovered in eryth-

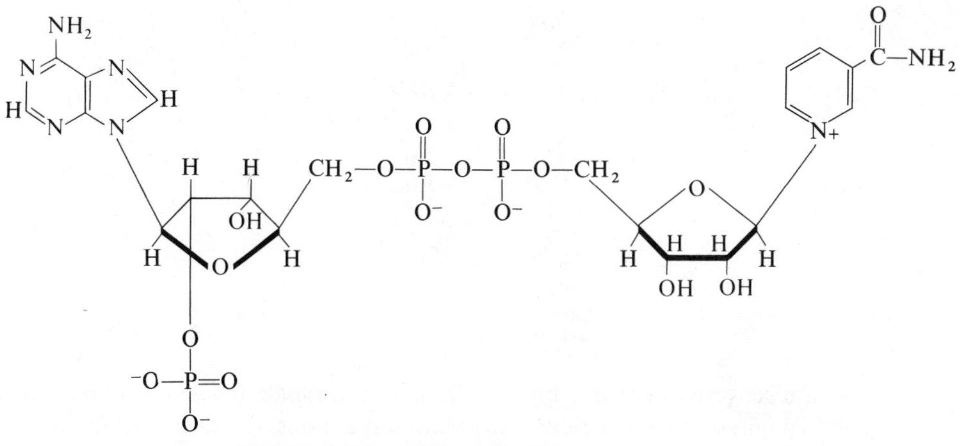

TPN (triphosphopyridine nucleotide)
NADP (nicotinamide adenine dinucleotide phosphate)

rocytes (red blood cells) and identified as an essential cofactor in the oxidation of glucose-6-phosphate.

Yet another series of nucleotides, adenosine triphosphate (ATP), adenosine diphosphate (ADP), and adenylic acid (AMP)

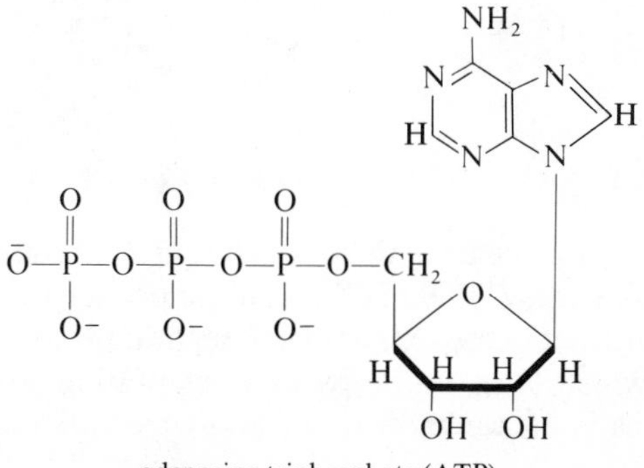

adenosine triphosphate (ATP)

19

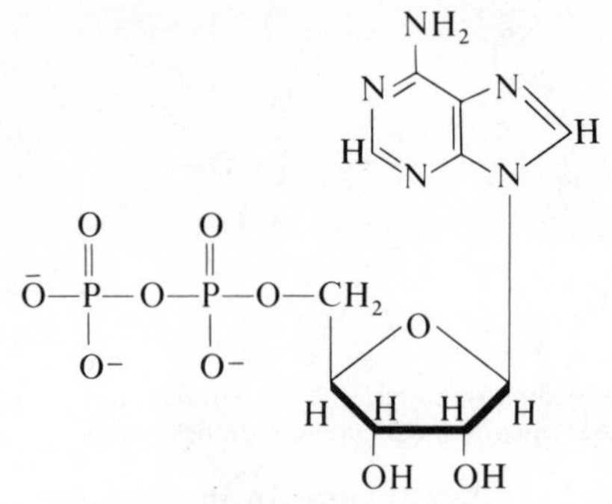

adenosine diphosphate (ADP)

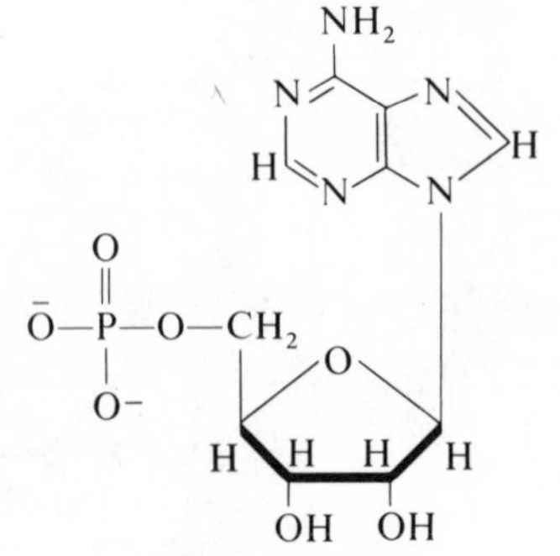

adenylic acid (AMP)

were discovered in yeast and muscle. These compounds were also required in fermentation to drive phosphorylation reactions, for example, the phosphorylation of glucose to glucose-6-phosphate

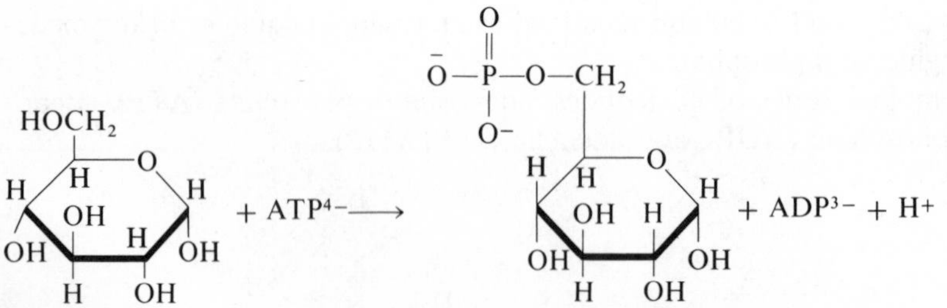

$$\text{glucose} + ATP^{4-} \longrightarrow \text{glucose-6-phosphate} + ADP^{3-} + H^+ \qquad (12)$$

With the availability of the sugar phosphates as substrates, the nucleotide cofactors (DPN, TPN), and the phosphate donors (ATP), it became possible to fractionate extracts into separate enzymatic steps and to purify each enzyme. Thus the steps of fermentation were ordered into the chain of 12 reactions we know today and which are considered in detail in Chapter 4.

2.4   BLOCKS—INHIBITOR TYPE AND GENETIC

Many metabolic sequences were elucidated by using specific blocking agents which allowed a portion of the sequence to be studied. Selective chemical poisons or inhibitors as well as specific genetic blocks have permitted this subdivision. Chemical blocking agents are most valuable if they are highly specific. Iodoacetate

$$
\begin{array}{c}
\mathrm{H} \\
| \\
\mathrm{I-C-COO^-} \\
| \\
\mathrm{H}
\end{array}
$$

iodoacetate

and fluoride are cases in point. They were of very great importance in working out of the reactions of fermentation and the pathways of glucose metabolism in muscle. Each acted to inhibit a specific enzyme (14, 16)

$$
\begin{array}{c}
\mathrm{CHO} \\
| \\
\mathrm{HC-OH} \quad\quad\quad \mathrm{O} \\
| \quad\quad\quad\quad\quad || \\
\mathrm{H_2C-O-P-O^-} \\
|\\
\mathrm{O^-}
\end{array}
+ \mathrm{HO-\overset{O}{\overset{||}{P}}-O^-} + \mathrm{DPN^+} \xrightleftharpoons[\text{dehydrogenase}]{\text{glyceraldehyde-3-phosphate}}
\begin{array}{c}
\mathrm{O} \quad\ \mathrm{O} \\
|| \quad\ \ || \\
\mathrm{C-O-P-O^-} \\
| \\
\mathrm{O^-} \\
\mathrm{H-C-OH} \\
| \\
\mathrm{O} \\
|| \\
\mathrm{H_2C-O-P-O^-} \\
| \\
\mathrm{O^-}
\end{array}
+ \mathrm{DPNH} + \mathrm{H^+} \quad (13)
$$

glyceraldehyde-3-phosphate   1,3-diphosphoglycerate

glyceraldehyde-3-phosphate
dehydrogenase
enzyme—SH + I—CH$_2$—COO$^-$ $\longrightarrow$ enzyme—S—CH$_2$—COO$^-$ + HI

$\hspace{16em}$ (14)

carboxymethylated enzyme

$$
\begin{array}{c}
\mathrm{COO^-} \\
| \quad\quad\ \ \mathrm{O} \\
| \quad\quad\ \ || \\
\mathrm{HC-O-P-O^-} \\
| \\
\mathrm{O^-} \\
\mathrm{H_2C-OH}
\end{array}
+ \mathrm{H_2O} \underset{}{\overset{\text{enolase}}{\rightleftharpoons}}
\begin{array}{c}
\mathrm{COO^-} \\
| \quad\quad\ \ \mathrm{O} \\
| \quad\quad\ \ || \\
\mathrm{C-O-P-O^-} \\
|| \quad\quad | \\
\mathrm{CH_2} \quad \mathrm{O^-}
\end{array}
+ \mathrm{H_2O} \quad\quad (15)
$$

2-phosphoglycerate   phosphoenolpyruvate

enolase + magnesium fluorophosphate $\longrightarrow$ inactive enzyme $\hspace{6em}$ (16)

in the sequence and allowed portions of the total sequence to be studied and the conversions involved placed in proper order. A large part of their utility lies in the fact that when a specific enzyme is blocked, the metabolite(s) which serve as its substrate(s) usually accumulate and can be isolated and characterized.

Carbon monoxide and cyanide inhibit respiration and act by combining with the iron coordinated in hemoglobin and in the respiratory catalysts. Arsenite was also identified as an inhibitor of the oxidation of pyruvate and α-ketoglutarate in the tricarboxylic acid cycle. Other poisons such as heavy metals, chelating agents, and compounds which can react with functional groups in proteins inhibit in a less specific manner.

The importance of another type of block, the genetic block, has developed extremely rapidly. Its utility in metabolic studies lies in its specificity and complete *independence* from other approaches. It is possible to cause mutations in bacteria by subjecting them to damaging radiation and to sort out the mutants produced so that those which lack a specific enzyme are obtained. Thus in a bacterium which converts A to K

$$A \xrightarrow{1} B \xrightarrow{2} C \xrightarrow{3} D \xrightarrow{4} E \xrightarrow{5} F \xrightarrow{6} G$$
$$\downarrow 7$$
$$K \xleftarrow{10} J \xleftarrow{9} I \xleftarrow{8} H \qquad (17)$$

it may be possible to produce mutants which lack enzyme 1, mutants which lack enzyme 2 and mutants which lack enzyme 3. The mutant lacking enzyme 1 grows when B,C. or D is provided but not with A. The mutant lacking enzyme 2 can grow with either C or D but not A or B; in fact, if A is given B will accumulate. The mutant lacking enzyme 3 requires D for growth and given A or B will accumulate C. Clearly the sequence of reactions A $\longrightarrow$ B $\longrightarrow$ C $\longrightarrow$ D is established by these studies. By these kinds of experiments, the pathway of histidine biosynthesis was worked out in *Escherichia coli* and *Salmonella* in a most elegant manner. The studies in microorganisms were rapidly extended to man, where genetic "inborn errors of metabolism" had been known since the work of Garrod (1908).

With such sophisticated techniques, not only were many new metabolic pathways worked out, but also the in vivo or intracellular function of enzymes could be approached for the first time. An example may serve to illustrate these points.

It was argued that the enzyme phosphorylase (the first enzyme shown to catalyze the synthesis of a biopolymer) catalyzed in vivo both the synthesis as well as the degradation of the α-1,4 linkages of glycogen

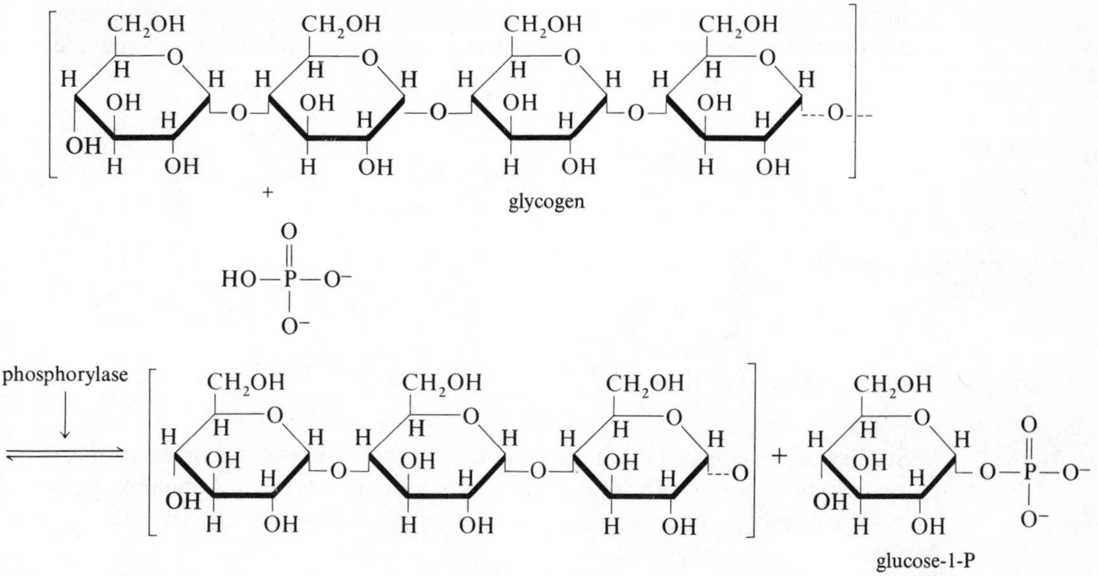

glycogen

$$HO-\overset{\overset{\textstyle O}{\|}}{\underset{\underset{\textstyle O^-}{|}}{P}}-O^-$$

phosphorylase

glucose-1-P

The reversibility of this reaction could be demonstrated in the test tube. The inescapable observation was present, however, that when phosphorylase became activated within the cell (in vivo), it was invariably associated with glycogen breakdown and not synthesis. Both the enzyme activation as well as the breakdown of glycogen were experimentally demonstrable. What, in fact, was the role of phosphorylase within the cell?

The answer was provided by studies of a human inborn error of metabolism, McArdle's disease. In this muscle disease, the breakdown of glycogen to lactate

$$(\text{glucose})_n \longrightarrow 2 \text{ lactate} + (\text{glucose})_{n-1} \tag{19}$$

was shown to be markedly impaired in vivo with the muscles forced to exercise, as well as in vitro, with samples of the patient's muscle ground up in the presence of a buffer. Further, it was shown that the glycogen level of the muscles was elevated even though breakdown of glycogen to glucose-1-phosphate (glucose—1—P) by phosphorylase was impaired (Eq. 18.) Since glycogen was present, it must have been synthesized by another reaction. The enzyme responsible for glycogen formation in these muscles was identified as glycogen synthase, which catalyzes the biosynthesis of the α-1,4 linkages of glycogen from an energetically more efficient donor than glucose—1—P, namely, uridine diphosphate glucose (UDPG).

$$UDPG^{-2} + (\text{glucose})_n \xrightarrow{\text{UDPG glycogen synthase}} UDP^{-3} + (\text{glucose})_{n+1} + H^+ \tag{20}$$

In this way, phosphorylase was assigned the in vivo role of glycogen degradation and McArdle's disease was shown to be due to a lack of that enzyme.

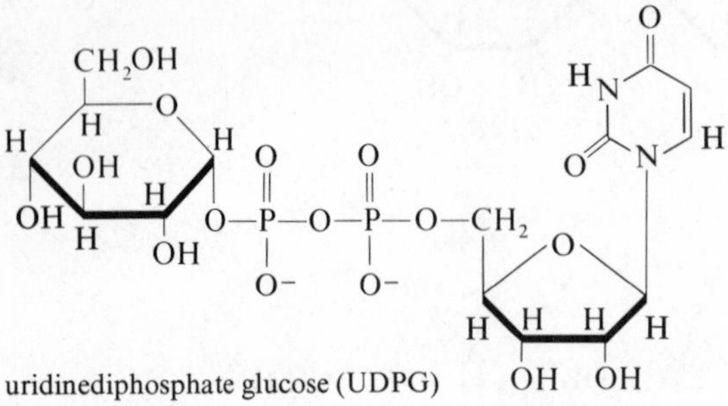

uridinediphosphate glucose (UDPG)

Studies of the altered metabolism in other human diseases has proved equally rewarding in terms of establishing in vivo significance. In Appendix Table A. 2 a number of the human genetic metabolic diseases known today are listed.

2.5 SERENDIPITY AND SHORTCOMINGS

As in all human endeavors, the elucidation of metabolic pathways has benefited from good fortune, chance, or serendipity. Claude Bernard stated this very clearly in 1865, "Experimental ideas are often born by chance, with the help of some casual observation. Nothing is more common; and this is really the simplest way of beginning a piece of scientific work. We take a walk, so to speak, in the realm of science, and we pursue what happens to present itself to our eyes." There are numerous examples of the successes achieved by this approach; one of the more recent is selected to illustrate the point.

In the study of phospholipid biosynthesis, it was discovered that ATP was required for the conversion of phosphoryl choline into lecithin

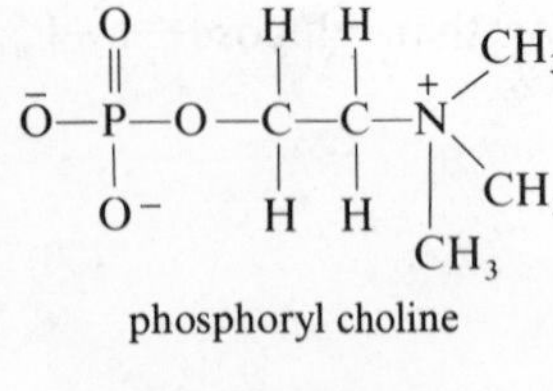

phosphoryl choline 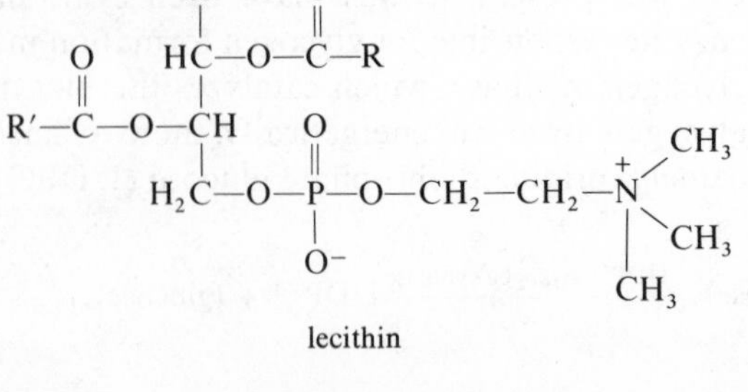   lecithin and that various ATP preparations varied markedly in their effectiveness. Closer scrutiny demonstrated that the most highly purified crystalline preparations of ATP were in fact the *least* active, whereas the cruder amorphous preparations were more active. This suggested that the actual activating substance was not ATP itself. It was soon discovered that the actual activating substance was cytidine triphosphate (CTP)

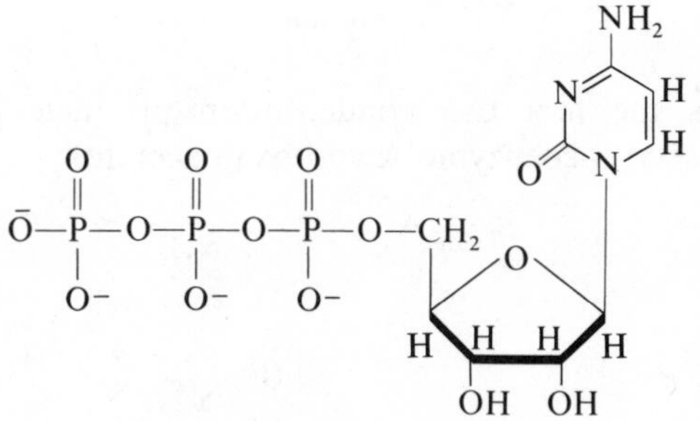

cytidine triphosphate (CTP)

present as a contaminant in the amorphous ATP, which reacted with phosphoryl choline to form cytidine diphosphate choline

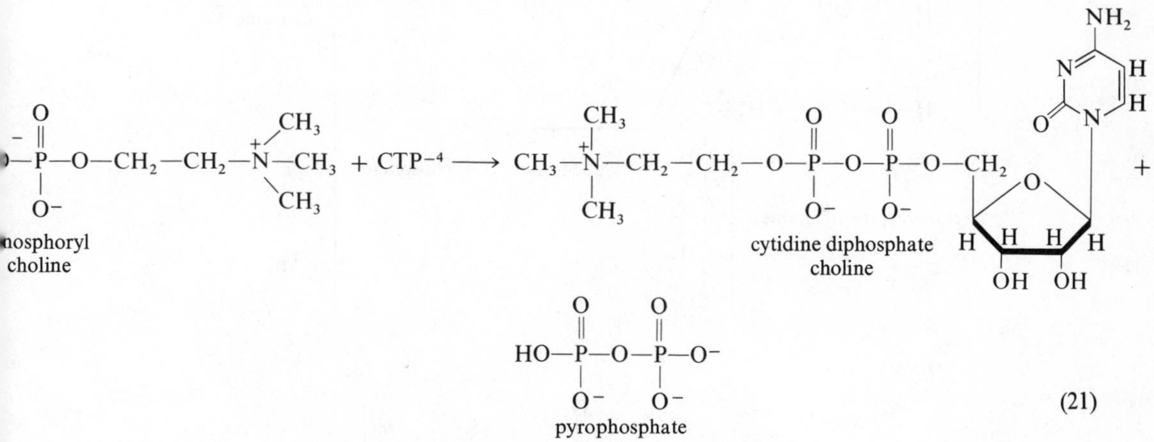

$$(21)$$

phosphoryl choline

cytidine diphosphate choline

pyrophosphate

Through serendipity, a new role for CTP was discovered, as well as the new intermediate cytidine diphosphate choline.

None of the methods described is completely foolproof and erroneous results can be obtained. It is useful to point out an example to illustrate this point.

From studies of oxidative metabolism with tracer techniques, it was deduced that a C-2 unit condensed with a C-4 unit to form a C-6 dicarboxylic acid. The asymmetry of the labeling pattern suggested the asymmetric compound isocitrate

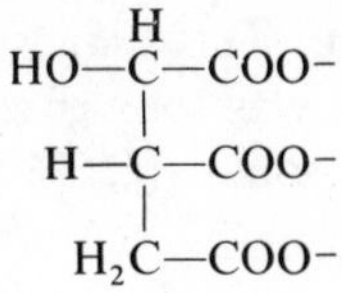

$$
\begin{array}{c}
\quad\ \ \ \text{H} \\
\text{HO—C—COO}^- \\
\quad | \\
\text{H—C—COO}^- \\
\quad | \\
\text{H}_2\text{C—COO}^-
\end{array}
$$

isocitrate

as the first C-6 condensation product. When the enzymatic substrates acetyl-S-coenzyme A and oxaloacetate

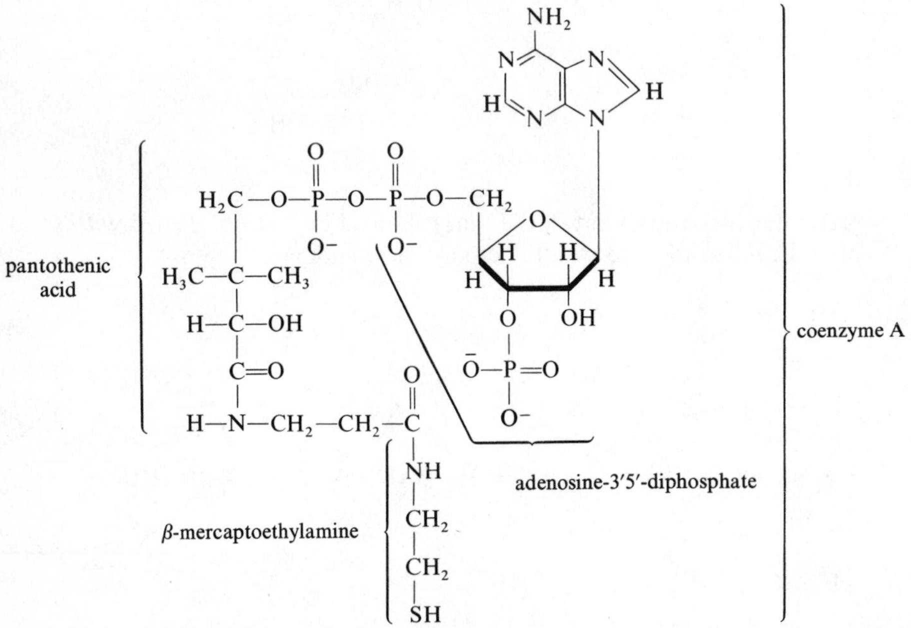

$$R = CH_3\overset{\overset{\textstyle O}{\|}}{C}\text{—(acetyl)}$$

acetyl—S—CoA

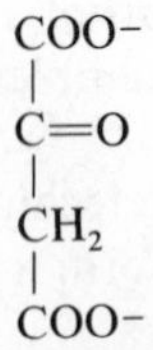

$$
\begin{array}{c}
\text{COO}^- \\
| \\
\text{C=O} \\
| \\
\text{CH}_2 \\
| \\
\text{COO}^-
\end{array}
$$

oxaloacetate

became known, the enzyme catalyzing the condensation was isolated from liver by Ochoa and coworkers and purified to the point where the condensation product was identified as citrate

$$
\begin{array}{l}
H_2C\text{—}COO\text{-} \\
\quad | \\
HO\text{—}C\text{—}COO\text{-} \\
\quad | \\
H_2C\text{—}COO\text{-}
\end{array}
$$

citrate

rather than isocitrate

$$
\begin{array}{l}
O \\
\| \\
C\text{—}S\text{—}CoA \\
\quad | \\
CH_3 \ \text{acetyl-S-CoA}
\end{array}
\quad + \quad
\begin{array}{l}
O=C\text{—}COO\text{-} \\
\quad | \\
HCH \\
\quad | \\
COO\text{-} \ \text{oxaloacetate}
\end{array}
\xrightarrow[H_2O]{}
\begin{array}{l}
H_2C\text{—}COO\text{-} \\
\quad | \\
HO\text{—}C\text{—}COO\text{-} \\
\quad | \\
H_2C\text{—}COO\text{-} \\
\text{citrate}
\end{array}
+ \text{CoASH} + H^+ \qquad (22)
$$

coenzyme A

A second enzyme aconitase catalyzed the conversion of citrate to isocitrate via *cis*-aconitate

$$
\begin{array}{l}
H_2C\text{—}COO\text{-} \\
\quad | \\
HO\text{—}C\text{—}COO\text{-} \\
\quad | \\
H_2C\text{—}COO\text{-} \\
\text{citrate}
\end{array}
\underset{+H_2O}{\overset{-H_2O}{\rightleftharpoons}}
\begin{array}{l}
HC\text{—}COO\text{-} \\
\| \\
C\text{—}COO\text{-} \\
\quad | \\
H_2C\text{—}COO\text{-} \\
\textit{cis}\text{-aconitate}
\end{array}
\underset{-H_2O}{\overset{+H_2O}{\rightleftharpoons}}
\begin{array}{l}
\quad\quad H \\
HO\text{—}C\text{—}COO\text{-} \\
\quad | \\
H\text{—}C\text{—}COO\text{-} \\
\quad | \\
H_2C\text{—}COO\text{-} \\
\text{isocitrate}
\end{array}
\qquad (23)
$$

How could the isotopic data be explained? The principle of an asymmetric reagent (in this case, the condensing enzyme) reacting with a *meso-carbon* atom (defined as C_{aabc}) came to be appreciated and readily explained the *apparent* discrepancy between the tracer and enzymatic approaches (see also the volume in this series by Barker). In this case, the enzyme aconitase could carry out the conversion of citrate, which is symmetric, to isocitrate, which is asymmetric. Citrate was ordered prior to isocitrate in the oxidative metabolism of carbon. If only tracer techniques had been used, the wrong conclusion regarding the role of citrate in metabolism would have survived.

2.6   BIOCHEMICAL CHAIN OF SYSTEMS

All of the methods just outlined have made use of a sequence of systems of increasing simplification (Figure 2.4). This consists of (a) the *intact organism*

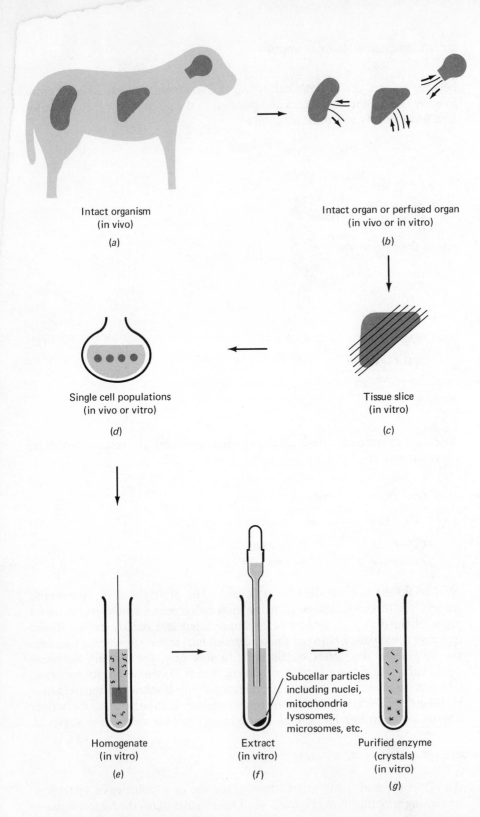

Intact organism
(in vivo)

(a)

Intact organ or perfused organ
(in vivo or in vitro)

(b)

Single cell populations
(in vivo or vitro)

(d)

Tissue slice
(in vitro)

(c)

Homogenate
(in vitro)

(e)

Extract
(in vitro)

(f)

Subcellar particles
including nuclei,
mitochondria
lysosomes,
microsomes, etc.

Purified enzyme
(crystals)
(in vitro)

(g)

(in vivo), the experiment is done in the whole animal; (b) the *intact organ* or *perfused organ* (in vivo or in vitro), the experiment is done in an isolated perfused organ whose cells are intact but which is removed from the other organs; (c) *the slice* (in vitro), the experiment is done with thin tissue slices in which barriers to diffusion are minimized by slice dimensions and where interior cells are intact but surface cells are of necessity damaged; (d) *single cell populations* (in vivo or in vitro), the experiment is done with a population of individual similar cells, e.g., bacteria, blood cells, or isolated or cultured tissue cells; (e) *homogenate* or *brei* (in vitro), the experiment is done with preparations where cell barriers are removed by breaking the cells by mechanical or other means in the presence of buffered solutions; (f) *extract* (in vitro), the particulate matter of the homogenate is removed, usually by centrifugation, and the experiment is done with the supernatant extract; from the extract the *organelles* or *subcellular particles* can be separated by differential centrifugation in relatively dense media and experiments can be performed with populations of purified particles; (g) *purified* or *homogeneous* enzyme (in vitro), the extract is fractionated to remove unwanted enzymatic contaminants and the experiment is done with the partially purified or highly purified enzyme. It is of obvious advantage to the investigator to have available such an ordered series with which to solve the problems of metabolism and it reflects a considerable development of the art.

Let us now discuss each of the systems more fully. The intact organism (a) has been of importance in studies of material balance and nutrition. In such studies, intake and output of a constituent are quantitatively monitored to assess whether the animal is in metabolic balance, in negative balance (a net loss is taking place), or in positive balance (a net gain is taking place). Examples include measurements of N, Na^+, K^+, and Ca^{2+} balances. This technique has also been used in another way, namely, to determine whether a substance must be fed in the diet or whether it can be synthesized in adequate amounts in the body. An example is the development by Rose and associates of the requirement for the *essential* amino acids in adult man (see Chapter 5). When the essential amino acid is fed in adequate amount, the patient is in N balance. When the amino acid is omitted from the diet, the patient rather rapidly goes into negative N balance. For many balance studies isotopic tracers have proven to be of great importance for analyzing the constituent under study.

Growth rate in the young animal, including man, has also served as a quantitative measure of nutritional adequacy. This has been especially useful in working out vitamin and other essential nutrient requirements. In many cases, there may be a rather specific *deficiency syndrome*, i.e., a set of

Figure 2.4   The chain of biochemical systems. (a) whole animal; (b) perfused organ; (c) tissue slice; (d) cell population; (e) homogenate; (f) extract; (g) purified enzyme. For a discussion of these systems and of the operational definition of *in vitro* and *in vivo* see the text.

signs and symptoms which appears with the altered growth rate during the development of the deficiency. This then provides an additional marker of considerable importance. When the chemical nature of the nutrient is known, chemical measurement of its concentration in body fluids such as blood (including blood cells), urine, sweat, bile, and lymph (obtained with surgical procedures) have been most valuable in following the metabolism in terms of balance. Similar considerations apply to the monitoring of toxic agents as well as therapeutic agents.

The metabolism of specific organs or regions of the body may be studied by selectively monitoring the blood supply to that organ. *Catheterization* (threading a thin hollow tube) of the heart or liver are particularly important examples. Direct sampling of the organ itself by *biopsy* techniques is perhaps the most important approach to the study of regional metabolism. The tissue sections are removed by needle aspiration or surgically under mild conditions (frequently under local anaesthesia) in order to obtain viable tissue for metabolic or other studies.

Information concerning the metabolism of specific organs in the body may be obtained by studies carried out in the entire animal through the use of surgical procedures such as the preparation of *fistulas* which drain the contents or secretions of organs, or organ extirpations where the function is studied by observing what happens to metabolism in the absence of the organ.

However, it has become increasingly clear that the detailed metabolism of an organ may be studied profitably by directly studying that organ in the isolated state, that is, removed from the influence of other organs. Remarkable advances have been made in the technique of perfusion (*b*). In this process, the organ is maintained for periods of time, of the order of hours, in a state approaching that in the body by pumping blood, or some simplified perfusion fluid, together with oxygen through the vascular tree under a set of carefully controlled conditions. Here, by sampling the fluid perfusing the organ, one can carefully monitor metabolism at the same time that one is able to follow a physiologic parameter of in vivo organ function. For example, with the perfused liver, bile flow can be measured; with the perfused kidney, urine output; with the heart, heart rate and pressure. Thus one has the opportunity to relate metabolism to organ function.

Up to this point, the organ may or may not function with intact physiological responses. From this point on, it no longer does so. With the slice technique (*c*), one can begin to examine the more detailed biochemistry of the system, at the expense, however, of the physiologic guideposts. For this reason, the slice system, and the remaining systems as well, are termed in vitro. Larger organs, such as liver, kidney, or brain are usually sliced free hand or mechanically with a tissue slicer. Slices so prepared consist essentially of ruptured cells on the surface, with intact cells in the slice center. Certain tissues are sufficiently thin so that no slicing is necessary. A particularly interesting example is the rat or mouse diaphragm, which is, in essence, a "natural slice" of skeletal muscle. Isolated adipose tissue preparations which are thin and only minimally damaged by cutting into sections are also available. These preparations have proved of great importance in studies of hormone action. With experience, slices can be prepared under standardized conditions such that from one organ or even a portion of an organ, many slices may be prepared sufficient for a number of flasks in a single experiment.

Various intact single cell preparations, a level of organization simpler than the slice, are now available (d). It has come to be recognized that single cells can be isolated following enzymatic digestion of minces of organs. An example has been the preparation of isolated fat cells by enzymatic digestion of adipose tissue minces with the crude enzyme collagenase which serves to separate the cells. These techniques may be combined with tissue and organ culture methods whereby the cells are maintained for prolonged periods of time in the isolated state and handled by microbiological methods. Such preparations are particularly valuable for studies of cell metabolism and have been used profitably in problems related to transport and hormonal control. Bacterial systems are natural single cell cultures and have been very widely used to study metabolism.

In the homogenate technique (e), the tissue, usually already minced, is homogenized with buffer (in a mechanical grinder) under conditions designed to insure cell rupture. A considerable number of techniques for rupturing cells have been developed, including grinding, rapid pressure change, sonic oscillation, freezing and thawing, etc., allowing a great flexibility for preparing homogenates. This is extremely useful since cells vary widely in the ease with which they rupture. The stabilities of the systems under study in the homogenate also vary widely.

The entire homogenate may be studied as such, or it may be further fractionated into its component subcellular particulate fractions by differential centrifugation or by other methods. In this way, nuclei, lysosomes, mitochondria, microsomes, cell membranes, and cytoplasm may each be separately studied. This technique has proven one of the most valuable in metabolism, especially in the problem of determining the subcellular site(s) of metabolic reactions within the cell.

The remaining techniques, the extract (f) and purified enzyme (g), are further simplifications of the homogenate. If the subcellular particles are removed, say by centrifugation, the cytosol remains and this contains the soluble cytoplasmic constituents. If cell particulates such as mitochondria or microsomes are collected, they may be solubilized or partially solubilized in order to initiate more detailed studies on the individual steps in a metabolic reaction sequence which has already been shown to be present in that particle. Thus if the sequence A $\longrightarrow$ $\longrightarrow$ P has been localized to a certain subcellular particle, it may then become useful to solubilize that particle in order to separately identify the partially separated segments

$$A \longrightarrow \longrightarrow F \qquad F \longrightarrow \longrightarrow L \qquad L \longrightarrow \longrightarrow P$$

Similarly, by protein fractionation procedures (Barker) it becomes possible to isolate individual enzymes and study individual reactions

$$A \longrightarrow B \qquad B \longrightarrow C \qquad C \longrightarrow D \qquad D \longrightarrow E \qquad E \longrightarrow F$$

For these sorts of studies two criteria of purity are in general operational use. The first criterion is relative purity, that is, freedom from interfering reactions, which permits the identification of a reaction. For example, in the simplest case in order to study the $A \xrightarrow{1} B$ transformation, enzyme 1 must necessarily be free of enzyme 2, which catalyzes the $B \xrightarrow{2} C$ conversion, since enzyme 2 would necessarily interfere with the identification of B as the product formed from A. On the other hand, enzyme 1 would not necessarily have to be free of enzyme 6, which catalyzes the $F \xrightarrow{6} G$ conversion, since it would not directly interfere with the reaction being studied. The second criterion used is purity in the usual sense, i.e., homogeneity of the enzyme as a protein. It is usual to examine the enzyme by several criteria, such as electrophoresis at several pH values, ultracentrifugation, etc.; if in all systems tested it appears homogeneous, its purity is assumed.

In this chapter we have discussed the principal approaches, techniques, and systems used to elucidate the pathways of metabolism. A key point has been the fact that when these basically *independent* approaches agree, there is assurance for the ordering of the reactions. When they disagree, further work is required to resolve the nature of the disagreement. From such further work new principles have usually developed within the individual approaches which have contributed significantly to scientific development. The rest of the book focuses on accumulated knowledge based on this type of thinking and experiment. The tenor will be to reassemble the individually well-studied reactions back into the cell, and to try to view them in the context of their in vivo roles as part of the intact cell or organism.

REFERENCES

Altman, P. L. and D. S. Dittmer (Eds.), *Metabolism,* Federation of American Societies for Experimental Biology.

Bernard, C., *An Introduction to the Study of Experimental Medicine,* Dover Publications, Inc., New York. 1957. Translated by Henry Copley Breen with an introduction by Lawrence J. Henderson.

Dixon, M. and E. C. Webb, *Enzymes,* 2nd ed., Academic Press, Inc., New York, 1964.

Schoenheimer, R., *The Dynamic State of Body Constituenets,* Harvard University Press, Cambridge, Mass., 1949.

Stanbury, J. B., J. B. Wyngaarden, and D. S. Fredrickson (Eds.), *The Metabolic Basis of Inherited Disease*, 2nd Edit. McGraw-Hill, New York, 1966.

Wolf, G., *Isotopes in Biology*, Academic Press, Inc., New York, 1964.

THREE | # ENERGY METABOLISM

In Chapter 1, it was stated that the maintenance of an energy balance was a process central to all living systems and that without a constant energy input, life ceases. In the present chapter, we will examine the ways in which chemical events in the cell participate in energy production and transfer. We will discover that nature has developed only a few chemical reactions for energy transfer and that many of these reactions involve compounds containing the element phosphorus in the form of phosphate esters or anhydrides.

In Chapter 2, we have already encountered several types of phosphates. In fermentation, for example, we have the sugar phosphates (esters) and the nucleotide, mono-, and polyphosphates (esters and anhydrides). In the present chapter, we will encounter acyl phosphates (mixed anhydrides) and N-phosphates such as creatine phosphate and arginine phosphate.

Three types of sulfur-containing compounds have also been recognized as important in energy transfer: the *acyl esters of thiols* such as acetyl-S-coenzyme A, the *mixed anhydrides of phosphoric and sulfuric acids* such as adenosine 5' phosphosulfate (APS), 3' phosphoadenosine 5' phosphosulfate (PAPS), and the *sulfonium compounds* such as S-adenosylmethionine. Finally, the N-compounds such as n-acetylimidazole complete the list of compounds involved in energy conservation and transfer.

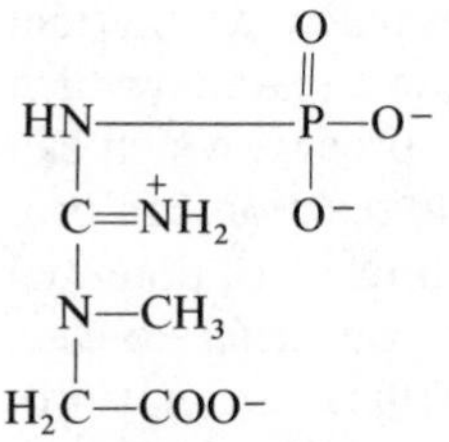

creatine phosphate

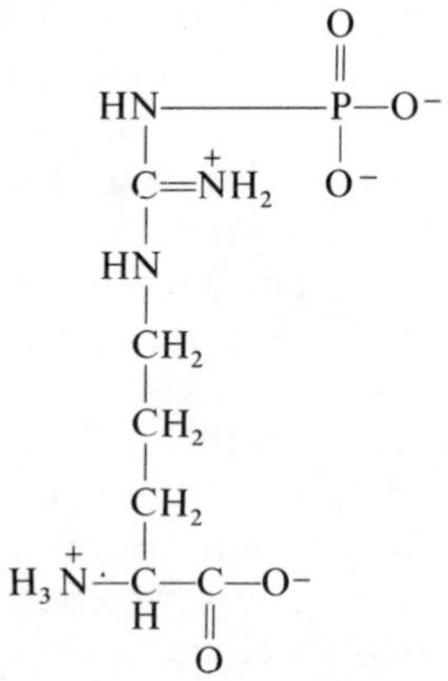

arginine phosphate

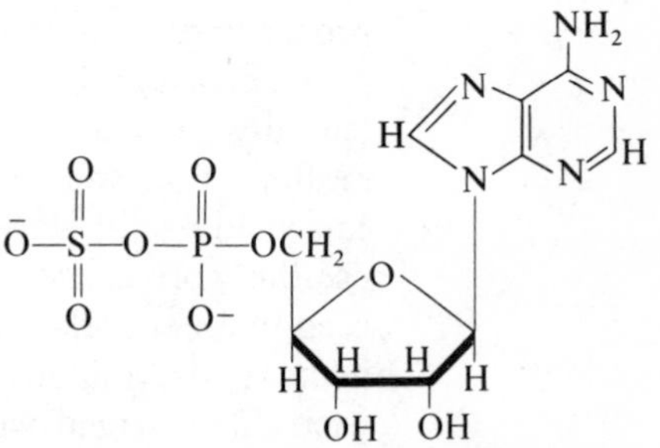

adenosine 5′ phosphosulfate
(APS)

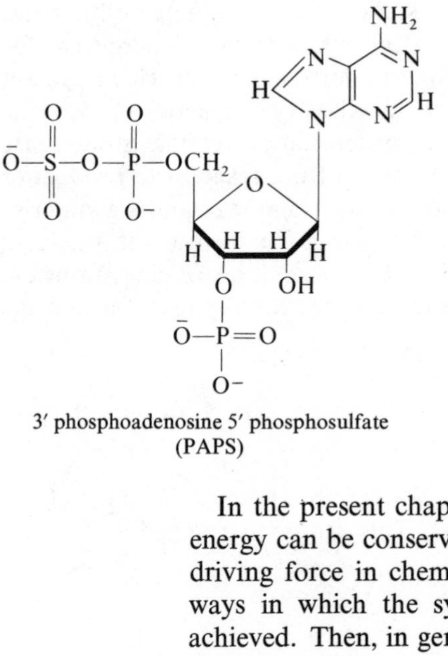

3′ phosphoadenosine 5′ phosphosulfate
(PAPS)

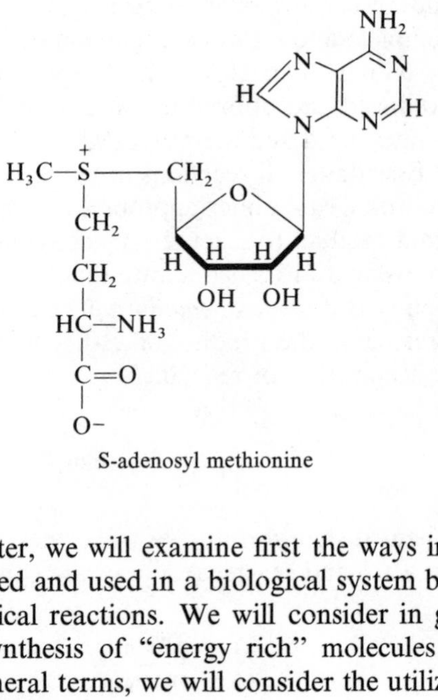

S-adenosyl methionine

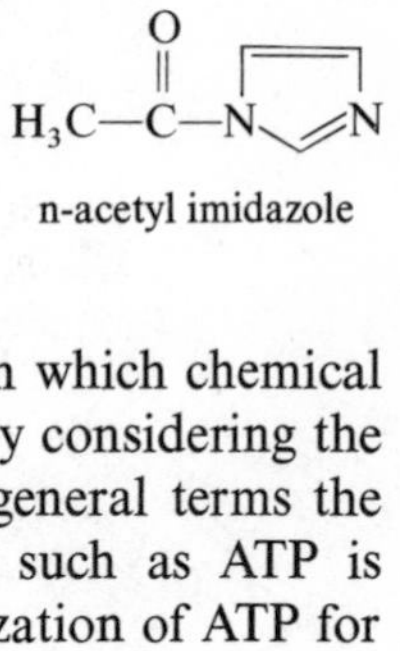

n-acetyl imidazole

In the present chapter, we will examine first the ways in which chemical energy can be conserved and used in a biological system by considering the driving force in chemical reactions. We will consider in general terms the ways in which the synthesis of "energy rich" molecules such as ATP is achieved. Then, in general terms, we will consider the utilization of ATP for energy-requiring processes.

3.1   THERMODYNAMIC BASIS

The Gibbs free-energy function (ΔG) expresses the maximum amount of work that can be obtained from a chemical reaction. It is this aspect that we must be concerned with in understanding how biochemical systems function. Knowledge of ΔG is useful in predicting whether or not a reaction will have a tendency to proceed in a given direction. ΔG is equal to the difference in work content between the initial and final states of a system; it specifies an amount of energy that must be absorbed or released when the reaction proceeds and its units are usually expressed in calories. For present purposes, ΔG may be considered as that fraction of total energy which is potentially available to do work rather than energy dissipated as thermal motion of the surroundings. However, to obtain work from a reaction which can yield useful work, the reaction must be coupled to a process which can use the work content. In the absence of this coupling, the reaction can proceed in an entirely wasteful fashion, with the release of all its work potential as heat. An analogy can be drawn to a waterfall which can generate electricity if provided with a water-wheel and a dynamo; if these are not provided, it dissipates its energies entirely as heat.

The study of the energetics of processes and the difference in energy content between states (such as reactants and products) is called *thermodynamics* and an exposition of its principles is beyond the scope of this book. For a complete and rigorous discussion of this subject see the volume in this series by Van Holde. However, to appreciate the way in which energy can be produced and utilized it is necessary to consider the ways in which ΔG can be measured and the way in which its value will vary as reactions proceed.

Essentially all reactions in biochemical systems are reversible in the sense that they can, under appropriate conditions, go from reactant to product or from product to reactant. Under conditions such that reactant is giving rise to product at the same rate that product is giving rise to reactant, the reaction is said to be in *equilibrium*. Recall that the rate of a reaction can be expressed as the product of a specific rate constant for the reaction and the concentration of reactant.

$$\text{rate} = k \text{ (reactant)}$$

Then at equilibrium, k_F (reactant) $= k_R$ (product), since the rate of the forward and reverse reactions are equal. This can be rearranged to

$$\frac{k_F}{k_R} = \frac{\text{(product)}}{\text{(reactant)}}$$

and k_F/k_R can be expressed as a single constant K_{eq}, the equilibrium constant.

Now when a reaction is at equilibrium, it is proceeding forwards and backwards at equal rates and the work (free-energy) content of reactants equals that of the products. This follows from the fact that the free-energy difference determines the tendency of a reaction to proceed in a given direction; at equilibrium the forward and reverse tendencies balance, the free energies are equal, and $\Delta G = 0$. At any ratio of products to reactants smaller than the equilibrium ratio, ΔG is negative and the reaction will have a tendency to proceed from reactant to product. If the ratio is larger, ΔG is positive and the reaction will have a tendency to proceed in reverse, from products to reactants.

$\Delta G°$ and ΔG Calculations

Consider a reaction $A \rightleftharpoons B$ which has at equilibrium

$$\frac{(B)}{(A)} = 5 \quad \text{or} \quad K_{eq} = 5$$

If we prepare a solution which is 1 molar with respect to both A and B, we would immediately predict that the reaction would tend to proceed until the equilibrium ratio was achieved. In other words, ΔG would be negative. But how large would it be? How much energy would be available to do work? Although at equilibrium $\Delta G = 0$ and no work can be obtained, the ratio of $(B)/(A) = 5$ indicates that A has a greater potential for reaction than B. In a sense, it is chemically five times more potent; thus, the equilibrium constant K_{eq} expresses the relative chemical potentials of A and B and should relate to the ΔG for the reaction $A \rightleftharpoons B$. The relationship is

$$\Delta G° = -RT \ln K_{eq} \text{ cal mole}^{-1}$$

or

$$\Delta G° = -2.303RT \log K_{eq} \text{ cal mole}^{-1} \tag{1}$$

where R is the gas constant, 1.987 cal mole^{-1} deg^{-1}, and T is the absolute temperature. The significance of $\Delta G°$ is that it is the amount of free energy released (or absorbed) when one mole of the reactant is converted to one mole of product at 25° and 1 atm pressure, and under (hypothetical) conditions where all reactants and products are maintained at $1\ M$ concentration (standard state by definition).

In the case of the reaction $A \rightleftharpoons B$,

$$\Delta G° = -970 \text{ cal mole}^{-1}$$

In most practical circumstances we do not deal with molar amounts and the equation

$$\Delta G = G° + 2.303RT \log \frac{\text{(actual concentration of product)}}{\text{(actual concentration of reactant)}} \tag{2}$$

is used to calculate the work that can be done under a specific set of conditions. Clearly, when the actual concentrations of reactants and products are the equilibrium values, Eq. (2) reduces to Eq. (1), since $\Delta G = 0$.

$$0 = \Delta G = \Delta G^\circ + 2.303RT \log K_{eq}$$

or

$$\Delta G^\circ = -2.303RT \log K_{eq}$$

As an example, let us calculate ΔG° for the reaction catalyzed by phosphoglucomutase (25°).

$$\text{glucose-1-P (G-1-P)} \rightleftharpoons \text{glucose-6-P (G-6-P)}$$

$$K_{eq} \text{ of } \frac{\text{G-6-P}}{\text{G-1-P}} = 17$$

$$\Delta G^\circ = -2.303RT \log 17$$

$$\Delta G^\circ = -2.303(1.987)(298) \log 17$$

$$\Delta G^\circ = -1,680 \text{ cal mole}^{-1}$$

The value obtained for ΔG° is $-1,680$ cal mole^{-1}, indicating that the reaction can proceed from left to right under standard conditions.

Let us now calculate ΔG under physiological conditions. In diaphragm muscle tissue, concentrations of glucose-6-P of 1×10^{-4} M and glucose-1-P of 3×10^{-5} M have been recorded (38°). Substituting in Eq. (2), we find

$$\Delta G = 1,680 + 2.303(1.987)(311) \log \frac{(1 \times 10^{-4})}{(3 \times 10^{-5})}$$

$$\Delta G = -1,680 + 1,428 \log 3.3$$

$$\Delta G = -1,680 + 1,428 (0.522)$$

$$\Delta G = -1,680 + 700$$

$$\Delta G = -980 \text{ cal mole}^{-1}$$

Thus, under physiological conditions, ΔG is less than ΔG° by some 700 cal mole^{-1}. The tendency for the reaction to go from left to right and the work that could be done is reduced under these physiological conditions.

It is possible that conditions will exist in the cell such that this reaction will have a tendency to proceed in the reverse direction. If the reactant concentration is decreased or the product concentration is increased so that the ratio of G-6-P/G-1-P exceeds 17, the ΔG of the reaction G-1-P $\rightleftharpoons$ G-6-P will be positive. However, that of the reaction G-6-P $\rightleftharpoons$ G-1-P will be negative and of the same magnitude.

The above discussion should have made clear that $\Delta G°$ values can be evaluated most readily by determining values for equilibrium constants.

3.2   COUPLED REACTIONS AND GROUP TRANSFER POTENTIALS

Metabolism consists of sequences of reactions. Some sequences yield free energy, others require it. How are these reactions arranged to allow coupling of the energy-yielding steps to the energy-requiring steps? First, let us consider the energetics of coupled reactions. An important use of $\Delta G°$ values derives from the fact that if two reactions can be coupled, their $\Delta G°$ values can be summed arithmetically and one can decide whether the sequence can proceed or not. As an example, let us consider the two reactions (3) and (4),

$$\text{ATP} + \text{H}_2\text{O} \rightleftharpoons \text{ADP} + \text{P}_i, \quad \Delta G° = -7{,}000 \text{ cal mole}^{-1} \tag{3}$$

$$\text{glucose} + \text{P}_i \rightleftharpoons \text{glucose-6-P} + \text{H}_2\text{O}, \quad \Delta G° = 3{,}000 \text{ cal mole}^{-1} \tag{4}$$

and ask what $\Delta G°$ would be for the sum of the reactions.

$$\text{ATP} + \text{glucose} \rightleftharpoons \text{ADP} + \text{glucose-6-P}, \quad \Delta G° = -4{,}000 \text{ cal mole}^{-1} \tag{5}$$

Summing the two reactions, we obtain a value of $-4{,}000$ cal mole^{-1}, indicating that if the reaction shown in (5) can be carried out it will proceed with the release of energy. Thus if we wish to produce glucose-6-phosphate, it would be feasible to do it by reaction (5) but not by reaction (4). What we have done in effect is to tap off the energy in the ATP for a biosynthesis which would not have taken place in its absence. The reaction involves transfer of a phosphate group and it is useful to consider the tendency of a variety of phosphate derivatives to transfer their phosphates to the common acceptor, water. A list of these group transfer potentials is given in Table 3.1. They are actually values for the $\Delta G°$ of hydrolysis of the compounds. The higher up the list, the greater is the potential of the compound; and substances higher on the list can transfer groups to acceptors lower on the list.

Reactions which occur in sequence can also be coupled, so that a reaction with a high value of $\Delta G°$ can "pull" preceding reactions, even though they have low or even positive values for $\Delta G°$. For example, consider the reaction sequence A $\overset{a}{\rightleftharpoons}$ B $\overset{b}{\rightleftharpoons}$ C $\overset{c}{\rightleftharpoons}$ D catalyzed by the enzymes a, b, and c so that the equilibria are rapidly established. Let us assume that the $\Delta G°$ values are $+3$ kcal mole^{-1} for A $\rightleftharpoons$ B, -0.5 kcal mole^{-1} for B $\rightleftharpoons$ C, and -7 kcal mole^{-1} for C $\rightleftharpoons$ D. $\Delta G°$ for the overall process is -4.5 kcal

TABLE 3.1 ΔG°_{hyd} **VALUES OF PHOSPHATE COMPOUNDS**

ΔG°_{hyd} kcal mole^{-1} at pH 7	Direction of Group Transfer	Group Transferred
14 — Acetylimidazole		Acetyl
Phosphoenolpyruvate		Phosphate
12 — 1,3-Diphosphoglycerate		Phosphate
Creatine phosphate		Phosphate
10 — Acetylphosphate		Phosphate or acetyl
S-Adenosylmethionine		Methyl
8 — Acetyl-S-Coenzyme A		Coenzyme A-SH or acetyl
Adenosine triphosphate		Phosphate
Uridine diphosphate glucose		Glucose
Arginine phosphate		Phosphate
Sucrose		Glucose or fructose
6 — Glucose-1-phosphate		Glucose or phosphate
Glycylglycine		Glycine
4 — Glutamine		Ammonia
Glucose-6-phosphate		Phosphate
Lactose		Galactose
Fructose-6-phosphate		
2 — Glycerol-1-phosphate		
— Peptide bond (in large polypeptide)		

mole^{-1} and at equilibrium more than 99 per cent of the reactants will be present as D. It should be apparent that there will be more of A at equilibrium than either B or C and that B will be present in the least amount.

In biological systems, the energy-requiring reactions are driven by reagents such as ATP and the energy-yielding metabolic reactions are concerned with the synthesis of ATP.

3.3 CHEMICAL CONSIDERATIONS

Now, we may inquire into the chemical reasons for the high group transfer potential nature of some compounds and not of others. The compounds with high group transfer potential fall into several classes, the anhydrides (ATP, ADP, acetyl phosphates, APS, PAPS, 1,3-diphosphoglycerate), the enol phosphates (phosphoenolpyruvate), the N-phosphates (arginine-P and creatine-P), the thioesters (acetyl-S-CoA), and the sulfonium compound (S-adenosyl-methionine).* The chemical reasons lying behind the high energy nature

* All of these have ΔG°_{hyd} values which are greater than about -7000 cal mole^{-1}.

or high group potential nature of these compounds are several:

1. There is an increase in the number of resonance forms in the split products when compared to the compound itself, so that there is an increase in resonance energy on hydrolysis. For example, the acetate carboxyl group and inorganic phosphate can exist in a larger number of resonance forms than can acetylphosphate.

2. Hydrolysis of many high energy compounds leads to a decrease in electrostatic repulsion in the split products, e.g., the hydrolysis of 1.3-diphosphoglycerate to 3-phosphoglycerate allows the highly negatively charged phosphate groups to be separated and the resonance of the system to increase.

$$
\begin{array}{c}
\begin{array}{cc} O & O \\ \| & \| \\ C{-}O{-}P{-}O^- \\ & | \\ & O^- \end{array} \\
| \\
H{-}C{-}OH \\
| \quad\quad O \\
\quad\quad \| \\
HC{-}O{-}P{-}O^- \\
| \quad\quad | \\
H \quad\quad O^-
\end{array}
\xrightarrow{\;H_2O\;}
\begin{array}{c}
COO^- \\
| \\
H{-}C{-}OH \\
| \quad\quad O \\
\quad\quad \| \\
H{-}C{-}O{-}P{-}O^- \\
| \quad\quad | \\
H \quad\quad O^-
\end{array}
\;+\;
\begin{array}{c}
O \\
\| \\
HO{-}P{-}O^- \\
| \\
O^-
\end{array}
$$

This is also true for ATP, which has the unusual distribution of charges shown below.

$$
\text{adenine-ribose}\ \overset{+0.153}{\underset{\downarrow}{\rule{0pt}{0pt}}}\!\!O\!\!-\!\!\overset{\overset{\displaystyle O\;{-0.809}}{\nwarrow}}{\underset{\underset{\displaystyle O\;{-0.809}}{\swarrow}}{\overset{+0.208}{\underset{+0.393}{P}}}}\!\!-\!\!\overset{+0.204}{\underset{\downarrow}{\rule{0pt}{0pt}}}\!\!O\!\!-\!\!\overset{\overset{\displaystyle O\;{-0.805}}{\nwarrow}}{\underset{\underset{\displaystyle O\;{-0.805}}{\swarrow}}{\overset{+0.204}{\underset{+0.397}{P}}}}\!\!-\!\!O\!\!-\!\!\overset{\overset{\displaystyle O\;{-0.821}}{\nwarrow}}{\underset{\underset{\displaystyle O\;{-0.821}}{\swarrow}}{\overset{-0.821}{\underset{+0.364}{P}}}}\!\!-\!\!O
$$

There is a main backbone made up of atoms carrying a net positive charge, surrounded by atoms which are negatively charged. When hydrolysis occurs, these repulsions are decreased and the resonance possibilities are increased.

3. In some cases, the *keto-enol* tautomerism in the split products, which is prohibited in the combined compound, is an extremely important factor. In the case of phosphoenol pyruvate, the major contribution to the $\Delta G°$ of hydrolysis comes from the conversion of the enol pyruvate into the keto form.

$$
\begin{array}{c}
\text{COO}^- \\
| \\
\text{C}-\text{O}-\overset{\overset{\displaystyle O}{\|}}{\underset{\underset{\displaystyle O^-}{|}}{\text{P}}}-\text{O}^- + H_2O \longrightarrow \quad
\begin{array}{c}
\text{COO}^- \\
| \\
\text{C}-\text{OH} \\
\| \\
\text{CH}_2
\end{array}
\rightleftharpoons
\begin{array}{c}
\text{COO}^- \\
| \\
\text{C}=\text{O} \\
| \\
\text{CH}_3
\end{array}
+ \;\text{HO}-\overset{\overset{\displaystyle O}{\|}}{\underset{\underset{\displaystyle O^-}{|}}{\text{O}}}-\text{O}^- \\
\| \\
\text{CH}_2
\end{array}
$$

enol   keto

4. Hydrolysis of many high energy phosphates leads to an increase in charge, as may be seen for the hydrolysis of ATP. The $\Delta G°$ of hydrolysis of ATP is extremely dependent on pH ($-$log of hydrogen ion concentration) and at physiological pH values, about pH 7, a significant portion of the $\Delta G°$ is due to the ionization reaction.

$$H_2O + ATP^{4-} \rightleftharpoons ADP^{3-} + P_i^{2-} + H^+$$

The free energy of ionization can be calculated from the equation

$$\Delta G_i = 2.303 RT \Sigma\, (pK_i - pH) - 2.303 RT \log\left(1 + \frac{[H^+]}{K_a}\right)$$

where $\Sigma\, pK_i - pH$ is the sum of each $pK_i - pH$ difference for each ionization (one for each pK_i), pH is the experimental pH, and K_a the constant for the dissociation which is incomplete, i.e., highest pK_a. If at the experimental pH, all dissociations are complete, the last term drops out and the equation becomes

$$\Delta G_i = 2.303 RT\, (pK_i - pH)$$

In the cited case, if the pK_i of the ADP is 6.2 and the operating pH is 7.4, we calculate at 38°

$$\Delta G_i = 2.303(1.987)(311)(6.2 - 7.4)$$

$$\Delta G_i = -1,700 \text{ cal mole}^{-1}$$

It can be seen that this ionization is an important added factor in favoring the hydrolysis of ATP, that is, in favoring the reaction from left to right.

In Table 3.2 are tabulated the contributions of the chemical factors contributing to the "energy richness" of phosphate compounds.

3.4   THE GENERATION OF ATP

Much of the remainder of this book will deal with sequences of reactions whose utility to the cell (or organism) is the production of energy. At this

TABLE 3.2   FACTORS CONTRIBUTING TO "ENERGY RICHNESS" OF HIGH
ENERGY PHOSPHATE COMPOUNDS (KCAL MOLE^{-1})[a]

Compound	Experimental	Base Line	Resonance	Calculated Electrostatic Repulsion	Keto-Enol Tautomerism	Free Energy of Ionization	Total
ATP	7–8	3	2.6	2			7.6
ADP	7–8	3	2.6	1.4			7
Carboxyl-P	10–12	3	4.6	−0.7		3.2	10.1
Phosphoenol-pyruvate	11.5–12.5	3	1.0	−0.5	9		12.5
Guanidino-P	9–10	3	1.2	−0.7		?	?

[a] Modified from A. Pullman and B. Pullman, "From Quantum Chemistry to Quantum Biochemistry," *Horizons in Biochemistry,* Edited by M. Kasha and B. Pullman. Academic Press, New York, 1962.

point, though, we will consider the general problem of producing compounds having high group transfer potentials. What the cell must do is generate a metabolite which has in it the group to be transferred. In the case of ATP synthesis this would be the phosphate group. The metabolite must be rearranged so that it has a group transfer potential sufficient to accomplish the formation of ATP and the total sequence of reactions has to have a sufficiently negative $\Delta G°$ to proceed to completion. The $\Delta G°$ of hydrolysis of the phosphorylated metabolite must be two to three kilocalories greater than that of ATP if the formation of ATP is to be efficiently accomplished in one step. The excess energy will be liberated as heat, but its release ensures that the reaction proceeds to completion.

Similar mechanisms are involved in the production of other metabolites having high group transfer potentials. However, there are other quite different ways in which energy can be conserved. These are in the processes of oxidative-phosphorylation, in photosynthesis, and in the generation of reducing power for the production of saturated systems from unsaturated systems.

3.5   OXIDATIVE-PHOSPHORYLATION

It is possible to obtain energy from a chemical reaction in the form of electrical potential, and conversely it is possible to use electrical energy to drive a chemical reaction. Electrical energy can be generated when oxidations occur by the removal of electrons which are then used in a reduction process. If the electrons fall through a potential drop, energy is evolved.

The relationship between an oxidation-reduction potential difference and the standard free-energy change is

$$\Delta G° = -nFE°$$

where n is the number of moles of electrons transferred in the reaction, F is Faraday's constant, 23,061 calories per volt per equivalent, and $E°$ is the standard oxidation-reduction potential difference, i.e., the potential that exists when a solution, one molar with respect to both the oxidized and reduced forms of a compound, is coupled to the standard hydrogen system

$$H \longrightarrow H^+ + e$$

For example, for the reaction in which cytochrome c is oxidized from the ferrous to the ferric state with oxygen, $E°$ being $+ 0.56$ volt,

$$2 \text{ cytochrome c Fe}^{2+} + \tfrac{1}{2}O_2 \rightleftharpoons 2 \text{ cytochrome c Fe}^{3+} + O^{2-}$$

$$\Delta G° = -2(23,061)(0.56)$$

$$\Delta G° = -25,853 \text{ cal mole}^{-1}$$

Thus, the reaction can occur with the release of energy in sufficient amount to generate ATP from ADP + P_i.

Figure 3.1   Diagram of pathways of carbon flow (left hand portion) and electron flow (right hand portion) in metabolism. The specific pathways of glycolysis and the tricarboxylic acid cycle will be discussed in Chapter 4. The electron transport chain catalysts are shown in boxes. The principal direction of flow is indicated by the arrows. The sites of conversion of ADP^{-3} + Pi^{-2} + H^+ to ATP^{-4} are as indicated. DPN^+-diphosphopyridine nucleotide; FP-flavoprotein; UQ-ubiquinone; B, C, A + A_3-cytochromes B, C, A + A_3. Modified from A. L. Lehninger, *Bioenergetics,* W. A. Benjamin, 1965.

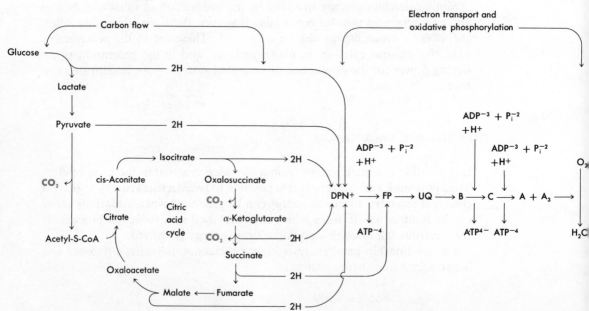

In most cells which obtain energy by oxygen-utilizing oxidation reactions there exist specialized organelles, the *mitochondria,* which contain a system known as the *electron transport system.* This complex system is supplied with electrons obtained from the oxidation of metabolites and channels them through a potential drop to oxygen. In the process, by a mechanism (or mechanisms) which is incompletely understood, the synthesis of 3ATP from 3ADP and $3P_i$ is accomplished. The overall reaction which occurs in the system is termed *oxidative-phosphorylation.*

The chain of respiratory carriers for the transport of electrons consists of a highly structurally organized system of colored iron-containing proteins, the cytochromes, together with several low-molecular-weight compounds, ubiquinone, flavin, and pyridine nucleotides, which can undergo reversible oxidation-reduction reactions (see appendix for structures). All are spatially arranged in the lipo-protein inner membranes of mitochondria. In Figure 3.1 is shown a diagram of the pathways of carbon flow, electron transport, and oxidative phosphorylation. The mitochondrion shown in Figure 3.2 is a

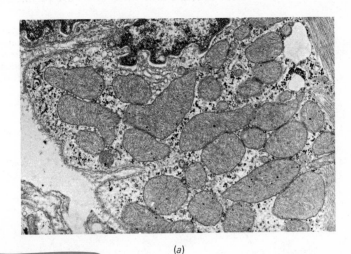

(a)

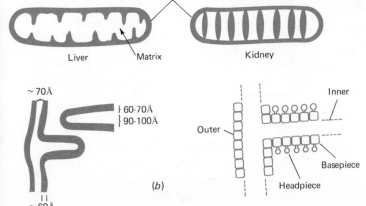

Cristae

Liver   Matrix   Kidney

~70Å

} 60-70Å
} 90-100Å

Outer

Inner

Headpiece

Basepiece

(b)

| |
~60Å

Figure 3.2

(*a*) Actual photograph of a mitochondrion from skeletal muscle (rat diaphragm). Courtesy of R. R. Cardell Jr., University of Virginia. (*b*) Schematic structure of a mitochondrion. The outer and inner membranes are as shown. The cristae are projections of the inner membranes.

fluid-filled, ovoid particle which is sometimes branched and located within the cell cytoplasm. The wall is a double layer made up of outer and inner membranes continuous with an array of closely packed vesicles or *cristae* as shown schematically in this figure. The inner membranes with the inner compartment contain all of the enzymes of the *citric acid (combustion) cycle*, (Figure 3.1) (see definition, chapter 4) the electron transport chain of respiratory carriers, and the apparatus for oxidative phosphorylation. The outer membrane, on the other hand, is similar in composition and function to the smooth membranes of the endoplasmic reticulum.

The chain of respiratory electron carriers is ordered by the oxidation-reduction potentials of the respective couples from substrate to oxygen as shown in Figure 3.3. The potentials become increasingly positive toward O_2. There is more than one entry into the system at the ubiquinone level: from the succinate-fumarate couple directly into flavin adenine dinucleotide (FAD), as well as from the malate-oxaloacetate couple through DPN and flavin mononucleotide (FMN). From fractionation studies it has become clear that the individual steps are physically as well as chemically related to

Figure 3.3   The respiratory electron transport chain. The numbers in parentheses indicate the approximate ratio of numbers of molecules of each component relative to each other: cytochrome (1), flavoproteins (2–3) and pyridine nucleotides (10–20). The values for the O–R potentials (E_0^1) are given in volts. The values for the voltage steps ΔE_0^1 are also pointed out.

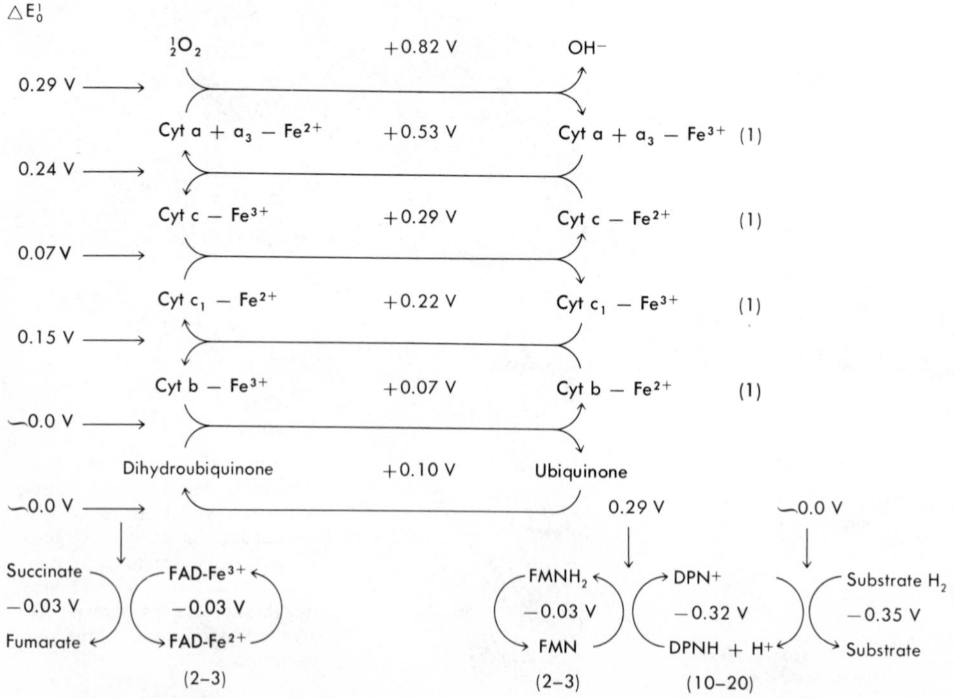

each other. Relatively mild disruptive procedures produce particles which catalyze the whole or sizable portions of the sequence. Further fractionation produces particles catalyzing smaller portions of the sequence. From these kinds of manipulations, the physical association of the carriers has been deduced. The molar ratios of the components, especially the molar equivalence of the cytochromes, is another important argument for this concept. DPN, ubiquinone, and possibly cytochrome c appear to be more soluble and therefore less intimately associated with the membranes.

For example, by fractionating submitochondrial particles with detergents, four kinds of particles have been obtained. These four particles each transport electrons separately through the following spans

$$\text{I} \quad \text{DPNH} \longrightarrow \text{ubiquinone}$$

$$\text{II} \quad \text{succinate} \longrightarrow \text{ubiquinone}$$

$$\text{III} \quad \text{ubiquinone} \longrightarrow \text{cytochrome c}$$

$$\text{IV} \quad \text{cytochrome c} \longrightarrow \text{O}_2$$

The complete chain of reactions by all four particles appears to be coupled by the three readily soluble components, DPN, ubiquinone, and cytochrome c.

Water, the final product, appears to be formed as follows: From substrate, hydrogen atoms are transferred to flavoprotein either directly or through DPN as an intermediate. Non-heme iron oxidizes the reduced flavin and protons are released

$$\text{FADH}_2 + 2\text{Fe}^{3+} \longrightarrow \text{FAD} + 2\text{Fe}^{2+} + 2\text{H}^+$$

to be taken up in the next reaction, the reduction of ubiquinone (UQ).

$$\text{UQ} + 2\text{H}^+ + 2\text{Fe}^{2+} \longrightarrow \text{UQH}_2 + 2\text{Fe}^{3+}$$

The ubiquinone is oxidized by cytochrome b with release of protons.

$$\text{UQH}_2 + 2 \text{ cyt b Fe}^{3+} \longrightarrow \text{UQ} + 2 \text{ cyt b Fe}^{2+} + 2\text{H}^+$$

In the final reaction, oxygen is reduced to OH^- by cytochrome oxidase.

$$\tfrac{1}{2}\text{O}_2 + \text{H}_2\text{O} + 2 \text{ cyt ox Fe}^{2+} \longrightarrow 2\text{OH}^- + 2 \text{ cyt ox Fe}^{3+}$$

OH^- together with H^+ form water.

$$\textit{Sum} \quad \text{UQH}_2 + \tfrac{1}{2}\text{O}_2 \longrightarrow \text{UQ} + \text{H}_2\text{O}$$

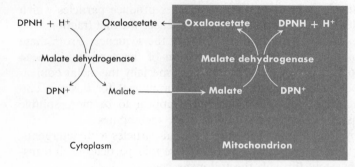

Figure 3.4

The mitochondrial-cytosol shuttle of reducing potential. In the cytoplasm oxaloacetate is reduced to malate via malate dehydrogenase. DPNH is oxidized to DPN+. Malate enters the mitochondrion where it is oxidized to oxaloacetate via malate dehydrogenase located within the mitochondrion. DPN+ is reduced to DPNH. The oxaloacetate leaves the mitochondrion and enters the cytoplasm. Then the process is repeated.

It is important to emphasize that reduced pyridine nucleotide formed in the cytoplasm does not readily enter mitochondria because of a permeability barrier. The reducing power of pyridine nucleotides can be transferred to mitochondria via substrates capable of reversible oxidation-reduction reactions catalyzed by enzyme systems present in *both* cytoplasm and mitochondria. Several are known, but malate dehydrogenase, which may be of significance in animal cells, will serve to illustrate (Figure 3.4). In the cytoplasm, reduced DPN is oxidized by malate dehydrogenase coupled with oxaloacetate reduction to malate. Malate enters the mitochondria and is reoxidized to oxaloacetate with reduction of DPN+ to DPNH + H+. This reaction is catalyzed by mitochondrial malate dehydrogenase. The oxaloacetate formed leaves the mitochondrion and reenters the cytoplasm to complete the cycle.

The oxidation-reduction potentials ($E°$ values) of the electron carriers, and the corresponding $\Delta G°$ values for the transfers are shown in Figure 3.3. Note that there are three large steps:

$$\text{DPN} \longrightarrow \text{FMN; cyt b} \longrightarrow \text{cyt c; and cyt a} \longrightarrow O_2$$

These steps are the sites of energy-conserving reactions of oxidative phosphorylation of electron transport.

Although the detailed mechanism of the oxidative phosphorylation of electron transport is not known, some chemical information is available. The oxygen in the newly formed anhydride bond of ATP has been shown to derive from ADP and not from P_i. This means that in the condensation of ADP and P_i to ATP, the P_i is activated rather than the ADP; i.e., mechanism II operates rather than mechanism I where ADP~X and P_i~X are hypothetical "high energy" compounds.

$$\text{I}\quad \text{ADP~X} + \quad P_i \longrightarrow \text{ATP} + \text{X}$$
$$\text{II}\quad\quad P_i\text{~X} + \text{ADP} \longrightarrow \text{ATP} + P_i$$

This fits in with the fact that if oxidative phosphorylation is carried out in the presence of P_i labeled with ^{18}O, it rapidly exchanges the label into H_2O.

There are three theories of oxidative phosphorylation that need to be considered. One states that there are covalent phosphorylated intermediates (involving P_i) of the type $P_i{\sim}X$. Another states that there is a direct reversal of ATP hydrolysis, namely, a condensation of ADP $+$ P_i to yield ATP. This could occur under circumstances such that

$$ADP^{3-} + P^{2-} + H^+ \longrightarrow ATP^{4-} + H_2O$$

the negative free energy of hydrolysis would be overcome by supplying protons to the system and by the removal of the water formed, using a highly organized cellular membrane to separate these reactions; this is discussed in Chapter 10. The third theory states that electron transport brings about a conformational change in the mitochondrial membranes, which can be observed microscopically as an alteration of structure. This "energy rich" conformation is discharged by an unknown mechanism on forming ATP.

The Electron Transport System

There are two pyridine nucleotides, DPN and TPN, which occur in cells. DPN is a component of the electron transport chain, whereas TPN is in-

TABLE 3.3   STEREOSPECIFICITY OF SOME PYRIDINE NUCLEOTIDE DEHYDROGENASES[a]

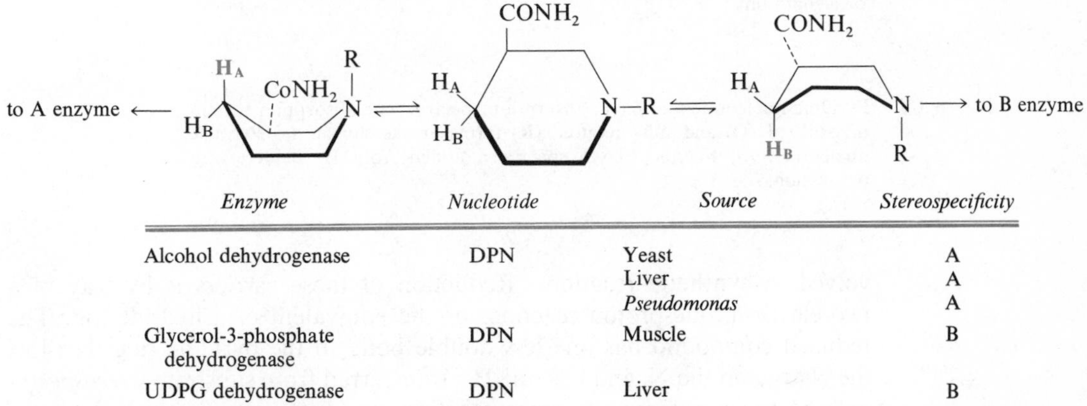

Enzyme	Nucleotide	Source	Stereospecificity
Alcohol dehydrogenase	DPN	Yeast	A
		Liver	A
		Pseudomonas	A
Glycerol-3-phosphate dehydrogenase	DPN	Muscle	B
UDPG dehydrogenase	DPN	Liver	B
Glyoxalate reductase	DPN	Spinach	A
	TPN	Peas	A
Lactate dehydrogenase	DPN	Muscle	A
	DPN	*Lactobacillus plantarum*	A
	DPN	Potato	A
Glycerate dehydrogenase	DPN	Parsley	A
	DPN	Liver (pig)	A
3-Hydroxyacyl-S-CoA dehydrogenase	DPN	Muscle	B

[a] Modified from R. Bentley, *Molecular Asymmetry in Biology*, Academic Press, New York, 1969.

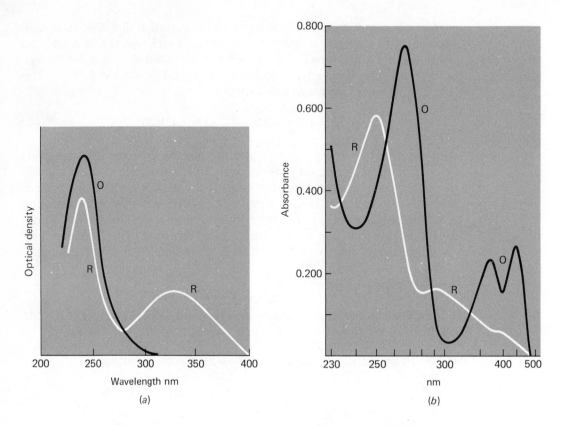

Figure 3.5   Pyridine nucleotide and flavin absorption spectra. The absorption spectra of oxidized (O) and fully reduced (R) forms are as shown. (*a*) Pyridine nucleotide; (*b*) Flavin. Flavin spectra modified from H. Beinert with permission.

volved in synthetic reactions. Reduction of these carriers is by way of a two-electron, one-proton reaction, or the equivalent of a hydride ion. The reduced compound has one less double bond in the pyridine ring, has lost the charge on the N, and has one H+ transferred from substrate *stereospecifically* to the 4 position. In some reactions the hydrogen is attached to one side of the ring, in others to the opposite side. The stereospecificity of a number of pyridine nucleotide-linked dehydrogenases (A or B) is illustrated in Table 3.3. It is of interest that the absolute configuration of the H in the A and B positions has been determined. The reduced forms of the pyridine nucleotides absorb strongly at 340 nm (Figure 3.5). They also exhibit fluorescence with maximal emission at about 465 nm when activated by light at 340 nm. These properties are extremely important since they are most widely used for analyzing systems in which DPNH (or TPNH) is formed or utilized.

Flavoproteins

Flavin compounds and flavoproteins are frequently yellow-colored and have distinct absorption spectra with maxima about 280, 380, and 450 nm (Figure 3.5). On complete reduction, the spectrum is markedly reduced, while on half-reduction to the semiquinone, a decrease is observed in the above mentioned bands (with the appearance of a broad band at 550–650 nm).

In Table 3.4, the components of a number of flavoprotein systems are listed. As can be appreciated, there is an astonishing diversity. The systems vary from no extra components to systems containing one or more metal ions, hemes, and other redox groups, such as ubiquinone.

The simple flavoproteins contain either FMN or FAD or both as redox molecules (Figure 3.3). Enzymes containing a single flavin appear to operate

TABLE 3.4 FLAVOPROTEIN ENZYME SYSTEMS

Enzyme	Substrate	Source	Electron Acceptor	Other Components
Monoamine oxidase	Various amines	Outer mitochondrial membrane of various organs, blood plasma	O_2	—
Diamine oxidase	Various diamines	Various organs, blood plasma	O_2	—
D-Amino acid oxidase	D-Amino acids	Liver, kidney	O_2	—
L-Amino acid oxidase	L-Amino acids	Kidney, snake venom, molds	O_2	—
Glucose oxidase	β-D-Glucose	Molds, liver	O_2	—
Hydrogenase	H_2	*Clostridium pasteurianum*	Various	—
Acyl-S-CoA dehydrogenase	Various acyl-S-CoA's (C6–C12)	Mitochondria of heart and liver	Flavoprotein	—
Butyryl-S-CoA dehydrogenase	Butyryl-S-CoA	Mitochondria of heart and liver	Flavoprotein	—
Dihydrolipoate dehydrogenase	Dihydrolipoic acid	Mitochondria of heart, liver E. coli	DPN+	—
Glutathione oxidase	Reduced glutathione	Liver, yeast E. coli	TPN+	
DPNH oxidase	DPNH, H+	Microsomes of liver	Cytochrome b_5	—
TPNH oxidase	TPNH, H+	Microsomes of liver	Cytochrome c	—
TPNH oxidase	TPNH, H+	Yeast		
TPNH oxidase	TPNH, H+	Yeast	O_2	
TPNH oxidase	TPNH, H+	Erythrocytes		—
Choline oxidase	Choline	Mitochondria of liver	Respiratory chain	Fe
Sarcosine oxidase	Sarcosine	Mitochondria of liver and kidney	Flavoprotein	Fe(?)
Dihydroorotate dehydrogenase	Dihydroorotate	*Zymobacterium oroticum*	DPN+	Fe

TABLE 3.4 **(Continued)**

Enzyme	Substrate	Source	Electron Acceptor	Other Components
DPNH oxidase	DPNH, H+	Mitochondria of heart	Respiratory chain	Fe
Pyridine nucleotide oxidase	DPNH, H+ TPNH, H+	Heart	Menadione	
Succinate oxidase	Succinate	Mitochondria	Respiratory chain	Fe
α-Glycerophosphate oxidase	Glycero-P	Mitochondria of liver	Respiratory chain	Fe
Xanthine oxidase	Various purines	Milk	O_2	Mo, Fe
Xanthine oxidase	Various purines	Chicken liver	O_2 DPN	Mo, Fe
Nitrate reductase or TPNH oxidase	TPNH, H+	Mold	NO_3^-	Mo
Sulfite reductase or TPNH oxidase	TPNH, H+	E. coli	SO_3^{2-}	Fe
D-Lactate oxidase	D-Lactate	Yeast	Cytochrome c	Zn
L-Lactate oxidase	L-Lactate	Yeast	Cytochrome c	Heme
D-α-Hydroxy-acid oxidase	D-α-Hydroxy acids	Yeast		Zn Heme
Sulfite oxidase	SO_3^{2-}		Cytochrome c, O_2	Heme
Aldehyde oxidase	Various aldehydes	Liver	O_2	Fe, Mo, ubiquinone
Nitrate reductase or DPNH oxidase	DPNH, H+	E. coli M. tuberculosis		
Nitrate reductase or DPNH oxidase	DPNH, H+	P. aeruginosa	NO_3^-	Cu, Fe, heme
Nitrate reductase or DPNH oxidase	DPNH, H+			
Formic oxidase or nitrate reductase	Formic acid	E. coli	NO_3^-	Vitamin K_3, cytochrome b_1

via the two hydrogen atom mechanism (two electrons, two H+). The reduced forms can frequently be reoxidized by oxygen to produce hydrogen peroxide. This does not occur in the electron transport system. Enzymes containing pairs of flavins appear to operate by free radical mechanisms in which the flavins alternate between fully oxidized and semiquinone forms,

$$
\text{enz} \begin{cases} -\text{FAD} \\ -\text{FAD} \end{cases} + \text{AH}_2 \longrightarrow \text{enz} \begin{cases} -\text{FA}\dot{\text{D}}\,\text{H} --- \dot{\text{A}}\text{H} \\ -\text{FAD} \end{cases}
$$

$$
\text{enz} \begin{cases} -\text{FA}\dot{\text{D}}\,\text{H} -- \dot{\text{A}}\text{H} \\ -\text{FAD} \end{cases} + \text{O}_2 \longrightarrow \text{enz} \begin{cases} -\text{FAD} \\ -\text{FAD} \end{cases} + \text{A} + \text{H}_2\text{O}_2
$$

or fully reduced and semiquinone forms (e.g., TPNH-cytochrome C reductase)

$$\text{enz}\begin{cases}-\overset{\bullet}{\text{FADH}} \\ -\underset{\bullet}{\text{FADH}}\end{cases} + \text{TPNH} + \text{H}^+ \longrightarrow \text{enz}\begin{cases}-\text{FADH}_2 \\ -\text{FADH}_2\end{cases} + \text{TPN}^+$$

$$\text{enz}\begin{cases}-\text{FADH}_2 \\ -\text{FADH}_2\end{cases} + 2\text{cyt c Fe}^{3+} \longrightarrow \text{enz}\begin{cases}-\overset{\bullet}{\text{FADH}} \\ -\underset{\bullet}{\text{FADH}}\end{cases} + 2\text{cyt c Fe}^{2+} + 2\text{H}^+$$

The metalloflavoproteins contain a metal, e.g., Fe or Mo, which also can be involved in oxidation-reduction reactions. The hemoflavoproteins contain heme.

Non-Heme Iron Proteins

It has become apparent recently that a new class of electron transport compounds exists, the non-heme iron proteins, called the *ferredoxins*. Some are listed in Table 3.5. These function in photosynthesis (*vide infra*), bacterial H_2 and N_2 fixation, as well as in oxidative phosphorylation.

TABLE 3.5 NON-HEME IRON PROTEINS

Source	Molecular Weight	Fe/mole	E'_0 (volts)
Clostridia ferredoxin	6,000	5–7	−0.42
Chromatia ferredoxin	6,000	3	−0.49
Spinach ferredoxin	13,000	2	−0.43
Adrenal microsomal adrenodoxin	22,000	2	+0.15

Cytochromes

The cytochromes are all heme-containing proteins. The only soluble cytochrome, cytochrome c, has been best studied. The amino acid sequence (molecular weight about 12,500) is known for the protein from a wide variety of bacterial, insect, and animal species. Variations in the sequence of amino acids in certain portions of the molecule have been used to trace evolutionary development. The sequence is constant in other portions; for example, in the heme-protein linkage region where the sequence is

$$-\text{cys}-\text{x}-\text{y}-\text{cys}-\text{his}$$
$$\boxed{\text{heme}}$$

the constant amino acids are underlined. The structure of the heme-iron protein complex (see Appendix) shows the two thioether linkages and the coordination of the Fe to four nitrogens of the porphyrin ring and to two nitrogens of histidine (imidazole rings) in the protein. This system accounts for the intense red color and the absorption spectra of cytochromes (and other heme proteins) (Table 3.6). The cytochromes undergo oxidation-re-

TABLE 3.6 PROPERTIES OF MAMMALIAN CYTOCHROMES

Cytochrome	Absorption Maxima of Reduced Forms		
	α_1 mμ	β mμ	γ mμ
a_3	600		445
a	605	517	414
c	550	521	416
c_1	554	523	418
b	563	530	430
b_5	557	527	423

duction by a one-electron mechanism in which the iron alternates between ferrous and ferric states.

The terminal member cytochrome oxidase (a + a_3) reduces O_2. It appears to be a polymer (monomer molecular weight about 72,000), containing one atom of copper in addition to the one heme per monomer.

3.6 PHOTOSYNTHETIC MECHANISMS FOR GENERATING ENERGY

Visible light is a small portion of the electromagnetic radiation spectrum. The energy content of photons as a function of wavelength is shown in Table 3.7. As can be seen, the energy of light in calories per Einstein varies inversely with the wavelength. An *Einstein* is a mole of photons (6.02×10^{23}).

Nature has developed mechanisms by which cellular enzymatic glycolysis and respiration reactions are coupled with the formation of the phosphate anhydride linkages of ATP as just discussed. ATP can also be generated by photosynthetic reactions carried out in green plants and certain bacteria. These reactions also result in CO_2 being reductively converted to sugar, and oxygen being formed as shown below:

$$6CO_2 + 6H_2O + 6nh\gamma \longrightarrow C_6H_{12}O_6 + 6O_2$$

where n is the quantum requirement per molecule of O_2 produced, γ is the light frequency (the reciprocal of the wavelength in centimeters) and h is Planck's constant.

TABLE 3.7   PHOTON ENERGY CONTENT[a]

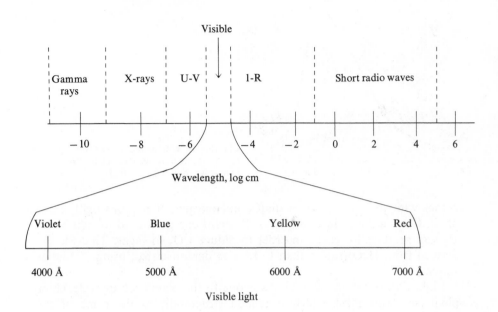

Visible light

Wavelength Å	Color	cal/Einstein
3,950	Violet	71,800
4,900	Blue	57,880
5,900	Yellow	58,060
6,500	Red	43,480
7,500	Far red	37,800

[a] Figure from A. L. Lehninger, *Bioenergetics,* W. A. Benjamin, New York, 1965.

Photosynthesis in purple bacteria involves a hydrogen donor other than H_2O, such as H_2, H_2S, or certain other inorganic or organic reductants,

$$6CO_2 + 12H_2A + 6n'h\gamma \longrightarrow C_6H_{12}O_6 + 12A$$

where n' is the quantum requirement per A produced.

It is frequently stated that photosynthesis is the reverse of respiration. It is true that the overall chemical reactions are the reverse of each other, but the energy relations are different and the fact that ATP is produced in both reactions should warn the reader that a simple reversal surely is not involved. Respiration produces energy as ATP and metabolic intermediates. It requires substrate and oxygen. Photosynthesis produces energy as ATP to-

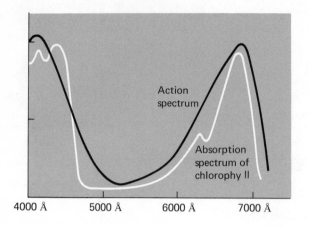

Figure 3.6

Chlorophyll action and absorption spectrum. For a discussion see the text. From A. L. Lehninger, *Bioenergetics,* Ibid.

gether with metabolic intermediates and oxygen. It requires light, chlorophyll, CO_2, and a reductant (H_2A). Radiant energy is used to split H_2O or H_2A to produce hydrogen in order to reduce CO_2 to sugar. That the O_2 is derived from H_2O (rather than CO_2) was demonstrated, using ^{18}O-labeled water.

Light absorption in green plants is due to the planar tetrapyrrole, chlorophyll (see Appendix), which is related structurally to the heme of cytochromes, hemoglobin, and myoglobin, but further reduced (dihydroporphyrin). Chlorophyll has a Mg^{2+} chelated to the tetrapyrrole structure in place of the Fe present in the other pigments. It also contains a long lipophylic phytyl side chain which enhances its solubility in lipid media.

That the chlorophyll is the main absorber of light energy is shown by an elegant experiment, which demonstrates that the spectrum of the efficiency of light in driving photosynthetic reactions (action spectrum) corresponds with the absorption spectrum of chlorophyll (Figure 3.6).

However, chlorophyll is not the only light absorber present. In algae and photosynthetic bacteria, light energy is absorbed by carotenoids (lipid-soluble colored compounds) and can be transferred to chlorophyll. In oxygen-producing plants, carotenoids also play a role, but in this case they appear to protect chlorophyll from photooxidation.

Just as respiratory oxidative phosphorylation is carried out in mitochondria, so photosynthetic oxidative phosphorylation is carried out in a highly organized efficient particle, the chloroplast [Figure 3.7(a)], which may or may not be arranged in highly ordered parallel membranous layers known as *grana,* shown diagrammatically in Figure 3.7(b). The *granum* has stacked layers of chlorophyll molecules encased in lipo-protein membranes which contain the electron transport and photosynthetic phosphorylation systems.

When chlorophyll is excited by light, an electron is promoted to an orbital of higher energy representing an excited state. In the test tube the electron may return to its original orbital, and energy is given off as fluorescence and heat. In the plant, however, the energy is not released but is conserved by

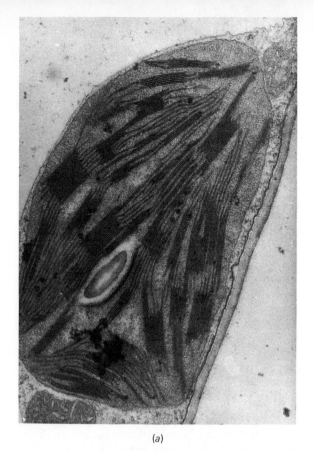

(a)

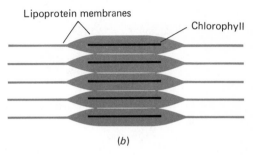

(b)

Figure 3.7

Structures of the (a) chloroplast and (b) grana. Note the high degree of organization present. Chloroplast and mitochondria of bean leaf (Phaseolus vulgaris) x2500 J. E. Weier.

reactions which lead to the formation of ATP. In the latter case, the electron in the higher energy orbital may be transported by a series of carriers along a new pathway to which ATP formation is coupled. Note the similarity at this point to the oxidative phosphorylation associated with electron transport in the mitochondrion. Finally, the electron, either directly or indirectly, is restored to its original orbital in the chlorophyll molecule. The electron transport chain in plants consists of the following simplified sequence

$$\text{ferredoxin} \longrightarrow \text{FP} \longrightarrow \text{cyt b} \longrightarrow \text{cyt f}$$

where ferredoxin (Table 3.5) is a non-heme iron protein capable of being oxidized and reduced through an $SH \rightleftharpoons S{-}S$ system. FP represents a flavoprotein carrier and cyt b and cyt f, two cytochromes. Cytochrome f is found only in green plants. For each electron pair travelling through the cycle, two molecules of ATP are formed.

Much evidence indicates that photosynthesis in plants takes place via two photochemical events with two different photochemical systems (normally occurring together) as shown in Figure 3.8. For each, a mechanistically similar function occurs but there is a distinct difference in the organization or arrangement. One system involves a specialized form of chlorophyll *a* (system I) and the other system involves chlorophyll *b* and other accessory pigments such as carotenoids or phycobilins (system II).

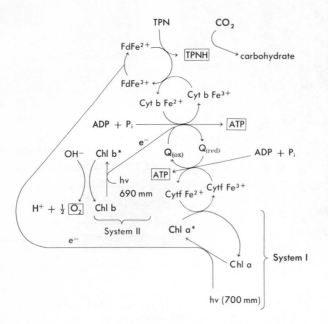

Figure 3.8

Electron transport and oxidative phosphorylation in chloroplasts (modified from Racker). System I is via chlorophyll *a* and system II is via chlorophyll *b*. The two sites of ATP formation are shown. Cyclic phosphorylation via ferridoxin and cytochrome b is indicated by the arrow, as is the non-cyclic which occurs via ferridoxin, flavoprotein, and TPN. Fd = ferredoxin. Modified from E. Racker, *Membranes of Mitochondria and Chloroplasts,* Van Nostrand Reinhold Co., New York, 1970.

Chlorophyll *a* is activated by light at 700 nm. Its electrons are promoted to higher energy orbitals and then may follow one of two pathways. They may pass to the electron transport chain (to the top in Figure 3.8) via ferredoxin, cytochrome b, and coenzyme Q (Ubiquinone), pass down the chain to cytochrome f, and then be restored to their original oribitals at the end of the chain of carriers. This closed pathway is called *cyclic* photosynthetic phosphorylation. On the other hand, they may pass to the top and, after ferredoxin reduction, pass on to reduce TPN^+ to $TPNH + H^+$. This reduced coenzyme can then be used in the reductive conversion of CO_2 to carbohydrate by the sequence of reactions shown in Figure 3.9. In the latter case, the electrons for

Figure 3.9   Pathway of carbohydrate synthesis in photosynthesis. Note the participation of the pentose pathway in the formation of ribulose-1,5P_2, the acceptor of CO_2, which is split into two 3 carbon fragments (3-phosphoglycerate). Note the requirements for two of the end products in photosynthesis (TPNH and ATP).

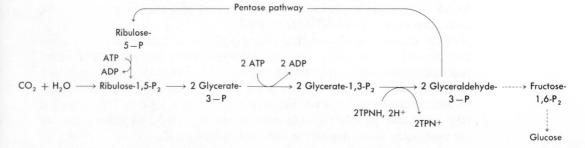

the electron transport chain are provided by the photosensitive pigments of system II. In this *non cyclic* system, electrons are also activated by light to occupy higher energy orbitals, then they may be transported to the same electran transport chain to reduce coenzyme Q. After passing down the chain, they reduce ferredoxin, and TPN. The electrons are restored to the pigments of system II from hydroxyl ions which are supplied from water. OH^- is split by an unknown reaction to two electrons, a proton, and an oxygen atom ($\frac{1}{2} O_2$).

This mechanism explains the two other portions of photosynthesis, namely, the splitting of H_2O to H and O, and the reduction of CO_2 to carbohydrate (Figure 3.9). Thus, we have seen how in oxidation-reduction reactions of glycolysis, respiration, and photosynthesis, energy is trapped as phosphate anhydride linkages of ATP. In glycolysis, the chemistry of these reactions is understood. Inorganic phosphate is incorporated into organic form and converted by a series of reactions to a high energy form. It is then transferred to ADP and ATP is formed. The chemistry of ATP formation from P_i and ADP associated with the oxidation-reduction reactions of electron transport or in photosynthesis is not yet understood. In principle, reactions similar to those of glycolysis might be involved. On the other hand, ATP may be formed by new reactions which are not analogous to those of glycolytic phosphorylation.

The unique role of the reduced pyridine nucleotides should be noted. If they are reoxidized via the electron transport system, they generate ATP in an efficient fashion. In other circumstances, the reducing power of the pyridine nucleotides (TPNH) is used directly to reduce unsaturated systems in the synthesis of cell constituents. Still other reducing agents ($FADH_2$) are utilized in an apparently wasteful fashion in the generation of H_2O_2.

3.7   UTILIZATION OF CHEMICAL ENERGY IN BIOSYNTHESIS

Now that we have discussed the energy conservation in glycolysis, respiration, and photosynthesis in the form of "quantal packets" of ATP, we can consider two examples of the ways in which this energy is used in synthesis.

The synthesis of glucose-6-phosphate has already been described in thermodynamic terms, and it was pointed out that using ATP as a phosphorylating agent gives a reaction with ΔG^0 of -4.0 kcal mole^{-1},

$$\text{glucose} + \text{ATP}^{4-} \rightleftharpoons \text{glucose-6-phosphate}^{2-} + \text{ADP}^{3-} + \text{H}^+$$

To have this reaction occur requires that the energy barrier which prevents the reaction be overcome and that the reactants meet in the proper geometry. This is accomplished by the enzyme hexokinase which catalyzes the reaction in a highly specific fashion. Apparently, it positions the reactants properly with respect to each other and lowers the energy barrier (activation energy).

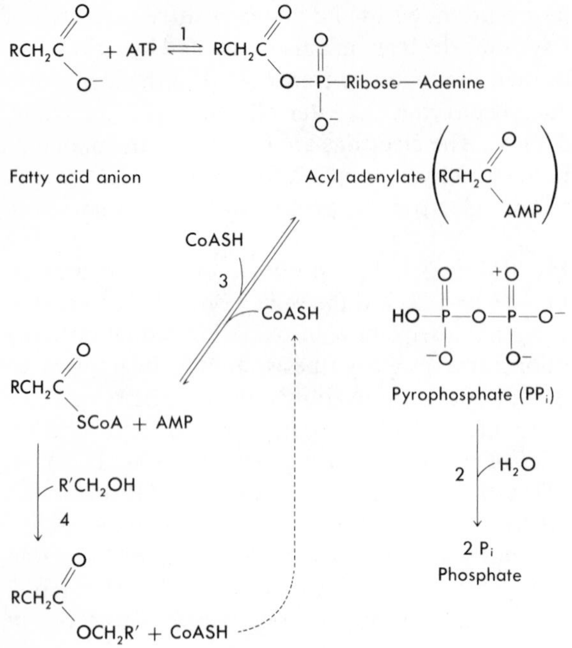

Total reaction RCOOH + R'OH + ATP + H₂O ⇌ RCOOR' + AMP + 2 Pᵢ

Reaction	Approximate $\Delta G°$ kcal mole^{-1}
1	+3
2	−7
3	0
4	−4
Total	−8 kcal mole^{-1}

Figure 3.10

Ester biosynthesis–thermodynamics. Note that the sequence is driven by reactions 2 and 4.

Its specificity is clearly illustrated by the fact that it protects ATP from reaction with water, a much more exothermic process (ΔG_{hyd}^{0} − 7,000 kcal mole^{-1}). This brings out an important point about "high energy" compounds. Although they have high negative ΔG_{hyd}^{0} values, they are usually quite stable in aqueous solution because of the activation energy which must be supplied before they can react. Reaction occurs only in the presence of enzymes and these are sufficiently specific to exclude reaction with water. However, there are specific enzymes present in some tissues which catalyze the hydrolysis of ATP.

Let us now examine how ATP can be used in the formation of a bond other than a phosphate ester bond. Other examples will be considered in subsequent chapters. The synthesis of ester bonds is important in the biosynthesis of lipids and proteins. The ΔG^{0} of hydrolysis of a typical ester bond is approximately 0 in water, so that the synthetic reaction starting from the acid and the alcohol

$$RCH_2-\overset{\overset{\displaystyle O}{\|}}{\underset{\underset{\displaystyle OH}{}}{C}} + R'CH_2OH \rightleftharpoons RCH_2-\overset{\overset{\displaystyle O}{\|}}{\underset{\underset{\displaystyle OR'}{}}{C}} + H_2O$$

would proceed to only a very limited extent because of the high concentration of water (55.6 M). This difficulty is overcome by the sequence of reactions shown in Figure 3.10. In reaction (1), an acyladenylate is formed which is similar in phosphate-donating potential to acetylphosphate (Table 3.1). In the absence of reaction (2), this would not proceed to completion, but in the presence of the catalyst for reaction (2), acyladenylate formation would be quantitative. This compound is a potent acylating agent and could chemically be used to form ester bonds. However, in a biological system the enzymes for ester bond formation specifically require the equally potent acylating agent acyl-S-CoA. Reaction (3), which generates this substance, cannot go to completion in the absence of reaction (4). The overall process has a very high negative ΔG^0 value and will proceed to completion without the accumulation of significant quantities of the intermediates.

3.8 ENZYMES

So far the subject of the catalysis of transformations that occur in biological systems has been dealt with only very casually. It will not be dealt with exhaustively in this book but some of the terminology needs to be introduced.

The role of a catalyst in any chemical reaction is to speed up the conversion of reactant to product. This is accomplished by lowering the energy barrier which the reactant must surmount before it can become product (Figure 3.11). The ways in which this is achieved are not understood. In equilibrium reactions, biological catalysts (enzymes) stimulate the forward and reverse reactions equally, so that their action is to speed up the attainment of equilibrium.

It is very well established that enzymes function by combining with their substrates (i.e., the reactant) to form a complex, that this complex passes through the transition state (Figure 3.11) into an enzyme-product complex which then dissociates into free enzyme and product. The enzyme usually comes out of the reaction in the same state in which it entered, but may undergo a series of very rapid rearrangements during the catalytic process. The sequence can be represented as follows:

$$E + S \rightleftharpoons ES \rightleftharpoons \overset{*}{EA} \rightleftharpoons EP \rightleftharpoons E + P$$

$\leftarrow$ binding$\rightarrow$ $\;$ $\leftarrow$ catalysis $\rightarrow$ $\;$ $\leftarrow$ unbinding $\rightarrow$

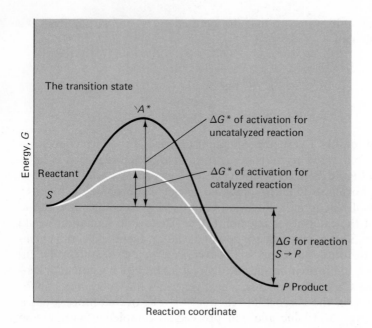

Figure 3.11

Enzyme thermodynamics. Note the difference in ΔG^0 for the uncatalyzed and catalyzed reactions.

Two aspects of enzyme action are particularly important to us in this book. These are their catalytic capability, i.e., the rate at which they can function, which can be expressed as the number of moles of substrate converted to product per mole of enzyme per minute or the *turnover number*. Some idea of the range of values that might be encountered for turnover numbers can be obtained from the fact that the enzyme catalase, which acts to convert H_2O_2 to $H_2O + \frac{1}{2}O_2$, has a turnover number of 5×10^6, whereas aldolase, which cleaves fructose-1,6-diphosphate, has a turnover number of 3×10^3 and D-amino acid oxidase, which converts D-amino acids to the corresponding α-keto acids, has a turnover number of 6. Turnover numbers are actually expressions of the maximum rate that can be achieved by the enzyme. In most physiological conditions, enzymes act at rates well below their maximum. This provides an opportunity for control of the reaction by manipulation of the enzyme's activity. Reaction rates can either be increased or decreased.

The rate at which an enzyme operates is also dependent on the amount of substrate available to it. The association of enzyme with substrate in the binding step $E + S \rightleftharpoons ES$ determines the rate, relative to the maximum rate. If the slowest step in an enzyme catalyzed reaction is the catalytic step $ES \rightleftharpoons EA^* \rightleftharpoons EP$, then the binding reaction $E + S \rightleftharpoons ES$ can be considered as a simple equilibrium and the proportion of enzyme existing in the ES form will determine the relative rate of the reaction. Knowledge of the equilibrium constant for the binding reaction can be useful in considering problems of metabolic control and an approximate value can be obtained by assuming that the rate-limiting step is the catalytic step and performing a series of experiments to determine the effect of substrate concentration on *initial* velocity. The data is plotted as shown in Figure 3.12 and the value of V_{max} (the turnover number) is obtained from the intercept on the ordinate and the value of K_m from the slope of the line. K_m is known as the *Michaelis constant*. It is formally equivalent to $k_{-1} + k_2/k_1$ from the following formalism for an enzymatic reaction.

$$E + S \underset{k_{-1}}{\overset{k_1}{\rightleftharpoons}} ES \xrightarrow{k_2} E + P$$

This is the simplification of the sequence discussed above. When k_2 is very small, $K_m = k_{-1}/k_1$, which is equivalent to K_{eq} for the reaction

$$ES \underset{k_1}{\overset{k_{-1}}{\rightleftharpoons}} E + S.$$

Thus K_m is a measure of the tendency of ES to dissociate. The smaller the value of K_m, the less tendency exists. When K_m is assumed to be a dissociation constant, we can write

$$K_m = \frac{(E)\,(S)}{(ES)}\,moles^{-1}$$

If we know the value of K_m, we can predict the relative rate of the enzymatic processes at all concentrations of substrate, since the proportion of E in the

Figure 3.12   In the double reciprocal plot $1/[S]$ = the reciprocal of substrate concentration and $1/v_0$ = the reciprocal of the *initial* velocity. The y intercept equals the reciprocal of V_{max} or maximum velocity, while the slope equals K_m/V_{max} or the Michaelis constant/maximum velocity. In the single reciprocal plot the y intercept equals V_{max}/K_m, while the slope equals $-1/K_m$.

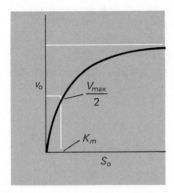

1. Direct plot

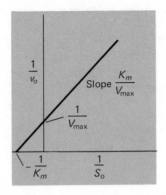

2. Double reciprocal plot

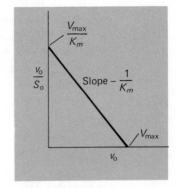

3. Single reciprocal plot

ES form can be calculated. When (E) = (ES), the reaction will be proceeding at one-half maximal velocity and (S) = K_m. This is a very useful reference point.

Knowledge of K_m and V_{max} values are of use in determining whether in vitro results fit with in vivo observations. For example, if a given in vivo conversion occurs much more rapidly than can be accounted for on the basis of the behavior of an isolated enzyme and the amount of that enzyme in the tissue, it is likely that alternate pathways exist. In other circumstances, we will find that many metabolites are substrates for several enzymes. Clearly, the K_m and V_{max} values of the various enzymes will determine the pathway through which the metabolite will be converted preferentially.

This very brief treatment of enzyme kinetics should serve the purposes of this text, but the more complete coverage of the topic in Wold's book in this series should be consulted also. In this chapter, the ways in which biological systems obtain energy for the maintenance of their integrity have been described in general terms. The process of "high energy" compound formation has been discussed at the substrate level, by oxidative phosphorylation, and by photosynthetic processes. The ways in which chemical reactions can be coupled so that energetically favorable reactions can be linked to energetically unfavorable ones have been described. In subsequent chapters, the actual systems involved will be detailed.

REFERENCES

Bentley, R., *Molecular Asymmetry in Biology*, Academic Press, Inc., New York, (1969).

Kasha, M., and B. Pullman, eds., *Horizons in Biochemistry*, Academic Press, Inc., New York, 1962. A clear discussion of energy-rich phosphates by Al Pullman and Bernard Pullman, p. 553.

Klotz, I. M., *Energy Changes in Biochemical Reactions*, Academic Press, Inc., New York, 1967.

Lehninger, A. L., *Bioenergetics*, W. A. Benjamin, Inc. New York, Amsterdam, 1965.

Racker, E., Ed., *Membranes of Mitochondria and Chloroplasts*, Van Nostrand Reinhold Co., New York, 1970.

West, E. S., Todd, W. R., Mason, H. S., and J. T. Van Bruggen, *Textbook of Biochemistry*, 4th ed., The Macmillan Company, 1966.

White, A., Handler, P., and E. L. Smith, *Principles of Biochemistry*, 4th ed., McGraw-Hill Book Company, New York, 1968.

METABOLISM OF THE FUELS: CARBOHYDRATES AND LIPIDS

In the present chapter, we will consider the metabolism of carbohydrates and lipids. This seems appropriate since the two constitute the principal energy fuels of the cell and are the major sources of ATP and DPNH. Figure 4.1 gives an overall view of this metabolic area and shows how the metabolisms of these fuels are integrated. The figure shows the key intermediates and the major branch points in the metabolism of materials for energy production.

Before proceeding with a detailed description of the events involved in the metabolism of carbohydrates and lipids, it is necessary to define some terms.

1. *Fermentation* is the metabolism of materials with the formation of gases, in this case, the conversion of carbohydrates to ethanol and carbon dioxide. No oxygen is required.

2. *Glycolysis* is the conversion of carbohydrates to pyruvate.

3. *Anaerobic glycolysis* is the conversion of carbohydrates to lactate via pyruvate. No oxygen is utilized.

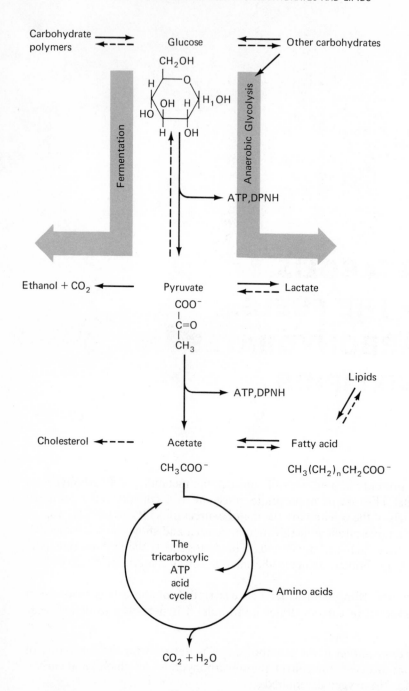

Figure 4.1   An overall view of the metabolism of carbohydrates, lipids and amino acids. Note that acetate is a common intermediate of carbohydrate and lipid metabolism and that the tricarboxylic acid cycle is the common pathway for oxidation of carbohydrates, lipids, and amino acids.

4. *Aerobic glycolysis* is the conversion of carbohydrates to carbon dioxide (CO_2) and water (H_2O) via pyruvate. Oxygen is utilized.

5. *Respiration* refers to the reactions which occur when a cell is consuming oxygen and forming CO_2 and water. The source of carbon is not specified.

6. The *tricarboxylic acid cycle* (Krebs cycle, citric acid cycle) is the enzyme system by which acetate is converted to CO_2 and water with the consumption of oxygen.

In Figure 4.1, we see that glucose, the key carbohydrate, is formed from and in turn is used to form carbohydrate polymers. These polymers may constitute energy reserves (glycogen or starch) or may serve a structural role within the cell (cellulose, chitin, hyaluronic acid, etc.). Glucose can also be formed from, and converted to, other carbohydrates.

Glycolysis is an *oxidative* process. Even when no oxygen is consumed, an internal oxidation-reduction reaction is carried out so that the carboxyl group of lactate is the product of oxidation and its methyl group a product of reduction. All metabolic energy is produced by oxidative processes and all oxidative processes require an oxidizing agent. In many cases oxygen serves the role of oxidizing agent, but it acts through many intermediate steps, the first of which involves DPN+ as an oxidizing agent. The key product of glucose metabolism is energy made available either as ATP or as the reducing power of DPNH or TPNH. In the tricarboxylic acid cycle also, the most important product is energy made available as reduced coenzymes.

Lipids may be *partially* converted to glycerol, which can then be further converted to carbohydrate and metabolized with the release of energy. The fatty acid components of lipids are also completely oxidized to CO_2 and H_2O via acetate in the tricarboxylic acid cycle. Even amino acids are oxidized by this much used pathway. Acetate, the key intermediate in lipid metabolism can be condensed to either fatty acids or cholesterol. Thus, the *two* functions of carbohydrate and lipid metabolism are: energy production and providing carbon compounds for synthesizing cellular substituents.

The chief difference between the two fuels (carbohydrates and lipids) is that carbohydrate $(CH_2O)_n$, which is already partially oxidized as compared to fat $(C_nH_{2n}O_2)$, yields less energy per unit weight on complete oxidation (4 kcal/gram as compared to 9 kcal/gram).

It is important to note some of the problems involved in these oxidative energy-producing reactions. In general, substances dissolved in the liquid phase are converted to gases, e.g., CO_2. Gaseous oxygen (O_2) is required for this process. The exit and entry processes of cells and problems of transport, especially of gases, are therefore important. In addition, the oxidations may produce acids (H^+), requiring the regulation of hydrogen ion concentration. Various portions of the metabolism are carried out in different subcellular locations and the transport of materials between compartments in the cell is important.

4.1 ANAEROBIC GLYCOLYSIS, GLUCONEOGENESIS, AND GLYCOGENESIS

Anaerobic Glycolysis

The overall stoichiometry of anaerobic glycolysis is given in Eq. (1):

$$\text{glucose} + 2ADP^{3-} + 2P_i^{2-} \longrightarrow 2 \text{ lactate}^{1-} + 2ATP^{4-} \tag{1}$$

For each mole of glucose converted, two moles of lactate are formed, and the energy yield is two moles of ATP. The pathway, composed of an *open* (*noncyclic*) sequence of reactions is detailed in Figure 4.2. In the figure, P stands for phosphate and the names of all enzymes and intermediates are given. All reactions are catalyzed by enzymes present in the *cytosol*. Those which are readily reversible in the cell are indicated by double arrows. In reactions (1–3) the six carbon hexose sugars are *derivatized* with phosphate to form hexose mono- and diphosphate; this requires that the cell supply energy, 2ATP for each glucose used. The other reactions are as follows: (4) *splitting* the C-6 chain into two C-3 triose phosphates; (5) *isomerization* by an enzyme, which catalyzes their interconversion; (6) *oxidation* of glyceraldehyde phosphate by DPN$^+$ coupled with the incorporation of inorganic phosphate into organic linkage as acyl phosphate, a "high energy" form capable of donating the phosphoryl residue to ATP; (7) *transfer* of P of acyl phosphate to ADP to form ATP; (8) intramolecular *transfer* of phosphate from C-3 to C-2; (9) *dehydration* to form enol phosphate; (10) phosphate transfer and ketolization; (11) reduction of pyruvate to lactate, which occurs with the concomitant oxidation of reduced DPNH + H$^+$ to DPN$^+$.

As shown in Figure 4.2, glucose-phosphate can be produced by the phosphorolysis of starch or glycogen by the action of phosphorylase (12) which splits off the terminal glucose residues incorporating inorganic phosphate to yield glucose-1-P. In reaction (13), glucose-1-P is converted to glucose-6-P so that this process requires less energy for the initiation of glycolysis than the pathway starting from glucose. As will be seen later, there is no real saving involved since the synthesis of the polymer requires the expenditure of energy. However, the requirement to expend ATP at the time that ATP demand is high is decreased. Two reactions which differentiate fermentation from anaerobic glycolysis and which occur in yeast and microorganisms are (14), in which pyruvate is *decarboxylated* to acetaldehyde (a reaction not present in animal tissues), and (15), in which acetaldehyde is reduced to ethanol with the concomitant oxidation of reduced DPNH + H$^+$

Figure 4.2   The pathway of glycolysis. Reactions 1 through 15.

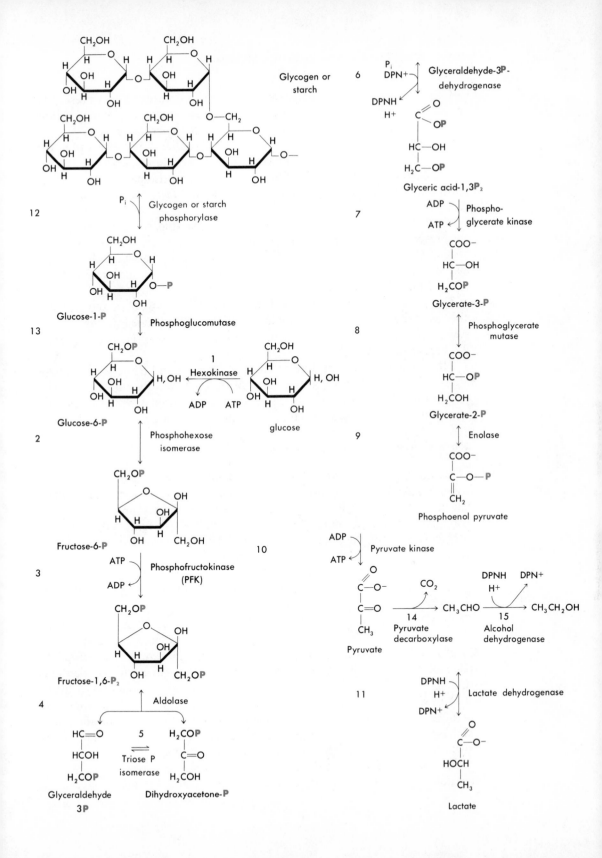

to DPN+. The enzyme responsible for this oxidation reaction is present in animal tissues but is used to catalyze the reverse reaction. Ethanol is thus the end product of *fermentation* in yeast and some microorganisms.

Note that the same types of reactions are utilized at the hexose and at the triose levels: (a) phosphoglucomutase (13) and phosphoglyceratemutase (8); (b) phosphohexoisomerase (2) and triose phosphate isomerase (5); and (c) phosphofructokinase (3), phosphoglycerate kinase (7), and pyruvate kinase (10).

In other reactions which are not entirely comparable, some similar aspects are present. For example, inorganic phosphate is converted into an organic form in (12), the phosphorylase reaction, by breaking the glycoside linkage, and in (6), where it is utilized in a very exothermic step to generate a "high energy" phosphate derivative.

The oxidation-reduction reactions involving DPN+, (6), (11), and (15), are also generally similar. Note that although DPN+ is consumed in step (6), it is regenerated in equal amount in either step (11) or step (15) depending upon the organism.

Other reactions are not duplicated at the hexose and triose levels. These include the C—C bond splitting reaction (4) catalyzed by aldolase and the dehydration reaction (9) catalyzed by enolase. Examples of these reaction types will be studied in connection with other metabolic pathways.

Gluconeogenesis (The Formation of Glucose)

Although glucose serves as an energy source when a demand for ATP arises, many cells can synthesize glucose and store it as a polymer, either starch or glycogen, when energy demands are low and a source of carbon is available. The formation of glucose via gluconeogenesis follows the pathway of glycolysis but in the opposite direction. The overall stoichiometry is given in Eq. (2):

$$2 \, \text{lactate}^{1-} + 6\text{ATP}^{4-} \longrightarrow \text{glucose} + 6\text{ADP}^{3-} + 6\text{P}_i^{2-} + 4\text{H}^+ \quad (2)$$

The reactions are outlined in Figure 4.3. To bypass the essentially irreversible steps of glycolysis *new* reactions are introduced and are also shown in Figure 4.3. Reactions (16) and (17) reverse the conversion of phosphoenolpyruvate to pyruvate by carboxylation of pyruvate to oxaloacetate (C-3 to C-4) and decarboxylation of oxaloacetate to phosphoenolpyruvate (C-4 to C-3) at the expense of ATP and GTP, respectively. Reactions (18) and (19) reverse the two ATP-dependent kinase reactions, by specific phosphatases. All of the other steps, as presently understood, are identical in glycolysis and gluconeogenesis and are used reversibly.

Gluconeogenesis has portions located in separate subcellular sites. As already discussed, the reactions of glycolysis (Table 4.1) are catalyzed by enzymes in the cytosol. Reaction (16), catalyzed by pyruvate carboxylase is present in mitochondria. As will be discussed in Chapter 8, this enzyme has an *absolute requirement* for acetyl-S-CoA, also made and found in the mitochondria. Thus the presence of the enzyme as well as its cofactor set up conditions which very much favor the production of oxaloacetate in mitochondria. Oxaloacetate is then reduced to malate via cytoplasmic malate dehydrogenase. Malate readily diffuses into the mitochondria where it is reoxidized

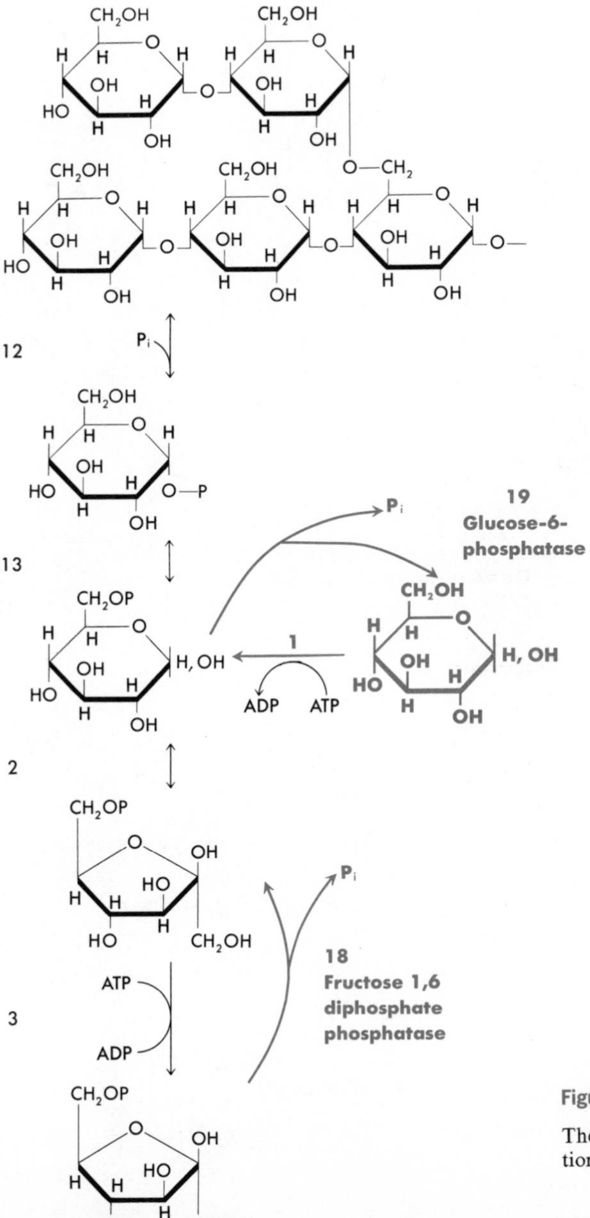

Figure 4.3

The pathway of gluconeogenesis. Note the new reactions 16, 17, 18, and 19.

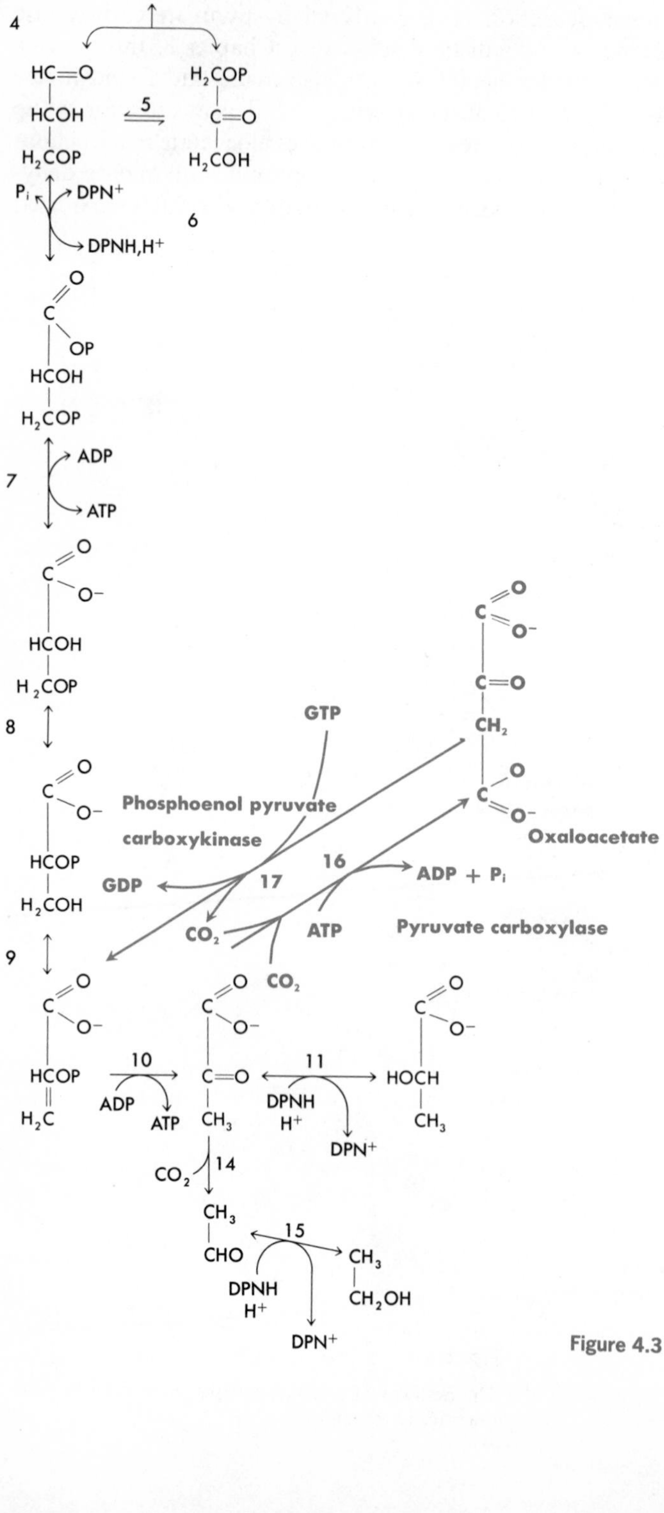

Figure 4.3   (Continued)

TABLE 4.1   SUBCELLULAR DISTRIBUTION OF ENZYMES

Metabolic Sequence	Principal Subcellular Distribution
Glycolysis (reactions 1 through 12)	Cytosol
(reaction 1)	May be glycogen bound
Gluconeogenesis (reaction 16)	Mitochondria
others	Cytosol
(reaction 19)	Microsomes
Pentose pathway	Cytosol
Tricarboxylic acid cycle	Mitochondria
(isocitrate dehydrogenase TPN requiring)	Cytosol
β-Oxidation	Mitochondria
Fatty acid synthesis	Cytosol
Cholesterol synthesis	Microsomes

to oxaloacetate via malate dehydrogenase (present in mitochondria). This shuttle system has already been discussed (Chapter 3, Section 3.5). The oxalo-acetate thus formed is decarboxylated to phosphoenolpyruvate (17) in the cytosol and the remaining reactions are also carried out in the cytosol. The final step of gluconeogenesis (19) is catalyzed by glucose-6-phosphatase present in the microsomes. The complete pathway thus requires the integration of reactions which occur in three different cell locations.

While glycolysis is general in animal cells, gluconeogenesis is more specialized, occurring only in certain organs such as the liver, the kidney, and the intestine. These organs carry out gluconeogenesis because they possess the enzymes which catalyze the four reactions required to reverse glycolysis. Other organs, such as skeletal muscle, which do not carry out any appreciable gluconeogenesis do not contain appreciable quantities of the enzymes catalyzing the reverse reactions.

Glycogenesis (The Formation of Glycogen)

Glycogen formation or *glycogenesis* takes place by two reactions (Figure 4.4). Glucose-1-phosphate is first converted to the more highly reactive nucleotide sugar, uridine diphosphate glucose (UDPG) or adenosine diphosphate glucose (ADPG) in the case of starch synthesis (20). The glucose moiety of the nucleotide sugar is then *transferred* to preexisting glycogen or starch called *primer* enlarging the existing polysaccharide (21). The newly synthesized polysaccharide is thus built up directly *on the outer chains* (nonreducing ends) of preexisting polysaccharide.

When we sum the reactions of glycogen α-1,4 bond synthesis and breakdown, we can observe a cyclic process, the glycogen cycle (Figure 4.4). This cycle is driven by an energy input from UTP, and it requires P_i. The P_i is

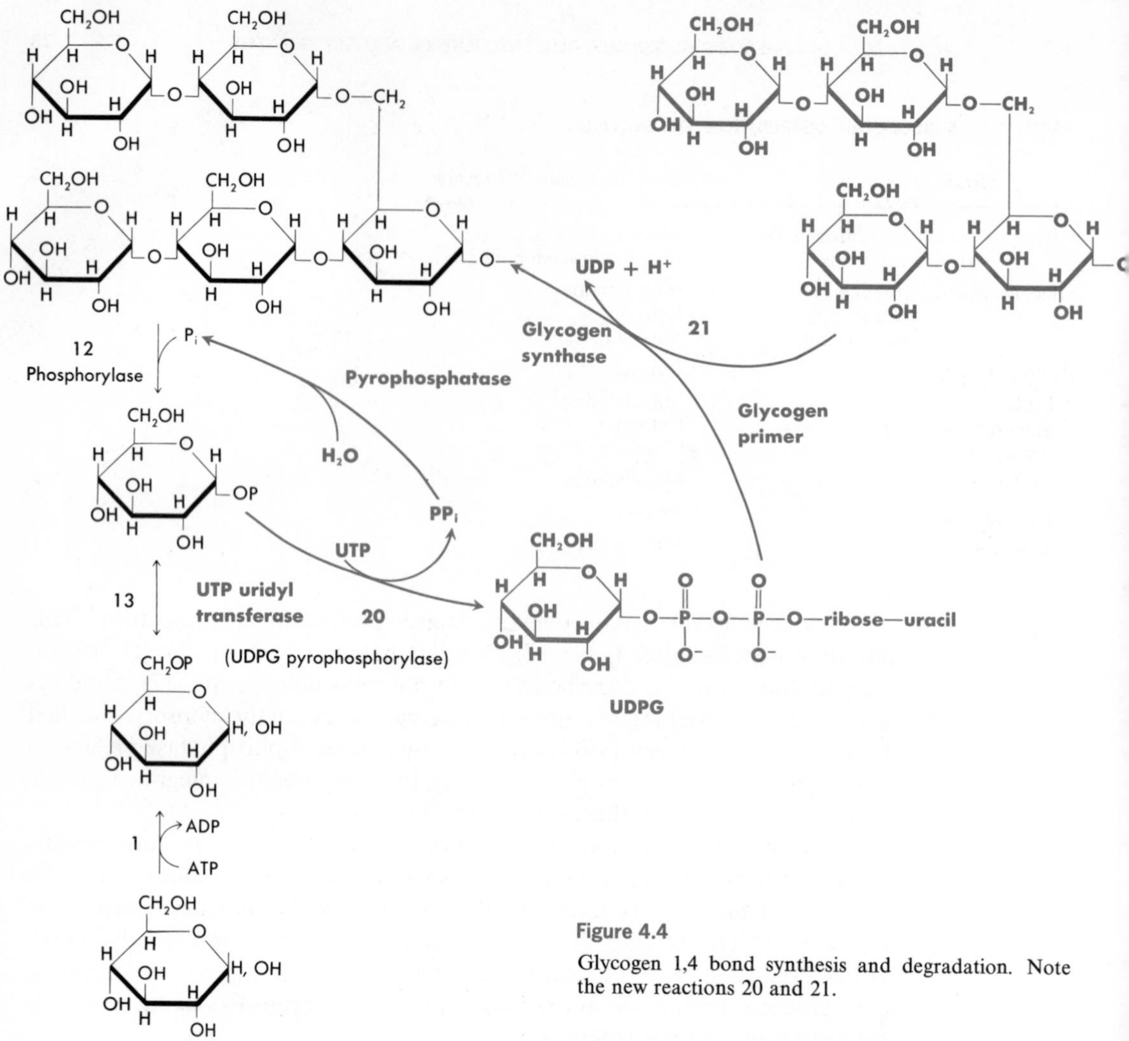

Figure 4.4

Glycogen 1,4 bond synthesis and degradation. Note the new reactions 20 and 21.

replenished by hydrolysis of pyrophosphate, the leaving group in the pyrophosphorylase reaction (20). Note that the polymerization reaction is an acid-forming one. If the cycle operated freely, it would result in the cleavage of UTP to UDP and P_i, a rather wasteful process. The system probably does not operate in a cyclic fashion, and glycogen (or starch) synthesis and degradation are regulated so as to occur separately, as described in Chapter 8.

Some properties of the enzymes and of the catalyzed reactions of glycolysis, gluconeogenesis, and glycogenesis are summarized in the appendix.

4.2 TRICARBOXYLIC ACID CYCLE

The cyclic series of reactions by means of which carbon of carbohydrate, lipid, or amino acids is *completely* oxidized to CO_2 with the release of energy is shown in Figure 4.5.

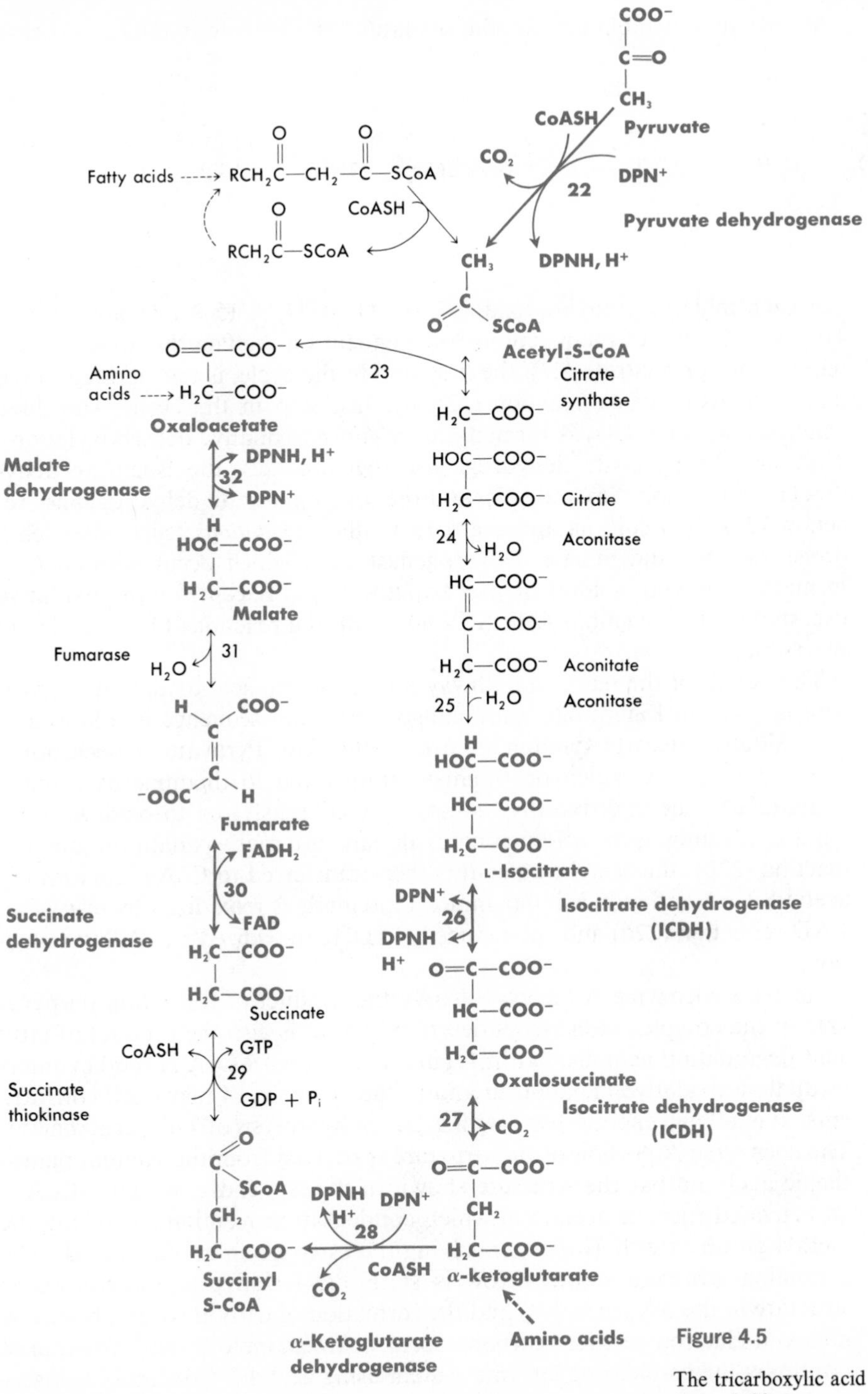

COO⁻
|
C=O
|
CH₃   Pyruvate

Fatty acids ----→
$$RCH_2\overset{\overset{\displaystyle O}{\|}}{C}-CH_2-\overset{\overset{\displaystyle O}{\|}}{C}-SCoA$$

CoASH

CO_2

CoASH

$$RCH_2\overset{\overset{\displaystyle O}{\|}}{C}-SCoA$$

CoASH   Pyruvate

DPN⁺

22

Pyruvate dehydrogenase

DPNH, H⁺

CH₃
|
$\overset{\overset{\displaystyle O}{\|}}{C}$
SCoA   Acetyl-S-CoA

Amino acids ----→
O=C—COO⁻
|
H₂C—COO⁻
Oxaloacetate

23   Citrate synthase

H₂C—COO⁻
|
HOC—COO⁻
|
H₂C—COO⁻   Citrate

Malate dehydrogenase

DPNH, H⁺
32
DPN⁺

24   H_2O Aconitase

H
|
HOC—COO⁻
|
H₂C—COO⁻   Malate

HC—COO⁻
‖
C—COO⁻
|
H₂C—COO⁻   Aconitate

Fumarase   31
H_2O

25   H_2O Aconitase

H
|
HOC—COO⁻
|
HC—COO⁻
|
H₂C—COO⁻
L-Isocitrate

H   COO⁻
\   /
C
‖
C
/   \
⁻OOC   H
Fumarate

DPN⁺
26
DPNH
H⁺

Isocitrate dehydrogenase (ICDH)

Succinate dehydrogenase

FADH₂
30
FAD

H₂C—COO⁻
|
H₂C—COO⁻   Succinate

O=C—COO⁻
|
HC—COO⁻
|
H₂C—COO⁻
Oxalosuccinate

CoASH   GTP
29
GDP + Pᵢ

Succinate thiokinase

27   CO_2

Isocitrate dehydrogenase (ICDH)

O=C—COO⁻
|
CH₂
|
H₂C—COO⁻   α-ketoglutarate

$$\overset{\overset{\displaystyle O}{\|}}{C}-SCoA$$
|
CH₂
|
H₂C—COO⁻
Succinyl S-CoA

DPNH H⁺   DPN⁺
28
CO_2 CoASH

α-Ketoglutarate dehydrogenase

Amino acids

Figure 4.5

The tricarboxylic acid cycle; reactions 22 through 32.

The overall stoichiometry for the oxidation of pyruvate is indicated below

$$
\begin{array}{c}
\text{COOH} \\
| \\
\text{C} = \text{O} \\
| \\
\text{CH}_3
\end{array}
+ 2\tfrac{1}{2}\text{O}_2 + 15\text{P}_i^{2-} + 15\text{ADP}^{3-} + 15\text{H}^+ \longrightarrow 3\text{CO}_2 + 17\text{H}_2\text{O} + 15\text{ATP}^{4-}
$$

For each mole of pyruvate oxidized to CO_2 + H_2O, 15 ATP's are formed. The cyclic nature of the reactions is dependent on the fact that oxaloacetate required to form citrate (23), the first step in the cycle, is regenerated in the malate dehydrogenase reaction (32), the last step in the cycle. The three reactions in which CO_2 is formed are *oxidative* (oxidative decarboxylation). They are the pyruvate dehydrogenase reaction (22), the isocitrate dehydrogenase reaction (26) and (27), and the α-ketoglutarate dehydrogenase reaction (28). In addition, there are two other *oxidations,* succinate dehydrogenase (30) and malate dehydrogenase (32), which occur without CO_2 formation, making a total of *five oxidative steps.* Except for the oxidative decarboxylation reactions (22), (27), and (28), the reactions of the cycle are reversible.

The details of the reaction pathway for the α-keto acid oxidation of pyruvate is given in Figure 4.6. An analogous reaction sequence is followed in the oxidative decarboxylation of α-ketoglutarate. Pyruvate is decarboxylated, and the 2-C aldehyde fragment transferred to thiamine pyrophosphate (22a). The hydroxyethyl moiety is next transferred to oxidized lipoamide, forming acetyl-S-lipoamide in an internal oxidation-reduction reaction (22b); the acetyl fragment is then transferred to CoA (22c) forming acetyl-S-CoA and reduced lipoamide. Lipoamide is reoxidized by way of an FAD reduction (22d) and the reduced $FADH_2$ reoxidized via DPN^+ reduction.

Acetyl-S-coenzyme A (acetyl-S-CoA), the product of the action on pyruvate of the complex of enzymes described above is also the product of fatty acid degradation as indicated in Figure 4.5. Acetyl-S-CoA is the key intermediate in oxidative metabolism and in the synthesis of many cell constituents. It is a "high energy" ester with a $\Delta G°$ of hydrolysis of -8.5 kcal mole^{-1}. The coenzyme A portion of the structure is derived from the vitamin pantothenic acid and has the structure shown in the Appendix. Acetyl-S-CoA is an activated form of acetate in which condensation reactions involving the methyl group as well as those involving the ester group are facilitated. The carbanion structure shown below is stabilized (relative to the equivalent structure in the oxygen esters) and the formation of carbon-carbon bonds by attack at electron deficient carbons occurs. An example is the formation of citrate by the condensing enzyme system using acetyl-S-CoA and oxaloace-

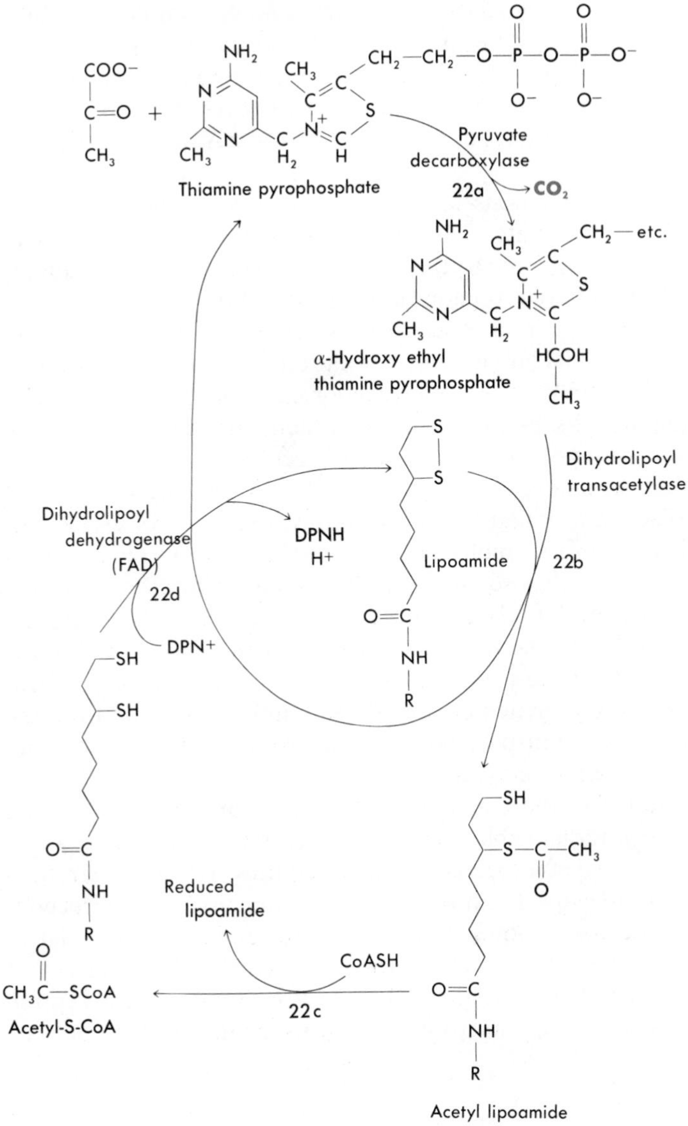

Figure 4.6

The α-keto acid oxidation pathway; reactions 22a, b, and c.

tate (Figure 4.5) (23). The condensation involves the relatively positive carbon of the keto group of oxaloacetate.

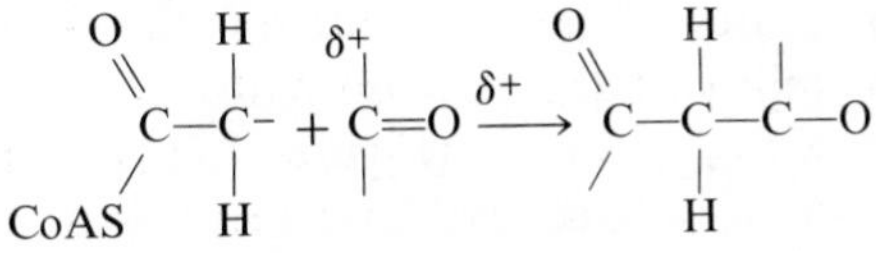

The chief function of the tricarboxylic acid cycle is the complete combustion of acetate to CO_2 and H_2O to provide energy in the form of ATP. Interestingly, another triphosphate product, GTP (guanosine triphosphate, see Appendix), is formed in one of the reactions of the cycle (29) which conserves the energy of the thiol ester bond of succinyl-S-CoA produced in reaction (28).

In addition, the cycle functions to synthesize such key intermediates as α-ketoglutarate and oxaloacetate. The amino acids glutamate and aspartate can be derived from or converted to the two α-keto acids and are in equilibrium with them. These interconversions are considered in Chapter 5.

The production of energy in the tricarboxylic acid cycle involves the electron transport system of oxidative phosphorylation described in Chapter 3. Each of the DPNH molecules produced (reactions 22, 26, 28, and 32) can be reoxidized by donating its electrons to the system. As the electrons are passed through the system to oxygen, three molecules of ATP are formed from ADP + P_i. In the oxidation of succinate (30) $FADH_2$ is produced and this can be reoxidized in a similar fashion with the production of 2ATP. Altogether, the oxidation of one molecule of pyruvate yields 15 molecules of ATP. In addition, when glucose is being completely oxidized via the tricarboxylic acid cycle, the DPNH produced in the oxidation of glyceraldehyde (6) can be shuttled to the mitochondrion and can yield an additional three molecules of ATP. Thus, the oxidative metabolism of glucose yields 38 ATP, two from the glycolytic part in substrate-linked steps, 34 from the operation of the electron transport system, and two as GTP from the conservation of the energy of succinyl-S-CoA.

The enzymes catalyzing the reactions of the tricarboxylic acid cycle are located in the mitochondria (Table 4.1). As is discussed in Chapter 8, a second form of isocitrate dehydrogenase which requires TPN+ rather than DPN+ is located in the cytosol and serves another function. The mitochondrial location, in close association with the enzymatic apparatus of oxidative phosphorylation and electron transport, serves to increase the efficiency of the reactions by virtue of propinquity. Almost all cells, with the exception of the mature erythrocyte and anaerobic organisms, contain mitochondria.

4.3   PENTOSE PATHWAY

Although glycolysis and the citric acid cycle are present in most cells, some cells have alternate ways of producing energy and useful metabolites from carbohydrates. One such system is the *pentose pathway*. The series of reactions comprising the pentose pathway form a cycle which is closely interlocked with glycolysis (Figure 4.7). It separates from glycolysis at the glucose-6-phosphate level and reenters at fructose-6-phosphate. A consideration of the overall stoichiometry will elucidate the scope of this aerobic

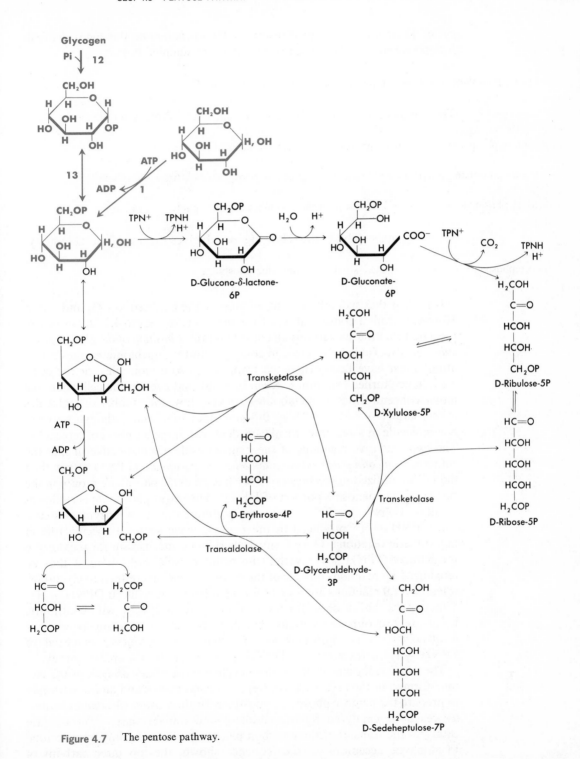

Figure 4.7   The pentose pathway.

cycle. There are two types of reactions, the *oxidative* and the *nonoxidative or transfer* reactions. The oxidative reactions are summed below:

6 hexose phosphate + $6O_2 \longrightarrow$ 6 pentose phosphate + $6CO_2$ + $6H_2O$

The nonoxidative or transfer reactions consist of three reactions:

4 pentose phosphate $\longrightarrow$ 2 hexose phosphate + 2 tetrose phosphate

2 tetrose phosphate + 2 pentose phosphate $\longrightarrow$ 2 hexose phosphate + 2 triose phosphate

2 triose phosphate + $H_2O \longrightarrow$ 1 hexose phosphate + inorganic phosphate

Summing up, we obtain the following, which gives the overall stoichiometry:

hexosephosphate + $6O_2 \longrightarrow$ $6CO_2$ + $6H_2O$ + inorganic phosphate

It is clear that six carbon atoms of glucose are oxidized to CO_2 and water. However, from a consideration of the reactions of Figure 4.7, it can be appreciated that the six carbons all come from the *1 position of the glucose molecule* (see also Table 6.9). Thus, to comply with the stoichiometry, the carbon atoms must have been originated from six glucose molecules, or the cycle must have "turned" six times. Keep in mind that even in the cell where the molar concentrations of metabolites are very low, the number of molecules is very large (10^{-3} M = 6.02×10^{20} molecules/liter) and, although we write one molecule in a reaction, we always deal with large numbers of molecules. The two oxidative reactions of the pentose cycle are distinctive in that the cofactor is *nicotinamide adenine dinucleotide phosphate* (TPN+) rather than the DPN+ utilized in glycolysis. TPN+ has an extra phosphate group on the ribose of the adenosine portion of DPN+. This extra phosphate is sufficient to allow DPN+ and TPN+ to be easily differentiated by enzyme systems. The TPNH + H+ produced in the pentose cycle serves a specific role in biosynthetic reactions. Once formed, there is no mechanism for reoxidizing the reduced TPNH + H+ within the pentose cycle itself. It must thus be reoxidized by reactions outside of the pentose cycle, in contrast to glycolysis, where several reactions are present for reoxidizing the reduced DPNH + H+. This implies that in order for the pentose cycle to operate with continuity, it must rely on outside reactions. The pentose cycle is not as independent as is glycolysis. It is important to note that if the reducing potential of TPNH + H+ is transferred to DPNH + H+, it can be a source of energy.

The other reactions of the pentose cycle consist of a *hydrolysis* of the lactone formed in the first oxidative step, an *epimerization* and an *isomerization* to prepare the pentose phosphate substrate for the various *C-2 and C-3 transfer* reactions catalyzed by transaldolase and transketolase. Transaldolase catalyzes the transfer of three-carbon pieces equivalent to dihydroxyacetone to aldehyde acceptors. In the sequence shown, the top three carbons of sedoheptulose-7-P are transferred to D-glyceraldehyde-P to form fructose-6-P and to leave erythrose-4-P. Transketolase catalyzes the transfer of the top two carbons of a keto sugar to an aldehyde acceptor as shown in Figure 4.7 for the reaction of xylulose-5-P (donor) with ribose-5-P (acceptor). The conversions are all reversible, and involve intermediates which vary in size from triose phosphate (C-3) to heptulose phosphate (C-7). The chief product to reenter glycolysis is fructose-6-phosphate. The stoichiometry of these nonoxidative reactions indicates that for every three pentose phosphates converted, two fructose phosphates and one glyceraldehyde phosphate are formed. This series of reactions serves to produce pentose, an essential component for nucleic acid biosynthesis. It also is of great importance in the photosynthetic conversion of CO_2 into carbohydrate (Figure 3.9). In addition, TPNH $+$ H$^+$, once formed, is a source of reducing power for fatty acid synthesis.

In spite of its great importance in metabolism, the pentose cycle is present with a rather wide but not universal distribution in nature. For example, skeletal muscle has little of the enzymatic machinery.

4.4 GLUCURONATE CYCLE

Another incomplete oxidative cycle, the *glucuronate* cycle, is shown in Figure 4.8. It, like the pentose pathway, is another system which bypasses glycolysis and the tricarboxylic cycle. Its function is to provide ascorbate (vitamin C) in plants and in those animals which are able to synthesize this vitamin. In addition, energy made available as DPNH $+$ H$^+$ is produced. Note here the striking fact that the oxidative reactions are specific for DPN$^+$, while the reductive reactions all require TPNH $+$ H$^+$.

4.5 NUCLEOTIDE SUGAR METABOLISM

A remarkable new chapter in carbohydrate metabolism was initiated by the discovery of the *nucleotide sugars*. The structure of one of them, uridine diphosphate glucose is shown.

uridine diphosphate glucose (UDPG)

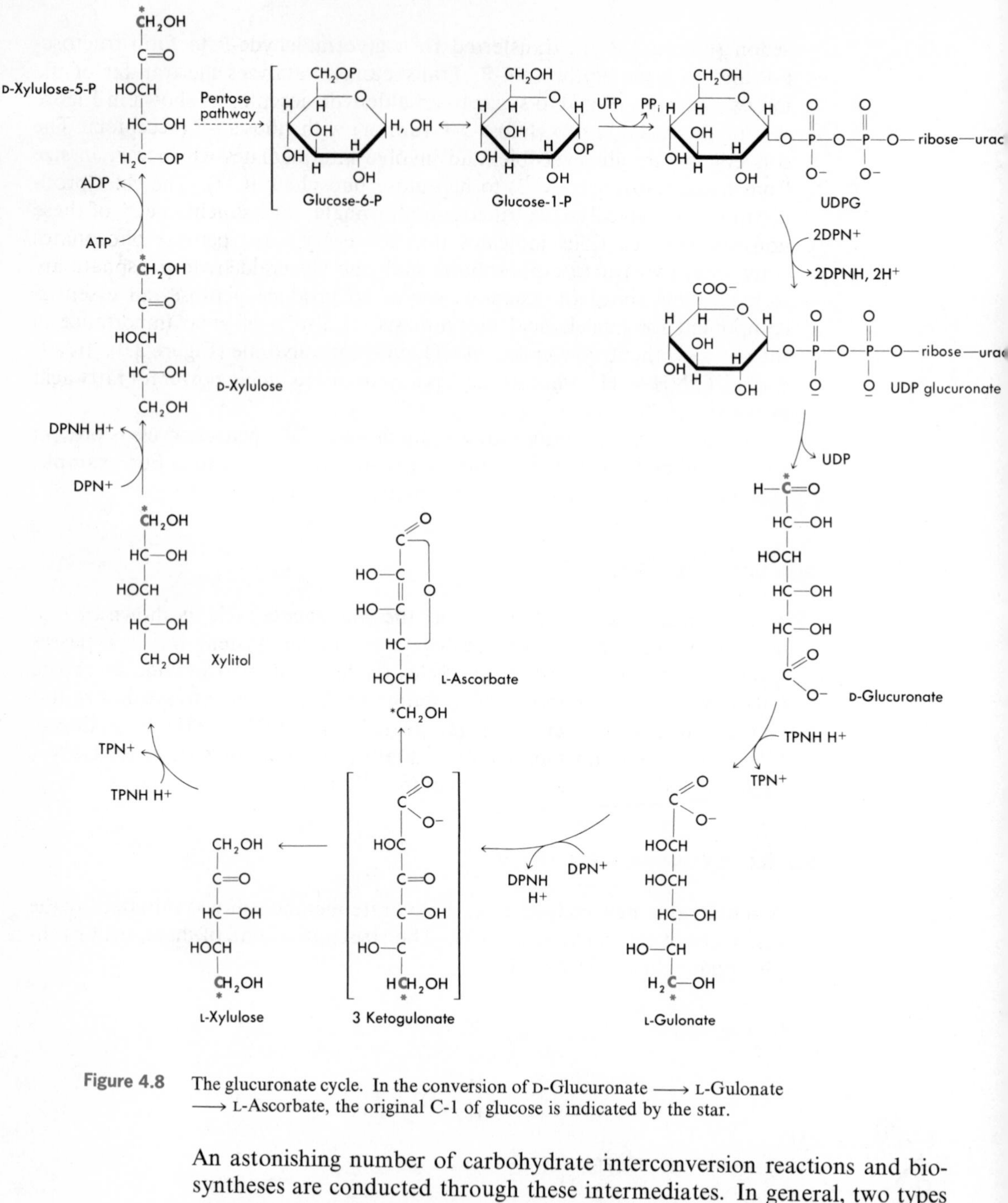

D-Xylulose-5-P

CH₂OH (starred)
|
C=O
|
HOCH
|
HC—OH
|
H₂C—OP

Pentose pathway

Glucose-6-P → Glucose-1-P → (UTP, PPᵢ) → UDPG

ADP / ATP

CH₂OH (starred)
|
C=O
|
HOCH
|
HC—OH
|
CH₂OH

D-Xylulose

DPNH H⁺ / DPN⁺

CH₂OH (starred)
|
HC—OH
|
HOCH
|
HC—OH
|
CH₂OH   Xylitol

2DPN⁺ → 2DPNH, 2H⁺

UDP glucuronate

UDP

H—C=O (starred)
|
HC—OH
|
HOCH
|
HC—OH
|
HC—OH
|
C—O⁻ (=O)   D-Glucuronate

TPNH H⁺ / TPN⁺

L-Ascorbate

TPN⁺ / TPNH H⁺

CH₂OH
|
C=O
|
HC—OH
|
HOCH
|
CH₂OH (starred)
L-Xylulose

←

3 Ketogulonate

DPNH H⁺ / DPN⁺

L-Gulonate

Figure 4.8   The glucuronate cycle. In the conversion of D-Glucuronate ⟶ L-Gulonate
⟶ L-Ascorbate, the original C-1 of glucose is indicated by the star.

An astonishing number of carbohydrate interconversion reactions and biosyntheses are conducted through these intermediates. In general, two types
of nucleotide sugar compounds are formed by the two types of reactions
shown in the equations below. The nucleotide *diphosphate* sugars are formed
from nucleoside triphosphates and the sugar-1-phosphates.

$$\text{nucleoside triphosphate}^{4-} + \text{sugar-l-P}^{2-} + H^+ \rightleftharpoons \text{nucleoside diphosphate sugar}^{2-} + PP_i^{3-}$$

A specific example, the formation of UDPG from UTP and glucose-l-P, has already been described. By a different and more common reaction, the nucleoside *monophosphate* sugars are formed from the nucleoside triphosphates and the *free* sugars. For example, CTP and N-acetylneuraminic acid condense to form cytidine monophosphate CMP-N-acetylneuraminic acid and pyrophosphate.

$$\text{cytidine triphosphate}^{4-} + \text{N-acetylneuraminic acid}^{1-} \rightleftharpoons \text{CMP-N acetylneuraminic acid}^{2-} + PP_i^{3-}$$

A large number of derivatives of the five bases, uridine, adenine, guanine, cytosine, and thymine have been discovered. Some of them are listed in Table 4.2 along with the type of condensation in which they are involved. In addition to serving as activators for the condensation of sugars, nucleotide sugars are interconverted and modified in a variety of important ways. The structures of the five bases are shown below.

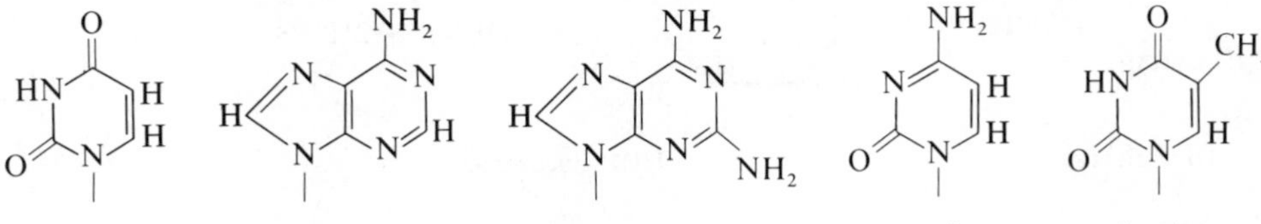

uracil   adenine   guanine   cytosine   thymine

TABLE 4.2 NUCLEOTIDE SUGARS AND BIOSYNTHESIS[a]

Donor Nucleotide	Acceptor	Products	Source
UDP glucose	Aglycone	Glucosides	Plants, insects
	Phenol	Phenyl-β-D-glucosides	Plants
	Phage DNA	Glucosylated DNA	Phage infected bacteria
UDP glucuronic acid	Aglycones	Glucuronides	Plants, animals
	Pneumococcal polysaccharides	Cell walls	Bacteria
UDP galactose	Glucose	Lactose	Animals
ADP glucose	Starch	Starch	Plants
CDP glycerol	Polyglycerol P	Teichoic acids	Bacteria
TDP L-rhamnose	Lipid	Rhamnolipid	Bacteria
CMP sialic acid	Glucose	Sialyl lactose	Animals

[a] From V. Ginsburg, *Adv. Enzym.* **26**, 35 (1964), and V. Ginsburg and E. F. Neufeld, *Ann. Rev. of Bioch., 38,* 371 (1969).

Epimerization

$$\text{UDP glucose} \rightleftharpoons \text{UDP galactose}$$

The enzyme UDP-D-galactose-4-epimerase catalyzes the inversion of the OH at the 4 position of the sugar interconverting UDP glucose and UDP galactose. It and other similar epimerases require catalytic concentrations of DPN+, suggesting that an oxidation-reduction mechanism may be operating. The suspected 4-keto intermediate has not, however, been detected—perhaps because it is tightly bound to the enzyme. This is an important interconversion for both the synthesis of lactose (a disaccharide containing glucose and galactose) and for the metabolism of lactose with the release of energy. In the lactating female mammal, lactose synthesis is important, while in the suckling infant its breakdown is essential.

Oxidation

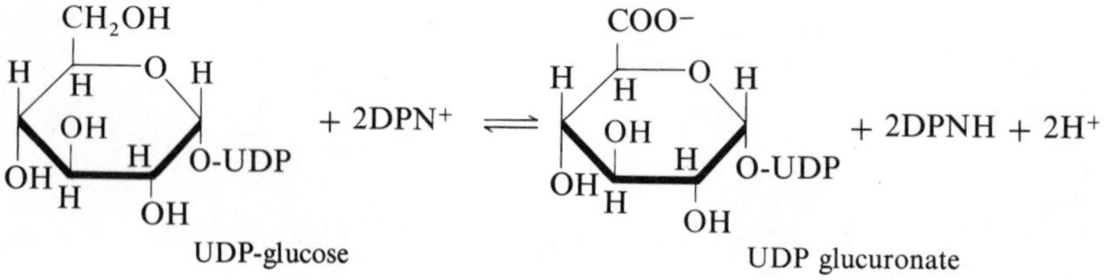

UDP-glucose   UDP glucuronate

In this two-stage oxidation of an alcohol to a carboxyl group, two equivalents of DPN+ are reduced with no evidence for an aldehyde intermediate in the reaction.

Reduction

This is accomplished by an interesting sequence. An example is the conversion of GDP-D-mannose to GDP-L-fucose.

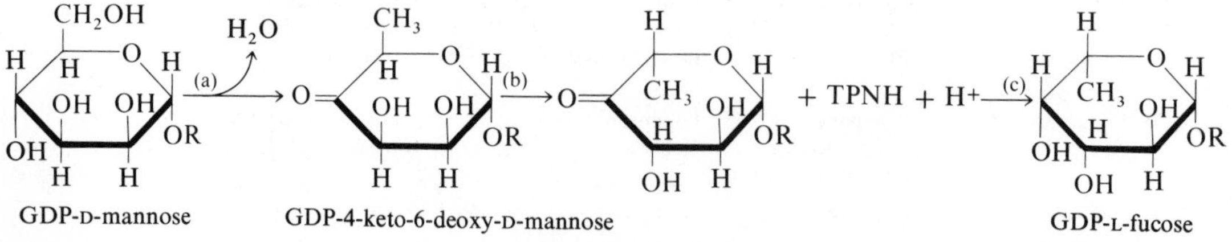

GDP-D-mannose   GDP-4-keto-6-deoxy-D-mannose   GDP-L-fucose

The initial reaction (a) is an internal oxidation-reduction accompanying a dehydration. Then, two inversions (b) occur at C-3 and C-5 and finally a stereospecific reduction occurs (c) with the TPNH + H+ at C-4. By an analogous reaction series, TDP-L-rhamnose is formed from TDP-D-glucose.

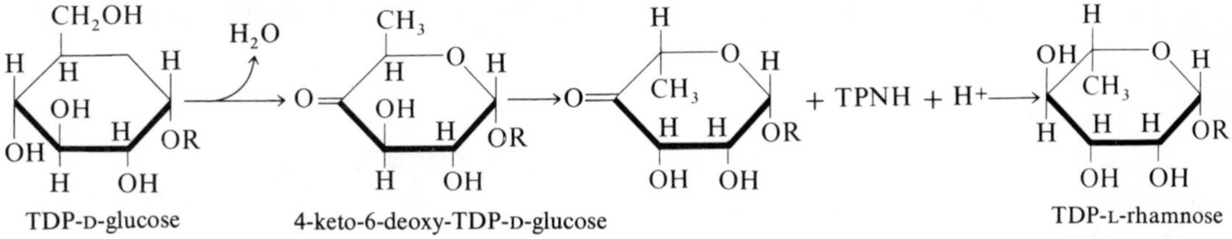

$$\text{CH}_2\text{OH} \quad \xrightarrow{\text{H}_2\text{O}} \quad \text{CH}_3 \quad \longrightarrow \quad \text{CH}_3 \quad + \text{TPNH} + \text{H}^+ \longrightarrow \quad \text{CH}_3$$

TDP-D-glucose   4-keto-6-deoxy-TDP-D-glucose   TDP-L-rhamnose

By further *reduction*, 3,6-dideoxy sugars are formed. An example is the formation of GDP colitose:

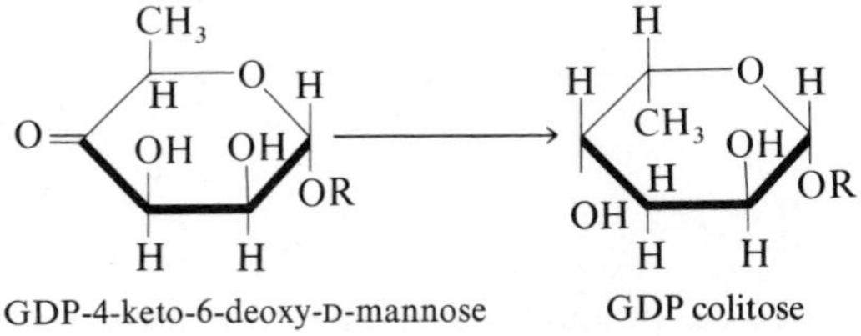

GDP-4-keto-6-deoxy-D-mannose   GDP colitose

C—C Bond Formation

This can also occur. An example is the formation of UDP-N-acetylmuramic acid from UDP-N-acetylglucosamine and phosphoenolpyruvate in a two-step reaction:

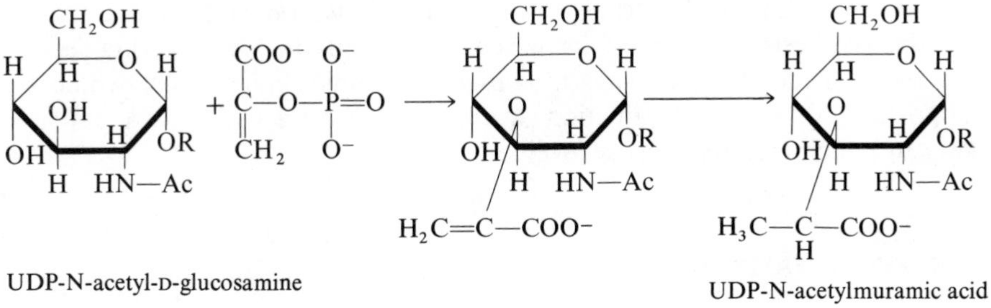

$$\text{CH}_2\text{OH} \quad + \quad \begin{matrix} \text{COO}^- & \text{O}^- \\ \text{C}-\text{O}-\text{P}=\text{O} \\ \text{CH}_2 & \text{O}^- \end{matrix} \longrightarrow \quad \text{CH}_2\text{OH} \longrightarrow \quad \text{CH}_2\text{OH}$$

UDP-N-acetyl-D-glucosamine $\text{H}_2\text{C}=\text{C}-\text{COO}^-$ $\text{H}_3\text{C}-\underset{\text{H}}{\text{C}}-\text{COO}^-$

UDP-N-acetylmuramic acid

The nucleotide sugars are precursors in disaccharide, oligosaccharide, and polysaccharide formation. These *transfer* reactions are catalyzed by transglycosylase enzymes which transfer the sugars from the nucleotide sugars to an appropriate acceptor to form the new sugar derivative as shown in the equation.

XDP-sugar + acceptor $\rightleftharpoons$ sugar-acceptor + XDP

A specific example, the glycogen synthase reaction, has already been given in Figure 4.4. Another example is the synthesis of sucrose from UDP glucose and fructose as the acceptor.

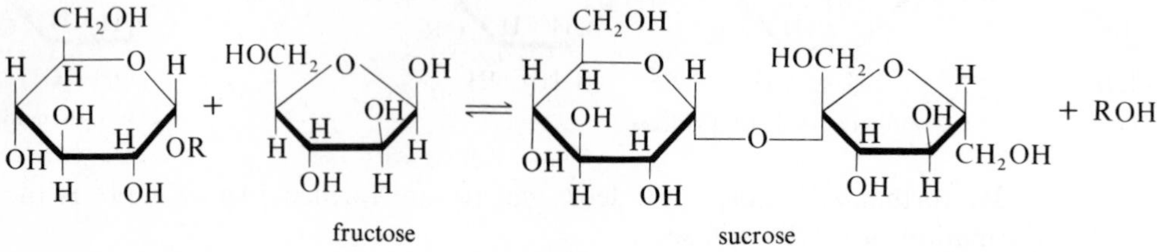

A number of oligosaccharides and polysaccharides synthesized from nucleotide sugars are listed in Table 4.2.

4.6 SUGAR INTERCONVERSIONS

The common hexoses, glucose, fructose, mannose, and galactose, as well as the amino sugars, deoxysugars, sugar acids, and sugar alcohols are all interconverted in metabolism. The more specialized sugar derivatives have specialized cellular structural functions, while the simpler sugars themselves serve as precursors. The common sugars can all be converted to glucose or to glycolytic intermediates and are thus made available for energy metabolism.

To this point in the chapter, the generation of energy from carbohydrates and the ways in which carbohydrates can be interconverted and activated for the synthesis of polymers have been described. In the following section we will consider the pathways by which the simple lipids, those which are important for energy production, are converted to acetyl-S-CoA, and the way in which that reaction is reversed.

4.7 HYDROLYSIS OF FATTY ACID ESTERS

Lipids (like carbohydrates) form important structural components as well as energy reserves for most living cells. Almost all lipids are composed in part of esters of long chain even-numbered fatty acids. Structures of three lipid molecules which contain such ester linkages are shown (p. 87). **a** is a triglyceride, **b** is phosphatidylcholine, a phospholipid, and **c** is a cholesterol ester. The ester linkages are marked by arrows which also indicate the bond susceptibility to enzymatic hydrolysis. The ester linkages of the triglyceride are hydrolyzed by lipases. The four linkages of **b** are subject to hydrolysis by four rather specific *phospholipases* known as phospholipase A, B, C, and D, respectively. The susceptable linkages are indicated by the letters next to the arrows. The ester linkage of **c** is cleaved by *cholesterol esterase*.

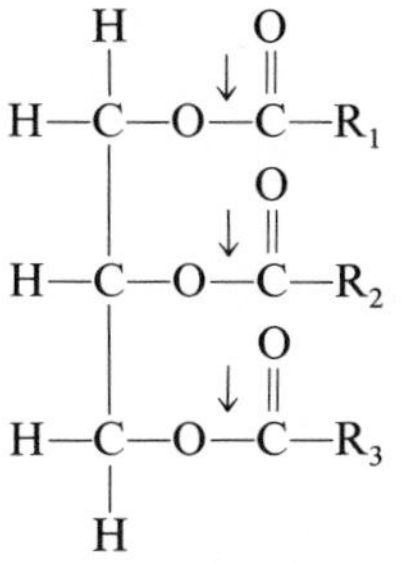

$$
\begin{array}{ll}
\text{a} & \text{b} \\
\end{array}
$$

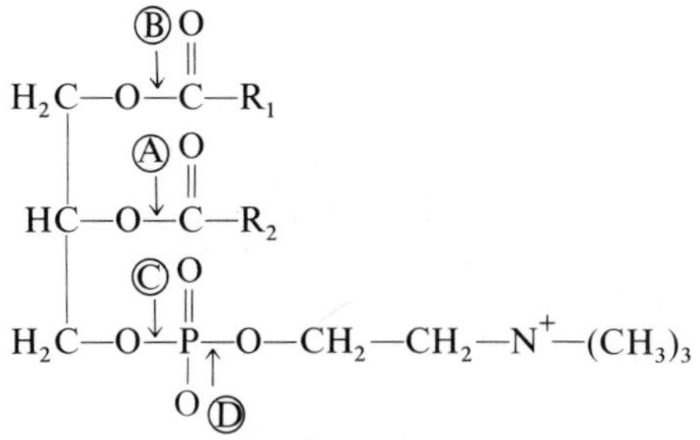

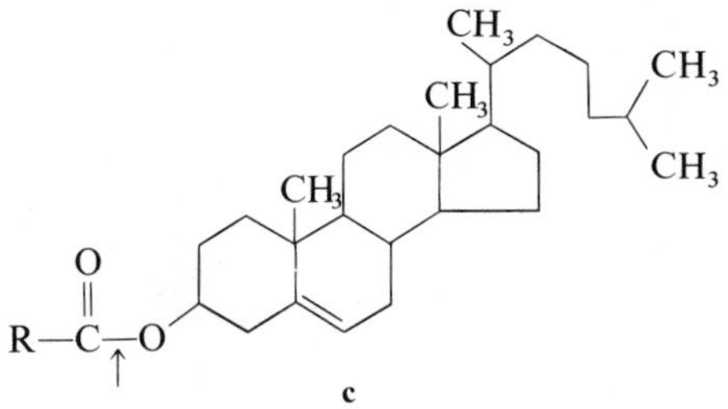

a (triacylglycerol structure with H–C–O–C–R$_1$, H–C–O–C–R$_2$, H–C–O–C–R$_3$ linkages)

b (phospholipid structure with positions Ⓑ, Ⓐ, Ⓒ, Ⓓ; H$_2$C–O–C–R$_1$, HC–O–C–R$_2$, H$_2$C–O–P–O–CH$_2$–CH$_2$–N$^+$–(CH$_3$)$_3$)

c (cholesteryl ester structure, R–C–O– with CH$_3$ groups)

None of these reactions yields energy, but they are necessary precursors to the metabolism of the fatty acids and other moieties in the molecules.

4.8 β-OXIDATION

The enzymatic reactions by which fatty acids are oxidized to form successive two-carbon acetyl-S-coenzyme A units are shown in Figure 4.9. The reactions all occur within the mitochondrion. The substrates are the CoA-SH derivatives of the fatty acids released from the lipids by *lipolysis.* After an initial *conversion* of the fatty acid to its CoA-SH derivative, at the expense of ATP, there occur two successive *oxidation* reactions, one the formation of a carbon-carbon double bond with reduction of FAD to FADH$_2$; and the other, the oxidation of a secondary alcohol to a β-keto group coupled to DPN+ reduction. The last reaction, a *thiolytic carbon-carbon bond cleavage* is essentially irreversible.

Except for the requirement for ATP in the first step, the other steps have ΔG^0 values below zero, especially when the reoxidation of FADH$_2$ and DPNH is coupled to the oxidative phosphorylation of electron transport. All steps are reversible to some extent. The series of reactions is such that when first started, it proceeds to generate C-2 units as acetyl-S-coenzyme A until the fatty acid is completely oxidized (with an even number of carbon atoms) or until propionyl-S-coenzyme A remains (with an odd number of carbon atoms). The sequence is essentially cyclic since the last step regen-

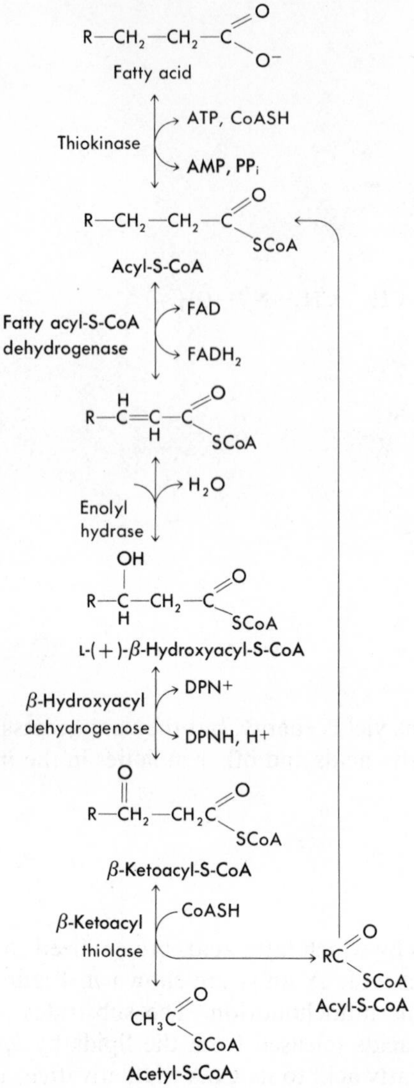

$$R\text{—}CH_2\text{—}CH_2\text{—}C\overset{\displaystyle O}{\underset{\displaystyle O^-}{}}$$

Fatty acid

Thiokinase
→ ATP, CoASH
→ AMP, PP$_i$

$$R\text{—}CH_2\text{—}CH_2\text{—}C\overset{\displaystyle O}{\underset{\displaystyle SCoA}{}}$$

Acyl-S-CoA

Fatty acyl-S-CoA dehydrogenase
→ FAD
→ FADH$_2$

$$R\overset{\displaystyle H}{\underset{}{}}{—}C{=}C\overset{}{\underset{\displaystyle H}{}}{—}C\overset{\displaystyle O}{\underset{\displaystyle SCoA}{}}$$

Enolyl hydrase
→ H$_2$O

$$R\overset{\displaystyle OH}{\underset{\displaystyle H}{}}{—}C{—}CH_2{—}C\overset{\displaystyle O}{\underset{\displaystyle SCoA}{}}$$

L-(+)-β-Hydroxyacyl-S-CoA

β-Hydroxyacyl dehydrogenose
→ DPN+
→ DPNH, H+

$$R{—}CH_2{—}CH_2C\overset{\displaystyle O}{\underset{\displaystyle SCoA}{}}$$
(with C=O)

β-Ketoacyl-S-CoA

β-Ketoacyl thiolase
← CoASH
→ RC$\overset{\displaystyle O}{\underset{\displaystyle SCoA}{}}$
Acyl-S-CoA

$$CH_3C\overset{\displaystyle O}{\underset{\displaystyle SCoA}{}}$$

Acetyl-S-CoA

Figure 4.9 β-oxidation of fatty acids.

erates an acyl-S-CoA derivative which can undergo further degradation without the expenditure of ATP.

It is of interest to compute the energy yield from the complete oxidation of a mole of palmitoyl-S-CoA, a sixteen-carbon fatty acid derivative.

1. In the generation of acetyl-S-CoA,

palmitoyl-S-CoA + 7O$_2$ ⟶ 8 acetyl fragments

$$7DPNH + H^+ \times 3 = 21ATP$$
$$7FADH_2 \quad\quad \times 2 = \underline{14ATP}$$
$$35ATP$$

2. In the operation of the citric acid cycle (12ATP per "turn"),

8 acetyl fragments + 16O$_2$ $\longrightarrow$ 16H$_2$O + 16CO$_2$

$$
\begin{array}{rl}
12\text{ATP} \times 8 & 96\text{ATP} \\
(\text{from 1 above}) & \underline{35\text{ATP}} \\
& 131\text{ATP}
\end{array}
$$

Assuming that the free energy of formation of a $\sim$P of ATP is about 7,000 cal, the efficiency of conservation of energy is:

$$
\frac{131 \times 7000}{2,400,000} \times 100 = 38 \text{ percent}
$$

a very high value, and comparable to the 42 percent yield from carbohydrate metabolism. 2,400,000 calories is the energy of complete combustion obtained from calorimetric measurements.

The intracellular site of β-oxidation is the mitochondria, but much of the thiokinase, which catalyzes the activation of free fatty acids, is located in the extramitochondrial portion of the cell. It has been discovered rather recently that carnitine (originally identified an insect growth factor) functions as a fatty acid carrier transporting fatty acids into the mitochondrion. The system is shown diagrammatically in Figure 4.10. After activation to their

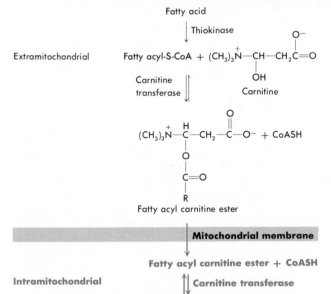

Figure 4.10

Transport of fatty acids into mitochondria as carnitine esters.

CoASH derivatives, fatty acids are transferred to carnitine by carnitine transferase. The fatty acyl carnitine passes through the mitochondrial membrane where it is reconverted to the fatty acyl-S-CoA ester by the carnitine transferase and then oxidized by the β-oxidation system just discussed.

4.9 SYNTHESIS OF TRIGLYCERIDES, PHOSPHOLIPIDS, AND SPHINGOLIPIDS

Triglycerides

The pathway of triglyceride synthesis is shown in Figure 4.11. It involves the expenditure of energy and requires L-α-glycerol-P, which is derived from dihydroxy acetone-P (an intermediate in glycolysis). In the first reaction, two equivalents of fatty acyl-S-CoA condense with L-α-glycerophosphate to form a phosphatidic acid. Hydrolysis by a specific phosphatase liberates P_i to form the diglyceride, which in turn condenses with another equivalent of fatty acyl-S-CoA to form the triglyceride.

Phospholipids

In general, phospholipids are synthesized by two-reaction pathways. In one series of reactions by which phosphatidyl choline (lecithin) is assembled, the choline is activated. These reactions are shown in Figure 4.12. Choline is *phosphorylated* with ATP to phosphorylcholine, which is, in turn, *con-*

Figure 4.11   Pathway of triglyceride synthesis.

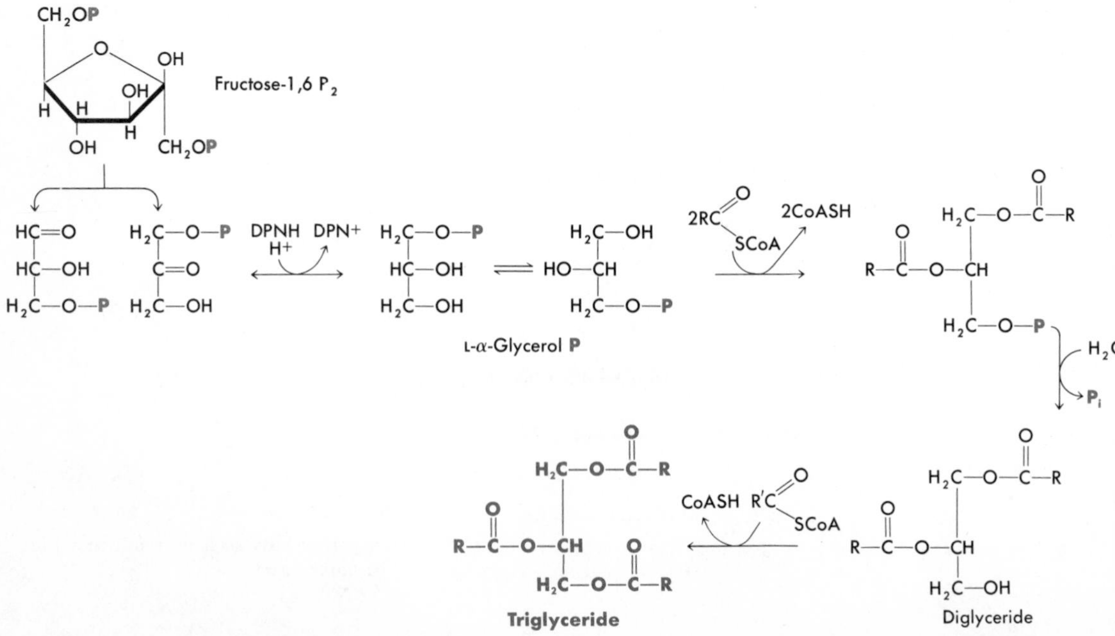

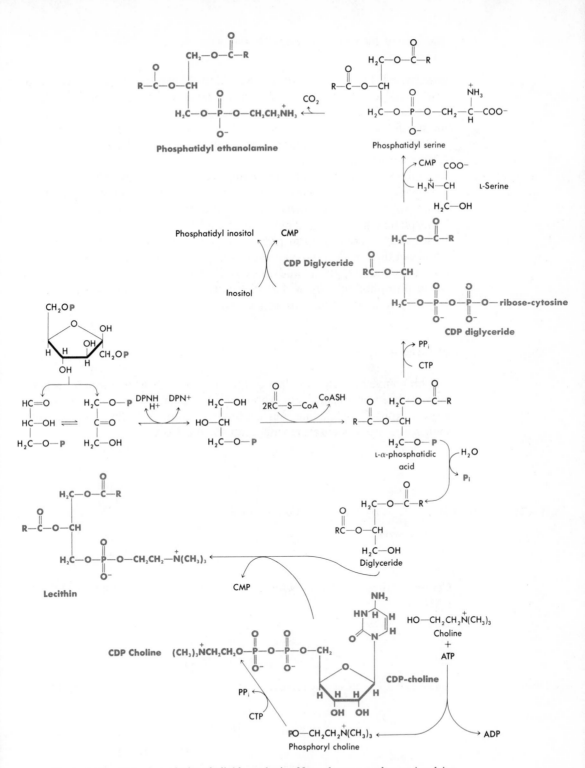

Figure 4.12 Pathways of phospholipid synthesis. Note the two pathways involving CDP choline and CDP diglyceride as intermediates.

densed with CTP to form CDP choline. CDP choline, in turn, condenses with an α, β-diglyceride, formed as shown in Figure 4.12 to give a lecithin. The total cost is 5ATP, one greater than the number of bonds synthesized, including the two for fatty acyl-S-CoA formation. An analogous pathway is available for phosphatidylethanolamine synthesis from ethanolamine via the CDP ethanolamine derivative.

A different route is used for the synthesis of phosphatidylserine. Here the phosphatidic acid is activated. The reactions are also shown in Figure 4.12. L-α-phosphatidic acid condenses with CTP to form the intermediate cytidine diphosphate diglyceride and pyrophosphate. The CDP diglyceride then condenses with L-serine to form phosphatidyl serine and CMP. Phosphatidylserine can then be decarboxylated to form phosphatidylethanolamine. In an analogous manner, phosphatidylinositol is formed.

The phospholipids are widely distributed in all cells and organs where they play vital structural roles in membranes.

Sphingolipids

Sphingomyelins, another class of lipid compounds whose structures have recently been established but whose precise functions are not known, are formed from CDP choline and ceramide. Ceramide is first formed from sphingosine by condensation with a fatty acyl-S-CoA.

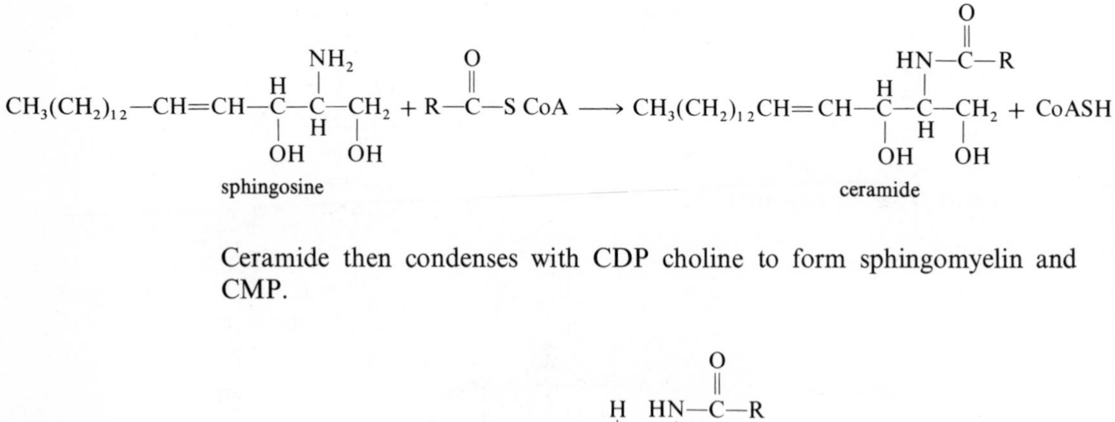

sphingosine   ceramide

Ceramide then condenses with CDP choline to form sphingomyelin and CMP.

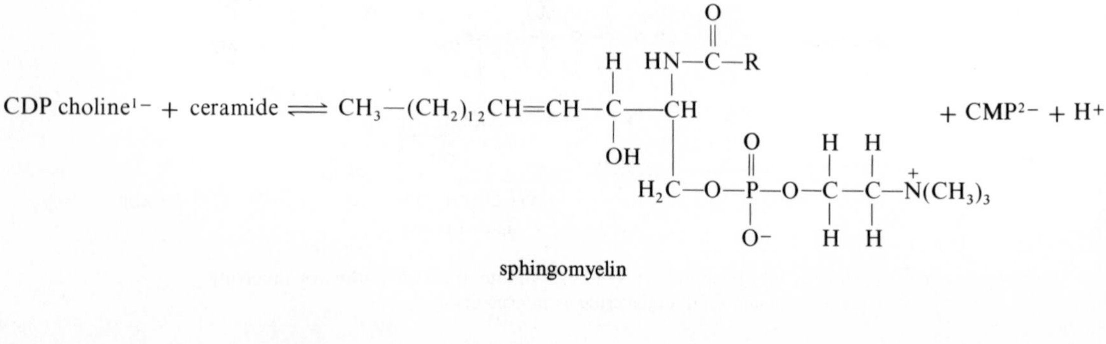

sphingomyelin

Glycosphingolipids are formed by carbohydrate transfer to ceramide.

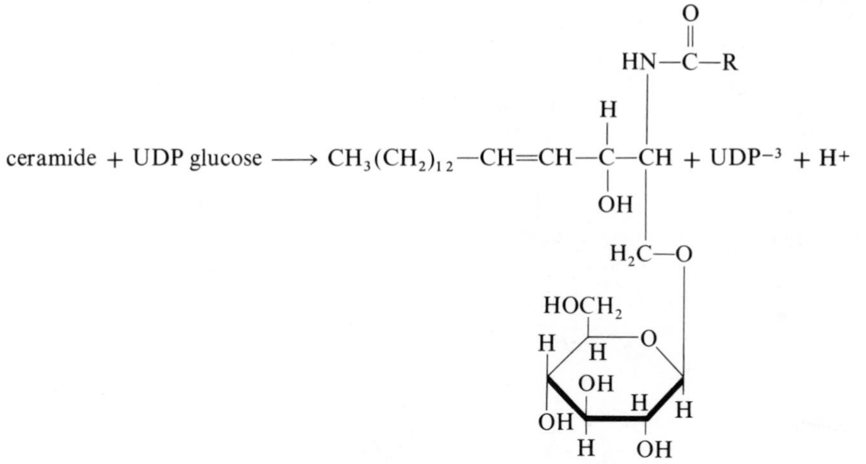

$$\text{ceramide} + \text{UDP glucose} \longrightarrow$$

$$
\begin{array}{c}
\text{O} \\
\parallel \\
\text{HN}-\text{C}-\text{R} \\
\text{H} \quad | \\
\text{CH}_3(\text{CH}_2)_{12}-\text{CH}{=}\text{CH}-\overset{|}{\text{C}}-\text{CH} + \text{UDP}^{-3} + \text{H}^+ \\
| \\
\text{OH} \quad | \\
\text{H}_2\text{C}-\text{O}
\end{array}
$$

ceramide glucose

$$\text{ceramide glucose} + \text{UDP galactose}^{2-} \longrightarrow \text{ceramide glucose galactose} + \text{UDP}^{3-} + \text{H}^+$$

$$\text{ceramide glucose galactose} + \text{CMP-N-acetylglucosamine}^{1-} \longrightarrow$$

$$\text{ceramide glucose galactose N-acetylglucosamine} + \text{CMP}^{2-} + \text{H}^+$$

These compounds are extremely important structural components of nervous tissue, but are also found in other sites as well.

4.10 FATTY ACID SYNTHESIS

The reactions of fatty acid synthesis are not those of β-oxidation. Instead, nature has devised a reaction series which is a modification of the reactions of β-oxidation but which provides several new features including irreversibility in the synthetic direction. The necessity of separate pathways for synthesis and degradation has previously been discussed and will be further considered in chapter 6. Their existence removes the possibility of wasteful cycling of materials. The sequence of reactions involved in fatty acid synthesis is shown in Figure 4.13. The driving force of fatty acid synthesis is that the new carbon-carbon bond is formed with the simultaneous liberation of CO_2, thus insuring irreversibility. An additional distinguishing feature is the fact that the condensation reactions occur utilizing an SH compound of higher molecular-weight than CoA-SH, namely, acyl carrier protein (ACP). The peptide or protein has a molecular weight of about 10,000. In ACP, the

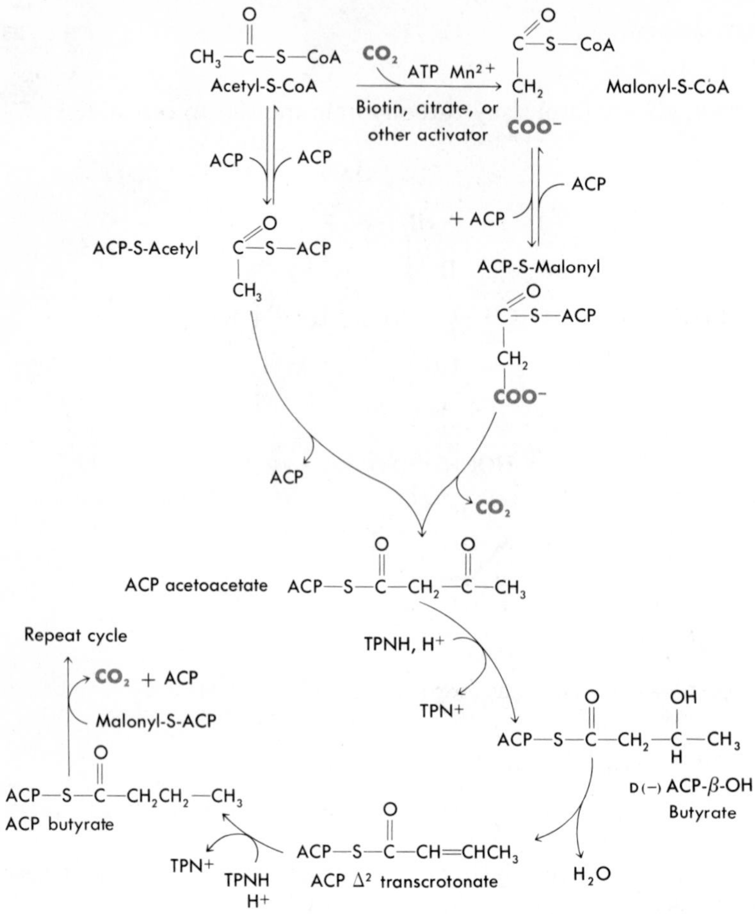

O
‖
$CH_3—C—S—CoA$ CO_2 $C—S—CoA$
Acetyl-S-CoA →ATP Mn^{2+}→ CH_2 Malonyl-S-CoA
                Biotin, citrate, or COO^-
                other activator

ACP ⇅ ACP   ⌐ ACP
                              + ACP ⌐

O   ACP-S-Malonyl
‖   O
ACP-S-Acetyl $C—S—ACP$ ‖
               CH_3 $C—S—ACP$
                                       CH_2
                                       COO^-

                    ACP ⌐   ⌐ CO_2

                         O   O
                         ‖   ‖
ACP acetoacetate $ACP—S—C—CH_2—C—CH_3$

Repeat cycle $TPNH, H^+$ ⌐

   ⌐ $CO_2 + ACP$ TPN^+ O   OH
   ⌐ Malonyl-S-ACP $ACP—S—C—CH_2—C—CH_3$
        O   H
        ‖ $D(-) ACP-\beta-OH$
$ACP—S—C—CH_2CH_2—CH_3$ Butyrate
ACP butyrate
                                 O
  TPN^+ ⌐   ‖
         $TPNH$ $ACP—S—C—CH=CHCH_3$ H_2O
         H^+ ACP Δ^2 transcrotonate

Figure 4.13   Pathway of fatty acid synthesis. Note the importance of ACP and of
              the carboxylation and decarboxylation as parts of the reaction sequence.

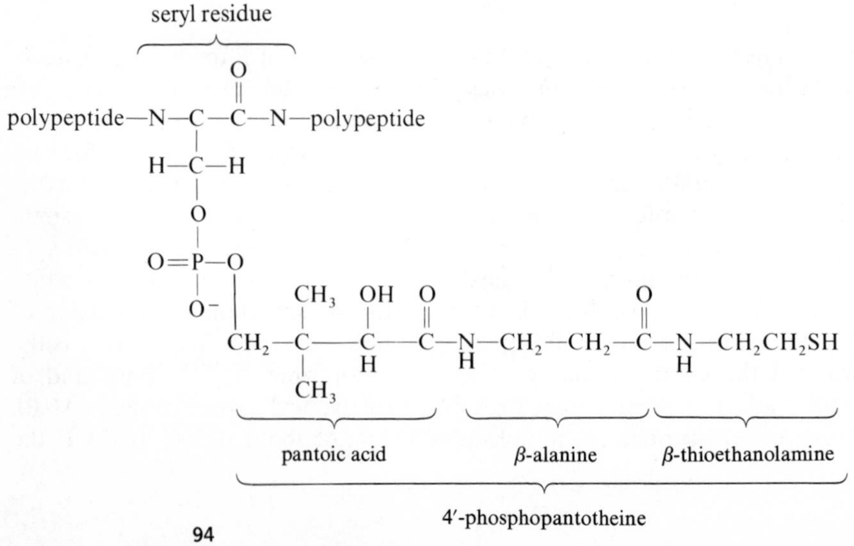

seryl residue
                    O
                    ‖
polypeptide—N—C—C—N—polypeptide
              H—C—H
                  O
              O=P—O
                O^- CH_3 OH O   O
                      $CH_2—C——C—C—N—CH_2—CH_2—C—N—CH_2CH_2SH$
                             | H   H   H
                            CH_3

                      pantoic acid β-alanine β-thioethanolamine

                              4'-phosphopantotheine

94

OH of a serine is derivatized with a 4'-phosphorylpantotheine. Thus, ACP is structurally related to coenzyme A-SH.

Following an initial *carboxylation* of some acetyl-S-CoA to malonyl-S-CoA, the two coenzyme A derivatives are converted to their respective acyl carrier protein derivatives. *The C—C bond is formed with the release of* CO_2 and the release of one ACP; next the *reduction* of the β-keto derivative to a β-hydroxyl group occurs with TPNH + H$^+$ as the reducing agent; the β-OH acid is *dehydrated* to the unsaturated acid, and lastly the *C—C double bond* is reduced with TPNH + H$^+$ as reducing agent. The overall sequence, after the condensation step, is very similar to the degradative pathway except that the two reduction steps in fatty acid biosynthesis are TPNH + H$^+$-requiring rather than FADH$_2$ and DPNH H$^+$-requiring. As has been previously mentioned (Section 4.3), the oxidation of the pentose pathway generates TPNH + H$^+$. Therefore, fatty acid synthesis is closely coupled to the pentose cycle and only occurs when glucose is available to generate TPNH + H$^+$. The reactions of fatty acid synthesis and the pentose cycle both occur in the cytosol.

The mechanism of the carboxylation reaction which produces malonyl-S-CoA is of interest. The enzyme catalyzing the reaction, acetyl-S-CoA carboxylase, contains biotin, which is covalently carboxylated in the reaction. The structure of the N-carboxy biotin enzyme is as shown:

In the two-step reaction, the biotin is first carboxylated at the expense of ATP,

$$HCO_3^- + ATP^{4-} + \text{biotin-enzyme} \rightleftharpoons {}^-OOC\text{-biotin-enzyme} + ADP^{3-} + P_i^{2-} + H^+$$

The CO_2 is then transferred to acetyl-S-CoA to form malonyl-S-CoA,

$$^-OOC\text{-biotin-enzyme} + \text{acetyl-S-CoA} \rightleftharpoons \text{malonyl-S-CoA} + \text{biotin enzyme}$$

The overall stoichiometry of fatty acid synthesis is such that for each malonyl-S-CoA required, two TPNH and two H$^+$ are also required. For the synthesis of one palmitoyl-S-CoA, the equivalent of 57ATP are required.

$$\text{acetyl-S-CoA} + 7\text{ malonyl-S-CoA} + 14\text{TPNH} + 14\text{H}^+ \longrightarrow$$
$$\text{palmitoyl-S-CoA} + 7\text{CO}_2 + 14\text{TPN} + 7\text{H}_2\text{O}$$

4.11 FATTY ACID MODIFICATIONS AND PROSTAGLANDIN SYNTHESIS

In addition to the pathway of fatty acid biosynthesis as outlined, there are additional pathways present in mitochondria and microsomes specifically for chain lengthening and shortening by C-2 addition and removal. Also, interconversions of mono to poly*unsaturated* fatty acids occur. In all cases, the stereochemistry of the double bonds is *cis*. In general, animals are able to synthesize monounsaturated fatty acids (palmitoleic, vaccenic, oleic, nervonic) and one series of polyunsaturated fatty acids (eicosatrienoic) *de novo* (Figure 4.14).

Biosynthesis of some of the cyclic prostaglandins from the unsaturated fatty acids is shown in Figure 4.15. These fascinating compounds, which

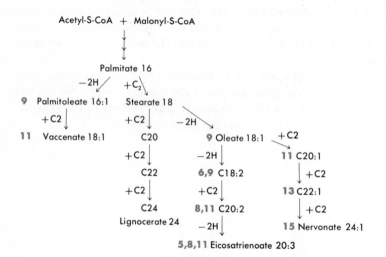

Figure 4.14

Fatty acid metabolic pathways in animals. Note the dehydrogenation and C-2 lengthening reactions. Numbers before the names indicate position of double bonds. Numbers after names indicate number of carbon atoms and number of double bonds before and after position of: Thus 20:1 represents 20 carbons and 1 double bond. Adapted from White, Handler & Smith, *Principles of Biochemistry*, McGraw-Hill, 1968.

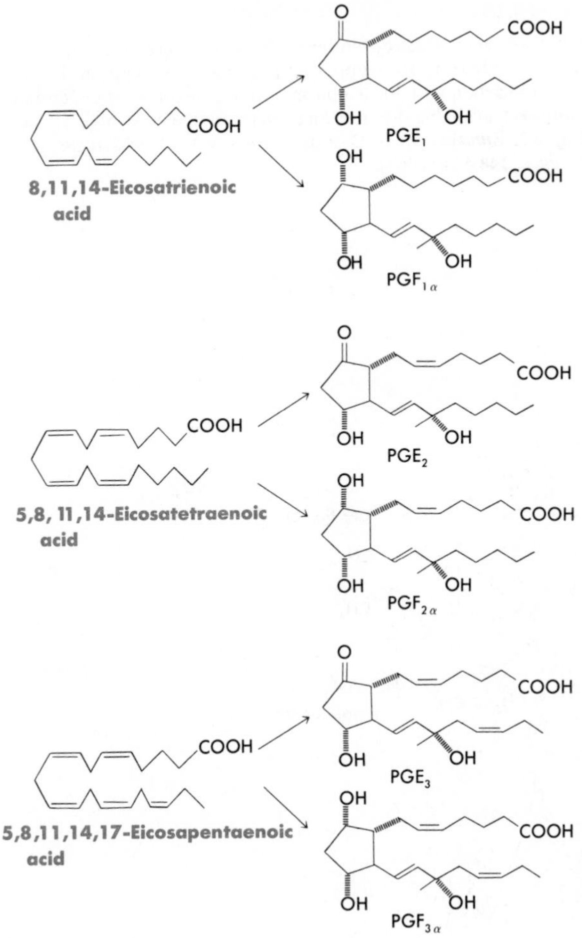

8,11,14-Eicosatrienoic acid

PGE₁

PGF₁ₐ

5,8,11,14-Eicosatetraenoic acid

PGE₂

PGF₂ₐ

5,8,11,14,17-Eicosapentaenoic acid

PGE₃

PGF₃ₐ

Figure 4.15

Pathways of prostaglandin synthesis. Note the number of prostaglandins made from the polyunsaturated fatty acids. From S. Bergstrom, L. A. Carlson & J. R. Weeks, *Pharmacological Reviews,* **20,** 1 (1968).

have important functions in control, will be referred to later in the book. Note the oxidized and reduced forms.

4.12   CHOLESTEROL SYNTHESIS

Some of the known reactions by which acetate is converted to cholesterol are shown in Figure 4.16. Three *C-2 units are converted to a C-6* unit β-hydroxy-β-methylglutaryl-S-CoA. This C-6 unit is reduced to *mevalonate*. *Mevalonate* is *phosphorylated* in two successive ATP-dependent reactions to form pyrophosphomevalonate. This C-6 intermediate is then *decarboxylated* with the hydrolysis of ATP to the C-5 unsaturated 3-isopentenylpyrophosphate, which is next *isomerized* to 3,3-dimethylallylpyrophosphate. One molecule of this intermediate *condenses* with one molecule of dimethyallyl-

Figure 4.16

Pathways of cholesterol synthesis. Note the successive buildup of the molecule from the isoprenoid precursor via 5 carbon, 10 carbon, 15 carbon and 30 carbon molecules; also note the alternate pathways available for the final steps in the biosynthesis. See Fig. 2.2. See also M. E. Dempsey, *Annals New York Academy of Science*, **148** 631 (1968).

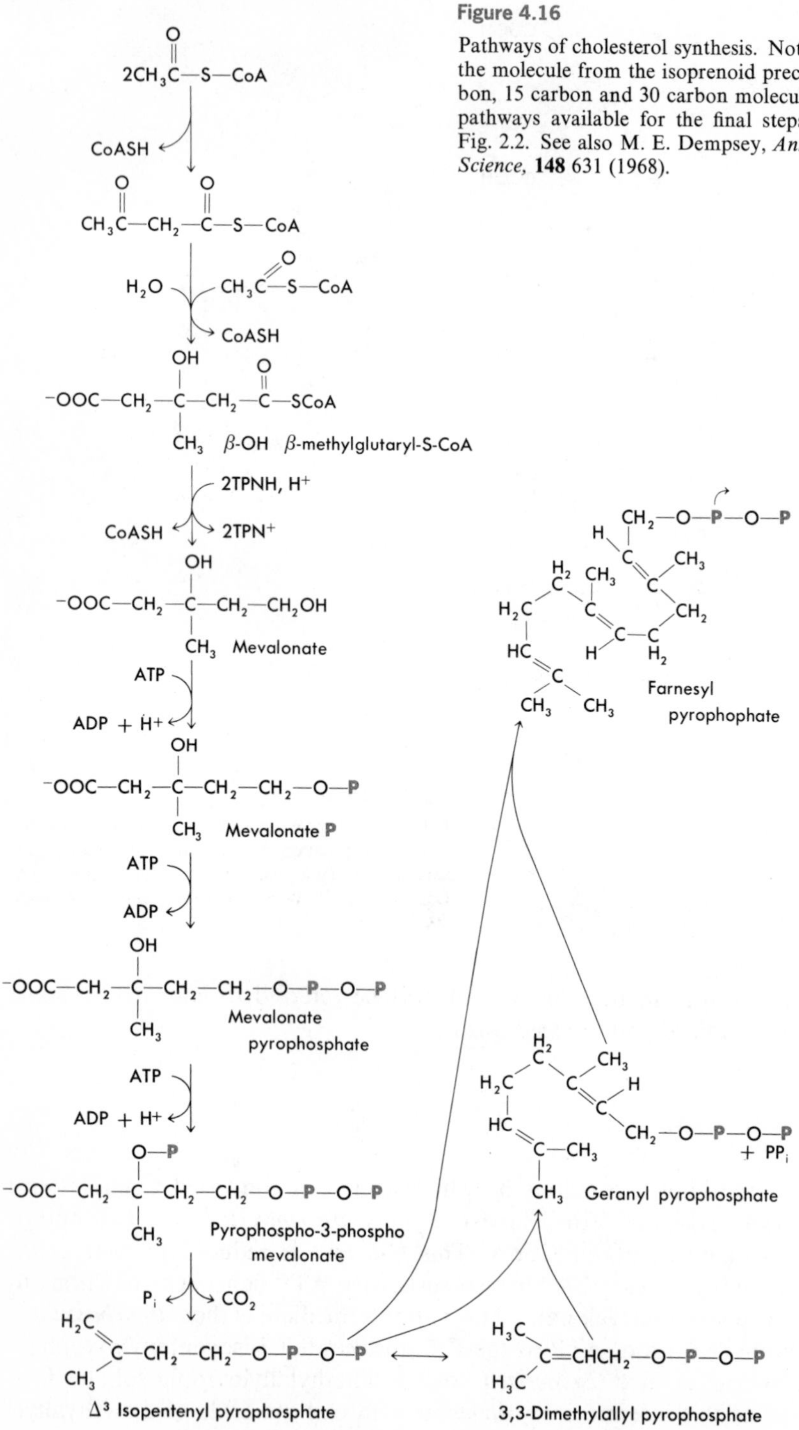

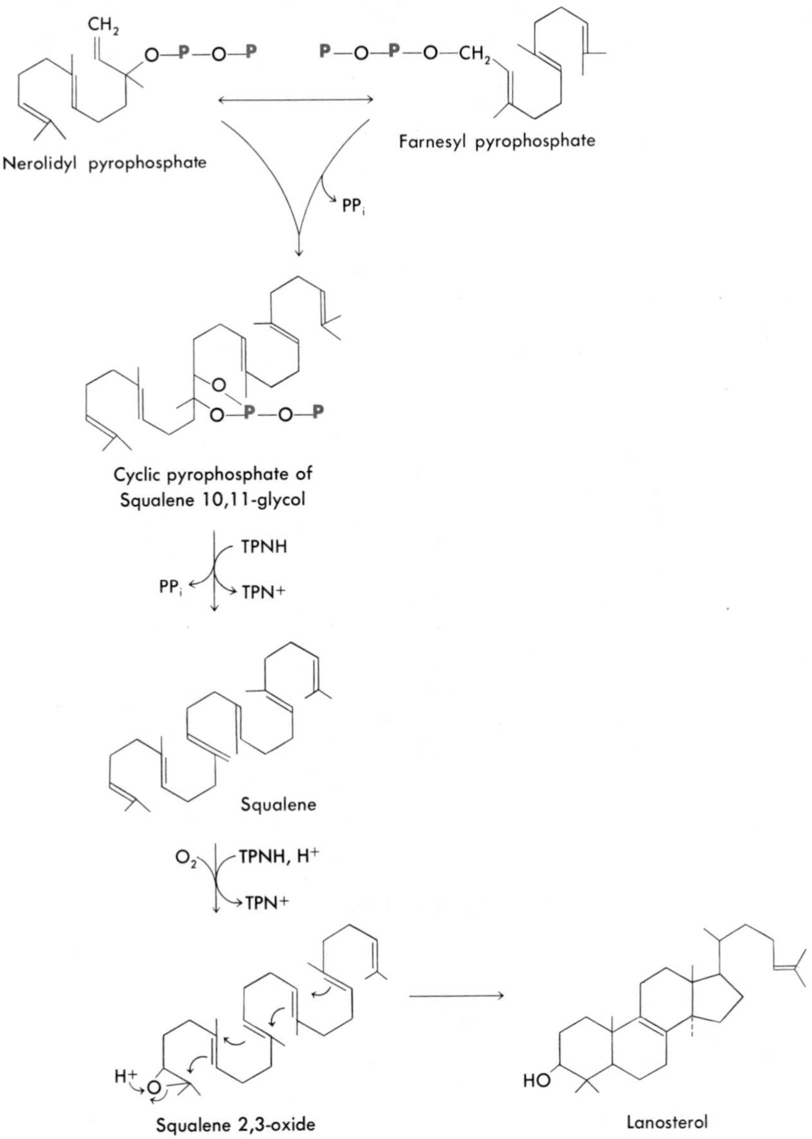

Nerolidyl pyrophosphate

Farnesyl pyrophosphate

PP$_i$

Figure 4.16 (Continued)

Cyclic pyrophosphate of
Squalene 10,11-glycol

TPNH

PP$_i$ ⟶ TPN+

Squalene

O$_2$ — TPNH, H$^+$

TPN+

H$^+$ ⟶ O

Squalene 2,3-oxide

HO

Lanosterol

pyrophosphate to form the C-10 geranylpyrophosphate, which in turn *condenses* with another C-5 unit (isopentenylpyrophosphate) to form the C-15 farnesylpyrophosphate. Two molecules of farnesylpyrophosphate *condense* tail to tail to form the C-30 intermediate squalene, which is *cyclized* in the presence of O$_2$ and TPNH + H$^+$ by way of the intermediate squalene 2,3-oxide to form the steroid lanosterol. Lanosterol ($\Delta^{8,24}$-cholestadienol) is con-

Figure 4.16 (Continued)

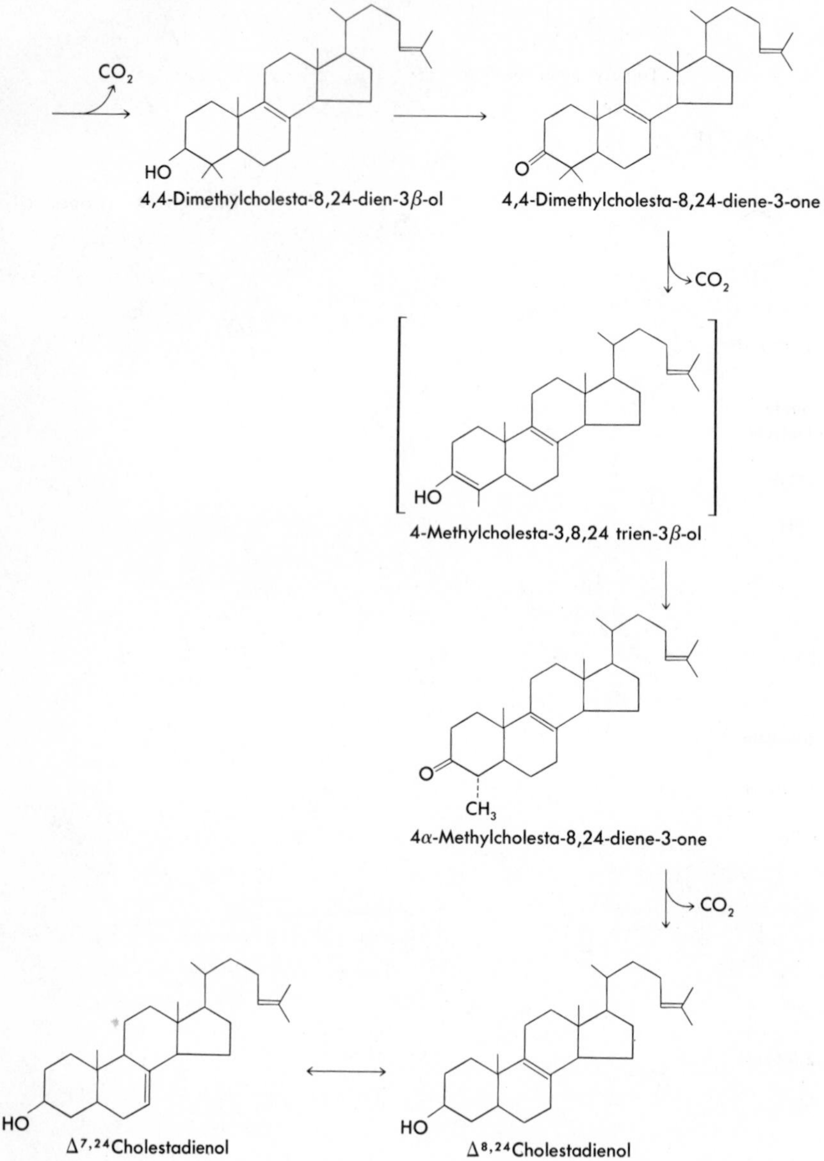
CO₂
HO
4,4-Dimethylcholesta-8,24-dien-3β-ol
O
4,4-Dimethylcholesta-8,24-diene-3-one
CO₂
HO
4-Methylcholesta-3,8,24 trien-3β-ol
O
CH₃
4α-Methylcholesta-8,24-diene-3-one
CO₂
HO
Δ7,24Cholestadienol
HO
Δ8,24Cholestadienol

verted in turn to cholesterol by a series of steps. In the overall process, the 14-α-methyl and the gem-dimethyl groups at the 3 position are removed oxidatively, the Δ^8 bond is isomerized to the Δ^7 position, the Δ^5 bond is introduced, yielding a $\Delta^{5,7}$ dienol, and the Δ^7 and Δ^{24} bonds are reduced.

In man, cholesterol is synthesized chiefly in liver but also in other tissues

Figure 4.16   (Continued)

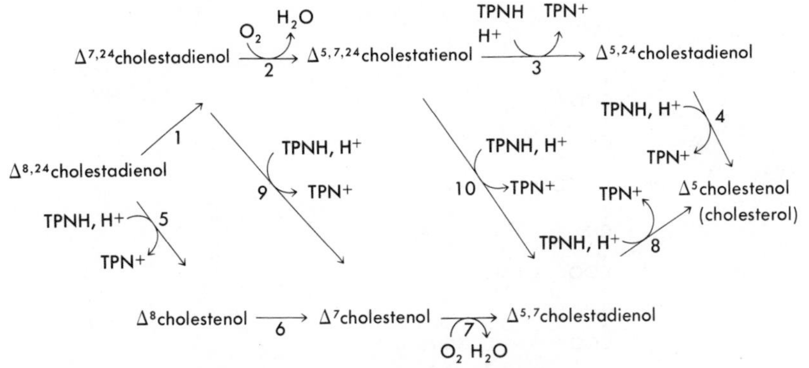

Reactions 4, 5, 9, 10 catalyzed by a Δ^{24}reductase
Reactions 3 and 8   catalyzed by a Δ^{7}reductase
Reactions 2 and 7   catalyzed by a Δ^{5}dehydrogenase
Reactions 1 and 6   catalyzed by a $\Delta^{7} \longleftrightarrow \Delta^{8}$isomerase

such as intestine, skin, adrenals, reproductive organs, blood vessels, and nerves. It is the starting material for the formation of all the other steroids, including the bile acids, the adrenal and gonadal steroids.

4.13   GLYOXALATE CYCLE

A discussion of the glyoxalate cycle is valuable in that it affords an opportunity to examine some interrelationships between the tricarboxylic acid cycle and gluconeogenesis. It has been recognized for some time that carbohydrates are readily converted into fats. The reverse process does not generally occur (in animal tissues), but it may occur in plants and microorganisms under special circumstances. In the case of seeds with a high fat content, for example, it has been shown that sugar (sucrose) is formed during germination. Since carbon is completely oxidized to CO_2 in the tricarboxylic acid cycle, a mechanism must exist for bypassing this oxidative cycle in order to synthesize carbohydrate from fat. This mechanism has been identified as the glyoxalate cycle (Figure 4.17.) Citrate formed by condensing oxaloacetate with acetyl-S-CoA is *isomerized* to isocitrate, as it is in the citric acid cycle. Isocitrate is then *cleaved* to glyoxalate and succinate, and glyoxalate is *condensed* with acetyl-S-CoA to form malate, which is then converted to oxaloacetate and is ready to accept another acetyl-S-CoA and reinitiate the cycle. In this way, the *net conversion* of two acetyl-S-CoA units into a C-4 unit, succinate, can take place. The succinate formed can readily be converted to glucose by gluconeogenesis. These two novel enzymes, malate synthase and isocitritase are found in systems where there is a *net conversion* of fat to sugar,

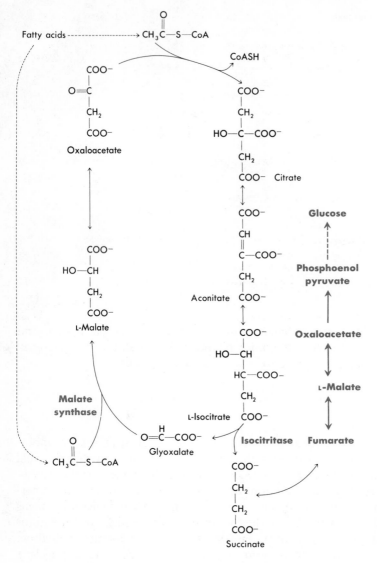

Figure 4.17

The glyoxalate cycle. By these reactions two carbon units may be converted to citrate, isocitrate $\longrightarrow$ succinate and via phosphoenolpyruvate to glucose, instead of being combusted to CO_2 via the tricarboxylic acid cycle.

and are not found where this conversion does not occur. Thus, it can be appreciated that the enzymatic apparatus of the cell determines the overall metabolic function.

In this chapter, we have discussed the main pathways in the metabolism of carbohydrates and lipids. We have seen that, in general, these carbon- and oxygen-containing compounds are metabolized as highly activated, charged, or ionized derivatives of phosphorus and sulfur. The reactions are arranged in sequences or cycles with many interrelationships through common intermediates. From the exergonic pathways of glycolysis, the pentose cycle,

β-oxidation of fatty acids and the tricarboxylic acid cycle, energy is made available *either* as ATP or as reducing power in the form of the reduced coenzymes DPNH + H⁺ and TPNH + H⁺. Key intermediates of vital importance to the cell are also produced in these pathways.

The biosynthetic pathways including gluconeogenesis, glycogenesis, fatty acid, cholesterol and lecithin biosynthesis, and the glyoxalate cycle coupled with gluconeogenesis all require a major energy input in the form of ATP with or without an accompanying supply of reducing power as DPNH + H⁺ or TPNH + H⁺ in order to drive these endergonic sequences. In general, all of these sequences generate protons because of the utilization of ATP. An exception is fatty acid synthesis, where the input of reducing power as TPNH and H⁺ is sufficiently high so as to overbalance the ATP utilization with the result of a net consumption of H⁺.

REFERENCES

Altman, P. L., and D. S. Dittmer (eds.), *Metabolism*, Federation of American Societies for Experimental Biology, 1968. This volume contains a wealth of collected information.

Bergstrom, S., Carlson, L. A., and J. R. Weeks, *Pharmacological Reviews* **20**, 1 (1968).

Dempsey, M. E., *Ann. N. Y. Acad. Sci.*, **148**, 631 (1968).

Ginsburg, V., *Advan. in Enzym.*, **26**, 35 (1964).

Ginsburg, V. and E. F. Neufeld, *Ann. Rev. of Biochem*, **38**, 371 (1969).

Masoro, E. J., *Physiological Chemistry of Lipids in Mammals,* W. B. Saunders Co., Philadelphia, 1968.

Scrutton, M. C., and M. F. Utter, "The Regulation of Glycolysis and Gluconeogenesis in Animal Tissues," *Ann. Rev. Biochem.*, **37**, 249 (1968).

Shapiro, B., "Lipid Metabolism," *Ann. Rev. Biochem*, **36**, 246 (1967).

Villar-Palasi, C., and J. Larner, "Glycogen Metabolism and Glycolytic Enzymes," *Ann. Rev. Biochem.*, **39**, 639 (1970).

THE METABOLISM
OF N COMPOUNDS

FIVE

In this chapter, the major metabolic reactions and pathways of the nitrogen-containing constituents of living matter are discussed. The nitrogen compounds include the extremely important informational biopolymers, DNA, RNA, and the proteins; structural biopolymers such as bacterial cell wall peptidoglycan; and a host of low-molecular-weight compounds, including the amino acids, peptides, the purine and pyrimidine bases, pigments such as heme, guanido compounds such as creatine, and the nitrogen-excretory products including urea, uric acid, and others. In contrast to the carbohydrates and lipids which serve as energy and carbon sources and which are stored in cells, the nitrogen compounds serve principally as constituents of dynamic systems which turn over and are not stored. When available in excess of cellular requirements, most nitrogen compounds can be utilized for energy production.

Since these compounds are not stored, their overall levels in animal cells are very well regulated in terms of balanced rates of synthesis and degradation. This is known as *nitrogen balance*. In adult humans, for example, under maintenance conditions, the nitrogen intake is exactly balanced by the nitrogen excretion in urine and feces. In growing children, more nitrogen is ingested than is excreted, the excess being laid down in cellular constituents. This is also the situation in a rapidly growing bacterial culture. This state is termed *positive nitrogen balance.* On the other hand, when tissues are being broken down, for example, during starvation, or after severe injury, or with a state of hormonal imbalance such as the diabetic state or adrenal cortical hypersecretion, an excess of nitrogen is excreted over that ingested. This state is termed *negative nitrogen balance.*

In contrast to the pathways of glycolysis and fatty acid synthesis and degradation which are widely distributed in nature, a number of pathways for the synthesis of nitrogen compounds have disappeared during evolution. Man and the higher animals, for example, have lost the ability to synthesize all the vitamins and the carbon chains of about half the amino acids. As a result, man has become parasitic, requiring that these molecules be supplied preformed in the diet and those amino acids which are no longer synthesized are termed "essential" (Table 1.2). This may actually be advantageous, since it allows a reduction in the number of enzymatic reactions within the cells.

In contrast to the carbohydrates and lipids, most nitrogen compounds have charged groups and are metabolized without derivatization.

The metabolism of the amino acids will be considered first in terms of the carbon chains and then of the nitrogen itself. The special metabolism of the *nonessential* and the *essential* amino acids will then be considered. This will be followed by a discussion of the metabolism of the nitrogen excretion products. The biosynthesis of the purine and pyrimidine nucleotides, the monomeric precursors of the nucleic acids, is then detailed, followed by a very brief discussion of the synthesis of DNA, RNA, and protein, the biosynthesis of heme, glutamine, and glutathione. Lastly, the synthesis of peptidoglycan is presented. (For a detailed discussion of the synthesis of the informational biopolymers, see the book by Wold in this series.)

5.1 AMINO ACID METABOLISM—GENERAL

Animals require protein or amino acids to be supplied in the diet. This is true for both young growing animals and for adults as well. In digestion, protein is hydrolyzed to its constituent amino acids. Proteolytic enzymes catalyze these reactions and their specificities of action are listed in Table 5.1. Many of these enzymes are released as inactive precursors from the tissues which synthesize them. Activation is achieved catalytically, in some cases autocatalytically, and involves cleavage of peptide bonds. After absorption from the intestine, the amino acids are built into the cellular proteins (or utilized as a source of energy). Nutritional experiments have permitted a classification of the amino acids into two groups, the *essential* and the *nonessential* amino acids. These are listed in Table 5.2. All essential amino acids must be supplied in the diet in order to maintain growth or nitrogen balance. Certain of the essential amino acids, however, can be replaced by others. Tyrosine, for example, can be formed from phenylalanine

TABLE 5.1   THE PROTEOLYTIC ENZYMES

Name	Origin	Type	Specificity	Molecular Weight	Approximate pH Optimum
Pepsin	Stomach, mucosa	Endopeptidase	Broad specificity	36,000	2
Trypsin	Pancreas	Endopeptidase	L-Arginine or L-lysine	23,000	8
Chymotrypsin	Pancreas	Endopeptidase	Aromatic L-amino acids + others	20,000–24,000	8
Papain	Papaya	Endopeptidase	Broad specificity	21,000	6
Ficin	Fig tree latex	Endopeptidase	Broad specificity	26,000	6
Subtilo-peptidase A	*Bacillus subtilis*	Endopeptidase	Broad specificity	26,700	8
Aspergillo-peptidase A	Various aspergilli	Endopeptidase	Bonds involving arginine and leucine especially	32,000–98,000	4–5
Carboxy-peptidase A	Pancreas	C-terminal exopeptidase	L-Amino acid at C terminus with free COOH (not on arg, lys or pro)	32,000–34,000	7.5
Carboxy-peptidase B	Pancreas	C-terminal exopeptidase	L-Amino acid at C terminus must be L-lys, L-arg or L-orn with free COOH	34,000	8
Aminopeptidase	Kidney	N-terminal exopeptidase	Broad specificity at N-terminal end for α-amino acid derivatives	28,000	7
Leucine aminopeptidase	Kidney	N-terminal exopeptidase	Broad specificity	300,000	8.5
Proline iminopeptidase	*E. coli*	N-terminal exopeptidase	N-terminal proline		
Dipeptidase	Liver	N-terminal exopeptidase	Variety of dipeptides		8
Iminodipeptidase	Kidney	N-terminal exopeptidase	Dipeptides N-terminal imino acids (pro or hypro)		
Prolidase	Kidney	N-terminal exopeptidase	N-terminal proline or hydroxyproline	150,000	8

and cysteine from methionine. Tyrosine *cannot* substitute for phenylalanine in protein biosynthesis. Indeed, no one amino acid can substitute for another in this process. Note that arginine and histidine are listed as essential amino acids which are stimulatory. This is because animals can grow on a diet lacking arginine or histidine. However, if they are added, the growth rate is increased. Presumably, they can be synthesized, but not at sufficient rate to supply optimal growth needs.

**TABLE 5.2 CLASSIFICATION OF AMINO ACIDS
ACCORDING TO NUTRITIONAL NEEDS**

Nonessential	Essential	
	Indispensable	Replaceable
Alanine	Arginine[a]	
Glycine	Histidine[a]	
Serine	Isoleucine	
Aspartate	Leucine	Tyrosine
Glutamate	Lysine	Cysteine, cystine
Proline	Methione	
Hydroxyproline	Phenylalanine	
	Threonine	
	Tryptophan	
	Valine	

[a]Stimulatory.

Nonessential amino acids can be synthesized and need not, therefore, be supplied in the diet. All of the amino acids, both essential and nonessential, must be on hand in order for protein synthesis to occur in cells. As was originally shown by the isotope experiments of Schoenheimer and his co-workers (Section 2.2), cellular proteins are in a constant state of dynamic turnover. It is now known that this turnover consists of *complete* breakdown to amino acids and *complete* resynthesis of protein from amino acids, molecule by molecule. In protein metabolism, there seems to be nothing analogous to the lengthening and shortening of the outer chains of glycogen or to the two carbon lengthening and shortening reactions of the fatty acids (see Chapter 4) which are *partial* rather than *complete* molecular replacements.

When amino acids are broken down, the carbon chains and the nitrogen of the amino acids part company. Nitrogen is excreted as one of a number of nitrogen excretory products. The carbon chains go one of two routes, being converted to carbohydrate or to fatty products.

The experiments which allow this conclusion are as follows: If an amino acid is administered to an animal in negative nitrogen balance, it is found that there is an increase either in the glucose excreted in the urine or in the ketone bodies

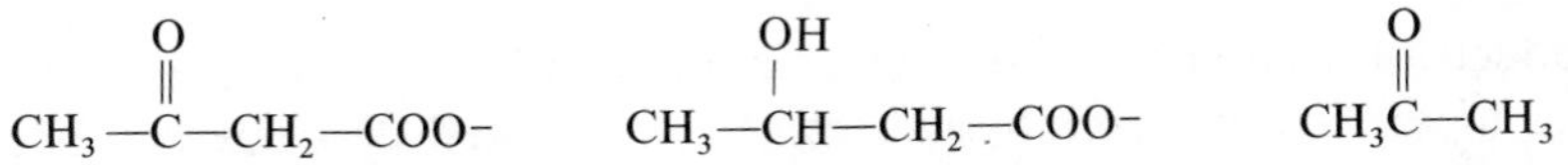

$$CH_3-\overset{\overset{\text{O}}{\|}}{C}-CH_2-COO- \qquad CH_3-\overset{\overset{\text{OH}}{|}}{CH}-CH_2-COO- \qquad CH_3\overset{\overset{\text{O}}{\|}}{C}-CH_3$$

acetoacetate   β-hydroxybutyrate   acetone

excreted. When the amino acids are so studied, some are found to be *glycogenic*, others *ketogenic*, and some both glycogenic and ketogenic. Interest-

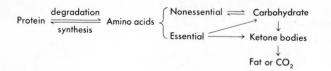

Figure 5.1

Overall metabolism of non-essential and essential amino acids. Note that only the essential amino acids are converted to ketone bodies.

ingly enough, all of the nonessential amino acids are glycogenic. This means that the conversion of these amino acids into carbohydrate is a *reversible* process. On the other hand, all of the ketogenic amino acids are essential. This means that these particular amino acids can be converted to fatty metabolites, but since they are essential, the reverse process does not occur. Fat thus differs from carbohydrate in that it does not contribute to amino acid biosynthesis. These important interrelationships are shown in Figure 5.1.

Before considering the pathways that are utilized for the degradation of amino acids to intermediates of the glycolytic pathway or the tricarboxylic acid cycle, an important reactant in many amino acid conversions should be considered. It is pyridoxal phosphate derived from vitamin B_6.

5.2 PYRIDOXAL PHOSPHATE REACTIONS—A SUMMARY

Pyridoxal phosphate is a key coenzyme in amino acid metabolism. It is involved in a wide variety of reactions which share a common chemical basis. In Figure 5.2, reactions involving seven different bonds are shown. The reactions corresponding to these bond cleavages and some enzymatic examples are also listed.

The amino acid condenses with pyridoxal phosphate on the enzyme surface and a *Schiff base intermediate* is formed. In this derivative, the bonds to the α-carbon atom are labilized and a variety of reactions are possible. The enzyme catalysts, however, guide specific reactions so that there is no tendency for side reactions. The common intermediate shown in Figure 5.2 is utilized in all cases.

In the following sections the general and specific ways in which amino acids are interconverted to CHO intermediates (and thus are utilized for energy) are presented.

5.3 AMINO ACID DEAMINATION

The products of deamination are ammonium ion and the α-keto acid corresponding to the specific amino acid, or an unsaturated derivative. While there are a number of specific reactions involving specific amino acids, we will be concerned with reactions which are general and apply to a number of amino acids.

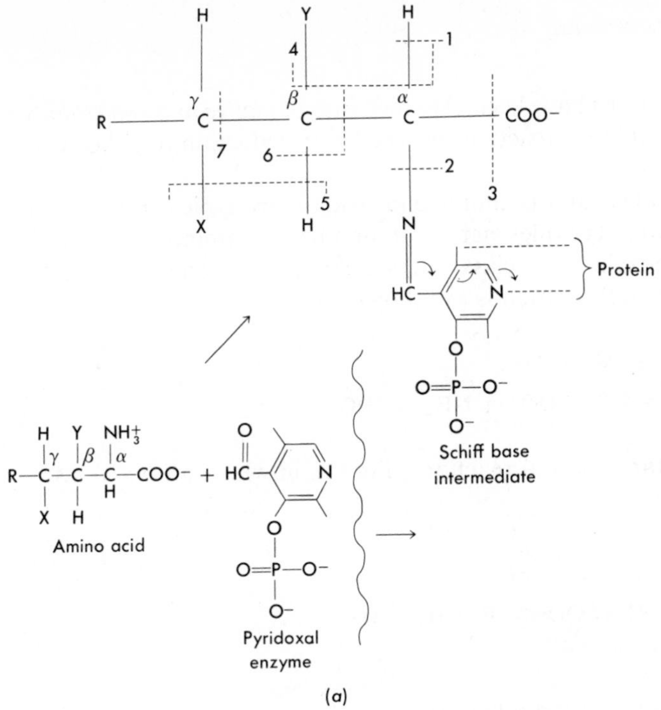

Figure 5.2

Pyridoxal phosphate reactions (*a*) of amino acid metabolism. The amino acid with specific carbon atoms labelled α, β, and γ combines with the pyridoxal phosphate bound to the enzyme to form the intermediate Schiff base as shown. The bonds at the α carbon are labelized and the reactions involving the seven different bonds (– – – –) are made possible. Specific examples are given in (*b*). Modified from A. E. Braunstein, *The Enzymes*, vol. 2, Boyer, Lardy, Myrback editors, Academic Press, Inc., 1960.

Schiff base intermediate

Amino acid

Pyridoxal enzyme

(*a*)

Bond Broken	Reaction Type	Enzyme
Removal and replacement of substituents on α-carbon atom		
(1) α-C—H	Dissociation of α-hydrogen Racemization of α-amino acids Condensations of glycine	Racemases Transaminases Δ-Aminolevulinate synthetase
(2) α-C—N α-C—H	Transamination Oxidative deamination	Transaminases Amino oxidases
(3) α-C—COOH	α-Decarboxylation	Amino acid decarboxylases
(6) α-C—β-C and β-C—H	α,β Cleavage of β-hydroxy amino acids	Serine and threonine deaminases
Removal and replacement of substituents on β-carbon atom		
(4) α-C—H and β-C—Y	Elimination of α-H and a polar substituent on β-C	Tryptophanase Serine and threonine dehydratase
	Replacement of a polar substituent on β-C	Tryptophan synthetase Cystathionine synthetase Serine desulfhydrase
(7) β-C—γ-C	β-Decarboxylation Hydrolytic cleavage of γ-keto, α-amino acids	Aspartate-β-decarboxylase Kynureninase
Removal and replacement of substituents on γ-carbon atom		
(5) γ-C—X and β-C—H	Elimination of β-H and polar substituent on γ-C	Homoserine dehydrase γ-Thionase Threonine synthetase Cystathionine synthetase

(*b*)

Deamination reactions have been classified into *oxidative* and *nonoxidative* or *hydrolytic*. The oxidative reactions proceed with reduction of either FAD or of DPN+ (TPN+).

L-Amino acid oxidase and D-amino acid oxidase are typical FAD oxidative deaminases. Both enzymes act on a number of amino acids of the α-amino monocarboxylic acid class but are specific for one or the other enantiomer. The overall reaction is as follows:

$$R—CH(NH_3)^+COO^- + O_2 + H_2O \longrightarrow R\overset{\overset{\displaystyle O}{\|}}{C}—COO^- + NH_4^+ + H_2O_2 \tag{1}$$

and is made up of three partial reactions, Eq. (2), in which an *imino* acid is formed,

$$R—CH(\overset{+}{N}H_3)^-COO^- + FAD \rightleftharpoons R—\overset{\overset{\displaystyle H}{\overset{\displaystyle N}{\|}}}{C}—COO^- + FADH_2 + H^+ \tag{2}$$

$$\text{imino acid}$$

and then (3) hydrolyzed to the α-keto acid.

$$R—\overset{\overset{\displaystyle H}{\overset{\displaystyle N}{\|}}}{C}—COO^- + H_2O + H^+ \rightleftharpoons R—\overset{\overset{\displaystyle O}{\|}}{C}—COO^- + NH_4^+ \tag{3}$$

The reduced flavin ($FADH_2$) of the enzyme is reoxidized (4) with the formation of peroxide. This is an irreversible step.

$$FADH_2 + O_2 \longrightarrow FAD + H_2O_2 \tag{4}$$

$$2H_2O_2 \xrightarrow{\text{catalase}} 2H_2O + O_2 \tag{5}$$

The H_2O_2 is rapidly destroyed by catalases in the cell, Eq. (5). In highly purified enzyme systems, H_2O_2 can oxidatively decarboxylate the keto acid nonenzymatically [Eq. (6)] as well as oxidizing many protein substitutents. This is unlikely to be an in vivo reaction.

$$R—\overset{\overset{\displaystyle O}{\|}}{C}—COO^- + H_2O_2 \longrightarrow CO_2 + R—COO^- + H_2O \tag{6}$$

The enzymes are present in those organs (chiefly liver and kidney) where amino acid deaminations occur. They are also found in other sources, for example, L-amino acid oxidase has been crystallized from snake venom. It is of interest that there is a high D-amino acid oxidase activity present in mammalian liver and kidney relative to the L-amino acid oxidase present. The D-amino acid oxidase will oxidize glycine to glyoxylic acid, Eq. (7).

$$O_2 + H\underset{\underset{NH_3^+}{|}}{\overset{\overset{H}{|}}{C}}COO^- + H_2O \longrightarrow O{=}\underset{\underset{H}{|}}{C}COO^- + NH_4^+ + H_2O_2 \tag{7}$$

glyoxylic acid

There is a wide variation in specificity of amino acid oxidases within the stereoisomeric group (D or L), depending on the source of the enzyme.

In some cases, such as alanine, glycine, glutamate, and aspartate, the α-keto acid can enter the energy-yielding reactions of the cell. In other cases, further processing is required. These events are described later in this chapter.

There are also present in tissues monoamine and diamine oxidases, which act by similar reactions involving FAD and a variety of amino substrates. The monoamine oxidase has received considerable attention because of its oxidation of such pharmacologically active amines as serotonin [Eq. (8)], tyramine [Eq. (9)], as well as dopamine, norepinephrine, and epinephrine.

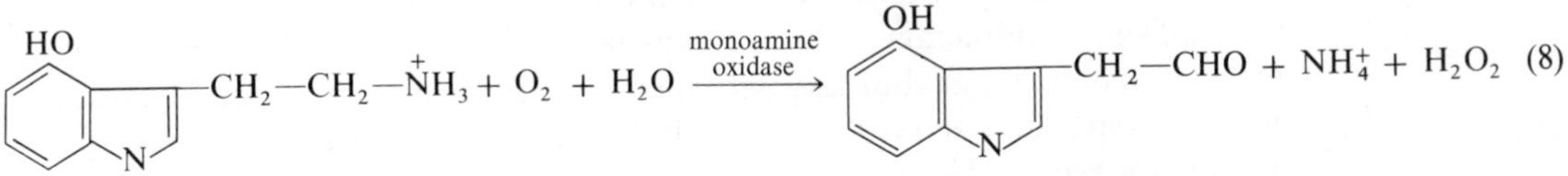

$$\text{5-hydroxytryptamine (serotonin)} \xrightarrow[\text{oxidase}]{\text{monoamine}} \text{5-hydroxytryptophal (serotonin aldehyde)} \tag{8}$$

$$HO\langle \bigcirc \rangle{-}CH_2{-}CH_2{-}\overset{+}{N}H_3 + O_2 + H_2O \xrightarrow[\text{oxidase}]{\text{monoamine}} HO\langle \bigcirc \rangle{-}CH_2{-}CHO + NH_4^+ + H_2O_2 \tag{9}$$

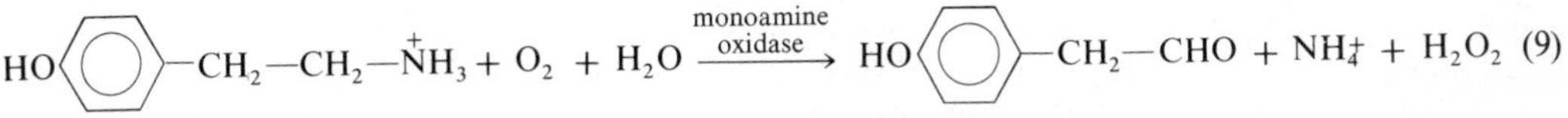

tyramine   tyramine aldehyde

A detailed study of the mechanisms of these reactions indicates that they proceed with partially reduced FAD intermediates, some of which are free radicals (see Chapter 3).

Glutamate dehydrogenase is an example of an enzyme catalyzing a pyridine nucleotide-dependent oxidative deamination. It has been prepared in crystalline form from liver and catalyzes the following reaction [Eq. (10)]:

$$\underset{\underset{\underset{\underset{\underset{COO^-}{|}}{CH_2}}{|}}{\underset{CH_2}{|}}}{\overset{\overset{COO^-}{|}}{\underset{H_3\overset{+}{N}{-}CH}{|}}} + DPN^+ + H_2O \underset{TPN}{\overset{or}{\rightleftharpoons}} \underset{\underset{\underset{\underset{\underset{COO^-}{|}}{CH_2}}{|}}{\underset{CH_2}{|}}}{\overset{\overset{COO^-}{|}}{\underset{C{=}O}{|}}} + DPNH + H^+ + NH_4^+ \tag{10}$$

As indicated, the enzyme reacts with either DPN+ and/or TPN+. DPN+-specific and TPN+-specific enzymes have been isolated from bacterial and other sources. The liver enzyme will oxidize a number of amino acids, including monocarboxylic as well as dicarboxylic amino acids. The reaction is freely reversible, in contrast to the FAD-linked reactions already discussed. Because of this reversibility, it provides a connection with the tricarboxylic acid cycle and allows glutamate to be oxidized or to be formed from α-ketoglutarate, depending on the needs of the cell.

In the *nonoxidative* reactions of α-deamination, the nitrogen is also removed as ammonium ion. An example is the histidase reaction [Eq. (11)].

$$
\begin{array}{c}
\underset{\substack{| \\ HN \quad NH \\ \diagdown \,\diagup \\ H}}{HC}\!\!=\!\!C\!-\!CH_2\!-\!\underset{\underset{H}{|}}{\overset{\overset{NH_3^+}{|}}{C}}\!-\!COO^- \xrightarrow{\text{histidase}} \underset{\substack{| \quad | \\ HN \quad N \\ \diagdown \,\diagup \\ H}}{HC}\!\!=\!\!\overset{\overset{H}{|}}{C}\!-\!\overset{\overset{H}{|}}{C}\!=\!C\!-\!COO^- + NH_4^+
\end{array}
\tag{11}
$$

histidine   urocanic acid

It has been recently shown that this enzyme is lacking in an inborn error of metabolism, histidinemia, a disease associated with elevated blood and urine levels of histidine and clinically with mental retardation, speech, and hearing defects. Aspartase, an enzyme found in bacteria, catalyzes a similar reaction in which aspartate is converted to fumarate in a reversible reaction. There exist additional α-deaminases which convert β-methyl aspartate, phenylalanine, and tyrosine to their respective unsaturated products and ammonium ion.

Finally, there are several types of serine- and threonine pyridoxal (vitamin B_6)-containing enzymes known as *dehydratases* which nonoxidatively deaminate by a mechanism in which pyridoxal phosphate is an intermediate. An example is the L-serine dehydratase reaction [Eq. (12)] in which serine is converted to pyruvate and ammonium ion.

$$
\underset{\underset{H_2C-OH}{|}}{\overset{\overset{COO^-}{|}}{\underset{\overset{+}{}}{H_3N}}}\!\!-\!\overset{}{C}\!-\!H \xrightarrow[\text{dehydratase}]{\text{L-serine}} \left[\underset{\underset{CH_2}{\parallel}}{\overset{\overset{COO^-}{|}}{HO}}\!-\!C \right] \xrightarrow[\text{dehydratase}]{\text{L-serine}} \underset{\underset{CH_3}{|}}{\overset{\overset{COO^-}{|}}{C}}\!\!=\!\!O + NH_4^+ + H_2O
\tag{12}
$$

Another enzyme has been found which acts specifically on D-serine. Similar reactions have been found for homoserine and threonine. In an analogous reaction, Eq. (13), L-cysteine is converted to pyruvate, ammonium ion, and H_2S.

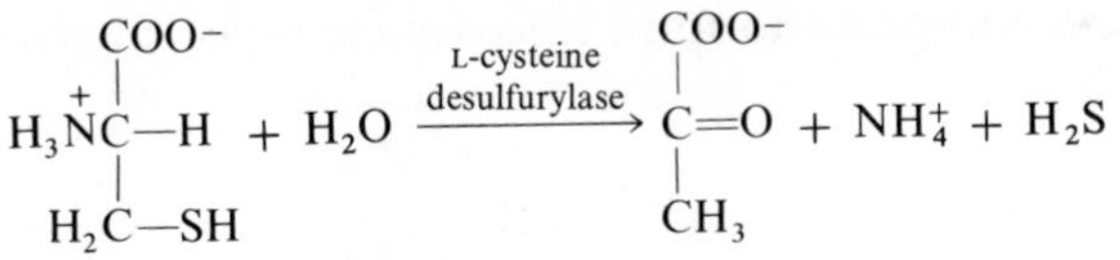

$$\underset{\underset{H_2C-SH}{|}}{\overset{\overset{COO^-}{|}}{H_3\overset{+}{N}C-H}} + H_2O \xrightarrow[\text{desulfurylase}]{\text{L-cysteine}} \underset{\underset{CH_3}{|}}{\overset{\overset{COO^-}{|}}{C=O}} + NH_4^+ + H_2S \qquad (13)$$

These latter reactions are all of the *β-elimination* type and mimic the non-enzymatic action of alkali on serine, threonine, and cysteine, Eq. (14).

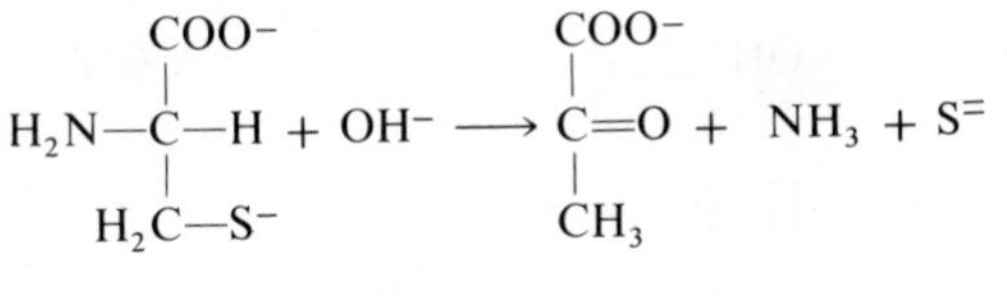

$$\underset{\underset{H_2C-S^-}{|}}{\overset{\overset{COO^-}{|}}{H_2N-C-H}} + OH^- \longrightarrow \underset{\underset{CH_3}{|}}{\overset{\overset{COO^-}{|}}{C=O}} + NH_3 + S^= \qquad (14)$$

5.4 TRANSAMINATION

Transamination provides for amino nitrogen transfer; is widespread in nature and involves the reversible transfer of the amino group from an amino acid to an α-keto acid. The glutamate oxaloacetate transaminase reaction catalyzed by aspartate aminotransferase, Eq. (15), is shown below.

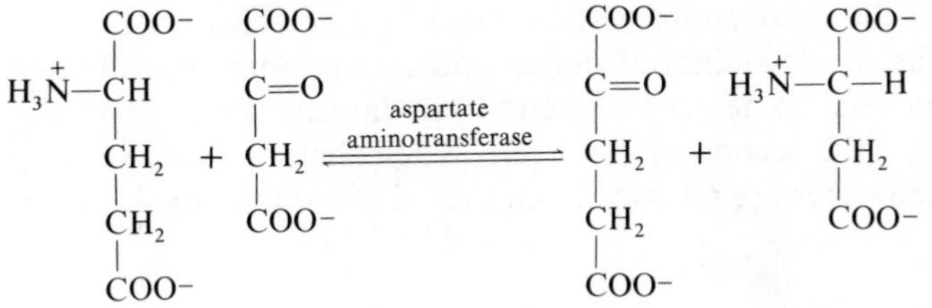

$$\underset{\underset{\underset{COO^-}{|}}{\underset{CH_2}{|}}}{\underset{CH_2}{|}}\overset{\overset{COO^-}{|}}{H_3\overset{+}{N}-CH} + \underset{\underset{COO^-}{|}}{\overset{\overset{COO^-}{|}}{C=O}}_{CH_2} \xrightleftharpoons[\text{aminotransferase}]{\text{aspartate}} \underset{\underset{\underset{COO^-}{|}}{CH_2}}{\overset{\overset{COO^-}{|}}{C=O}}_{CH_2} + \underset{\underset{COO^-}{|}}{\overset{\overset{COO^-}{|}}{H_3\overset{+}{N}-C-H}}_{CH_2} \qquad (15)$$

In this reversible reaction, as in all transaminase reactions, pyridoxal phosphate is required. A second transaminase reaction between α-keto-glutarate and alanine, Eq. (16), is catalyzed by alanine aminotransferase.

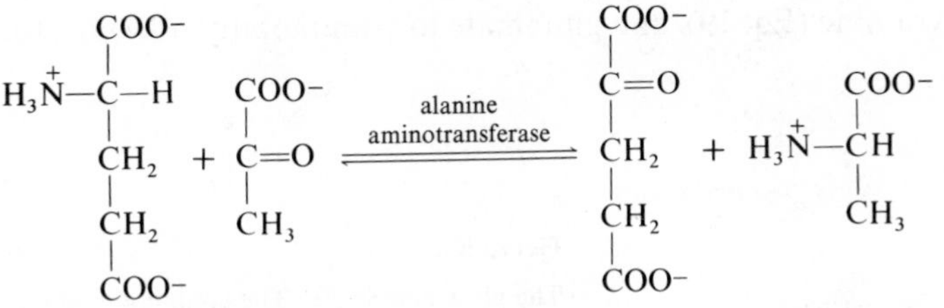

$$\underset{\underset{\underset{COO^-}{|}}{\underset{CH_2}{|}}}{\underset{CH_2}{|}}\overset{\overset{COO^-}{|}}{H_3\overset{+}{N}-C-H} + \underset{\underset{CH_3}{|}}{\overset{\overset{COO^-}{|}}{C=O}} \xrightleftharpoons[\text{aminotransferase}]{\text{alanine}} \underset{\underset{\underset{COO^-}{|}}{CH_2}}{\overset{\overset{COO^-}{|}}{C=O}}_{CH_2} + \underset{\underset{CH_3}{|}}{\overset{\overset{COO^-}{|}}{H_3\overset{+}{N}-CH}} \qquad (16)$$

Specific transaminations also occur with keto compounds which are not analogs of amino acids. For example, the amide nitrogen of glutamine transaminates with fructose-6-phosphate to form glucosamine-6-phosphate, Eq. (17).

$$\text{(17)}$$

The transamination reaction is the first step in the *degradation* of most of the amino acids including the branched amino acids, valine, leucine, and isoleucine, as well as the aromatic amino acids, tyrosine and phenylalanine. The coupling of transamination to reversible oxidative deamination leads to the cycle shown in Figure 5.3 in which the *synthesis* of amino acids proceeds from α-keto acids, NH_4^+, and reduced DPNH + H$^+$. The transamination reaction is thus used for the *synthesis* and *degradation* of the *nonessential* amino acids and for the *degradation* of the *essential* amino acids.

The activities of aspartate aminotransferase and alanine aminotransferases in serum have been used to detect heart and liver damage since the first is rich in the heart and the second in the liver. When there is heart or liver cell damage, these enzymes are released from the cells into the blood.

5.5 AMINO ACID DECARBOXYLATION

A general reaction of amino acids is their decarboxylation to amines. By this important reaction are formed a number of amines which are pharmacologically active. Histidine, for example, is decarboxylated to histamine (Eq. 18), tyrosine to tyramine (Eq. 19), and glutamate to γ-aminobutyrate (Eq. 20).

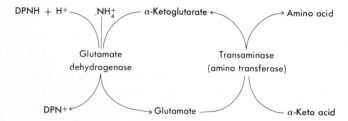

Figure 5.3

The glutamate cycle. The coupling of glutamate dehydrogenase and transamination can lead to the formation of amino acids reductively (run counter clockwise) or the formation of ketoacids, ammonia, and reducing potential from amino acids (run clockwise).

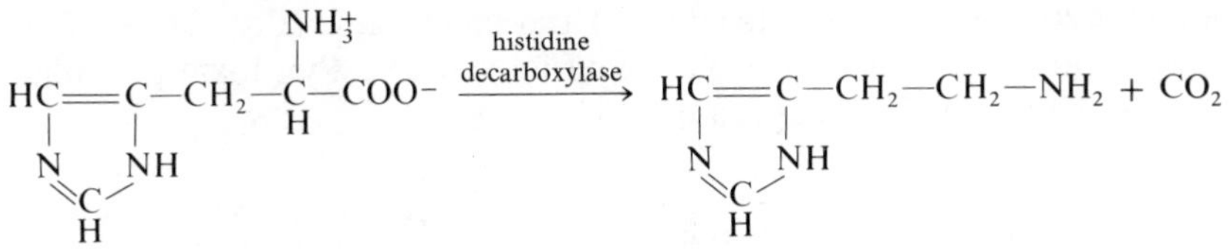

$$HC = C - CH_2 - \underset{\underset{H}{|}}{\overset{\overset{NH_3^+}{|}}{C}} - COO^- \xrightarrow[\text{decarboxylase}]{\text{histidine}} HC = C - CH_2 - CH_2 - NH_2 + CO_2 \qquad (18)$$

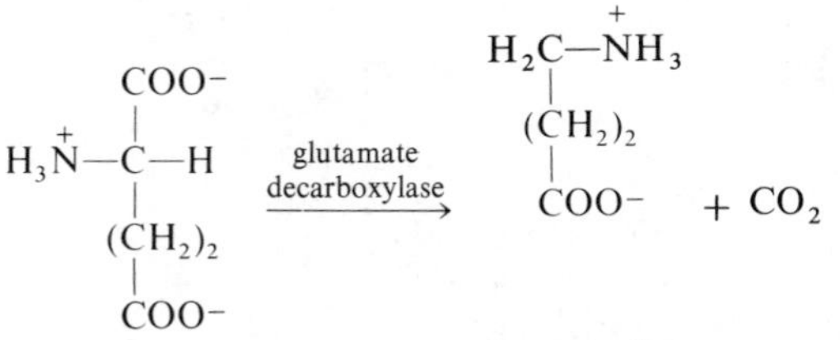

L-histidine   histamine

$$\langle O \rangle - CH_2 - \underset{}{\overset{\overset{NH_3^+}{|}}{CH}} - COO^- \xrightarrow[\text{decarboxylase}]{\text{tyrosine}} HO\langle O \rangle - CH_2 - CH_2NH_2 + CO_2 \qquad (19)$$

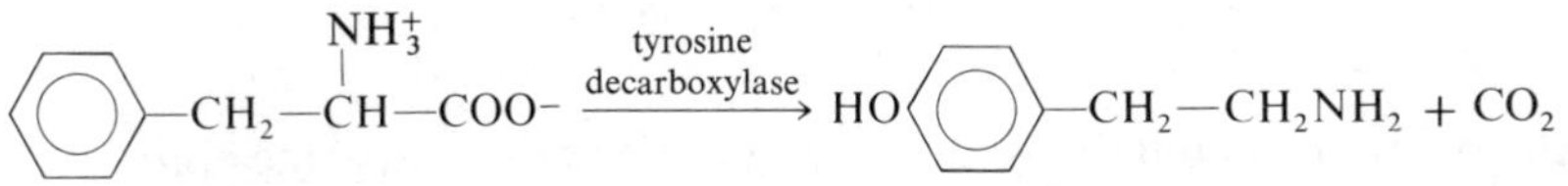

L-tyrosine   tyramine

$$\underset{\underset{COO^-}{|}}{\overset{\overset{COO^-}{|}}{\underset{(CH_2)_2}{H_3\overset{+}{N} - C - H}}} \xrightarrow[\text{decarboxylase}]{\text{glutamate}} \underset{\underset{COO^-}{|}}{\overset{\overset{H_2C - NH_3^+}{}}{(CH_2)_2}} + CO_2 \qquad (20)$$

γ-aminobutyrate

5.6   RACEMIZATION AND EPIMERIZATION

Nutritional studies have shown that certain D-amino acids can replace L-amino acids in supporting growth of certain microorganisms and animals. The D-amino acid is presumably converted to the L-amino acid by oxidative deamination, followed by L-specific transamination. This is consistent with the fact that the appropriate α-keto acids can support growth. In certain cases, however, with bacteria, there is a specific requirement for D-amino acids, which are components of cell structures or antimetabolites. Bacteria meet this requirement by conversion of L-amino acids to D-amino acids by *racemization* or *epimerization*.

These reactions are catalyzed by racemase and epimerase enzymes which are specific for single amino acids. For example, alanine racemase, purified from *S. faecalis* interconverts only D- and L-alanine (Eq. 21).

$$\text{D-alanine} \xrightarrow[\text{racemase}]{\text{alanine}} \text{L-alanine} \qquad (21)$$

The evidence indicates that there is a *direct* racemization *without* the formation of an α-keto intermediate. Pyridoxal phosphate participates in the reaction as a cofactor (see Section 5.2). Enzymes catalyzing similar racemization reactions with glutamate (Eq. 22) and methionine (Eq. 23) have been detected and purified from various bacterial sources. Pyridoxal phosphate appears to be required in these cases also.

$$\text{D-glutamate} \underset{\text{racemase}}{\overset{\text{glutamate}}{\rightleftharpoons}} \text{L-glutamate} \tag{22}$$

$$\text{D-methionine} \underset{\text{racemase}}{\overset{\text{methionine}}{\rightleftharpoons}} \text{L-methionine} \tag{23}$$

With compounds containing two asymmetric centers, specific epimerases have been detected which interconvert one center only. For example, an enzyme catalyzing the interconversion of L,L- and meso-α, ε-diaminopimelate has been purified from *E. coli*

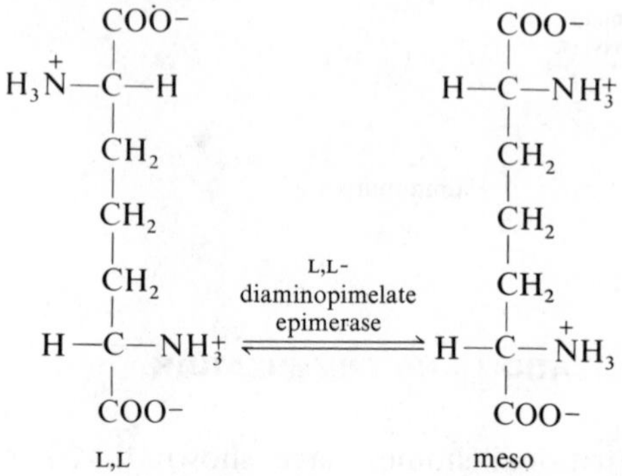

$$\tag{24}$$

The enzyme does not act on the D,D isomer.

In the conversion of L-hydroxyproline to α-ketoglutarate by a strain of *Pseudomonas* adapted to grow on L-hydroxyproline, the initial reaction is the epimerization of L-hydroxyproline to D-allohydroxyproline (Eq. 25).

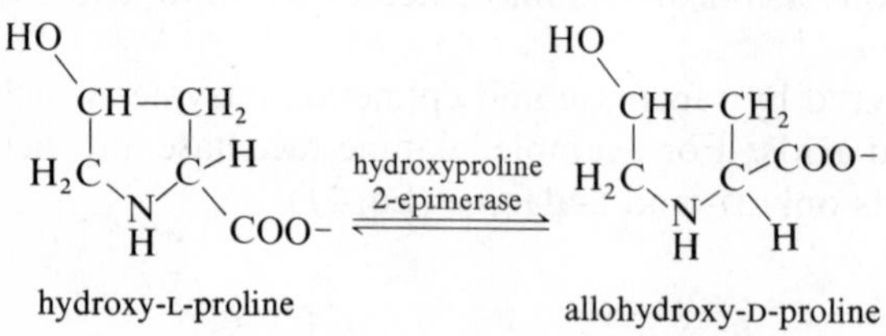

$$\tag{25}$$

The enzyme catalyzing the reaction has been high purified and does *not* require pyridoxal phosphate for its activity. Apparently, there is more than one chemical reaction mechanism by means of which the epimerization can proceed.

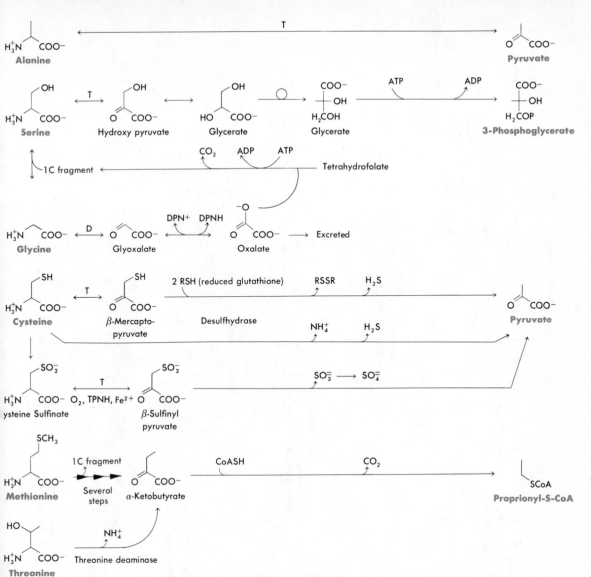

Figure 5.4 Pathways of amino acid degradation. Note that the structures are drawn to emphasize similarities between amino acids and between precursors and products. Stereochemistry (i.e. optical isomerism) has been ignored. Small arrows ▶ are used to indicate similar reactions and all amino acids are arranged in a column to the left and products in a column to the right. In some cases a few steps have been omitted but the number is indicated. The symbol ─○→ means that a structure has been rotated without changing its chemical composition. This is done to help emphasize similarities. T = transaminase; D = deaminase. (Cont. on pp. 118–20.)

5.7 AMINO ACID DEGRADATION

A. Nonessential Amino Acids

The nonessential amino acids can be synthesized from and degraded to intermediates that can be utilized for energy. α-Ketoglutarate is perhaps the most important of these intermediates. As shown in Figure 5.4 histidine,

117

Figure 5.4 (Continued).

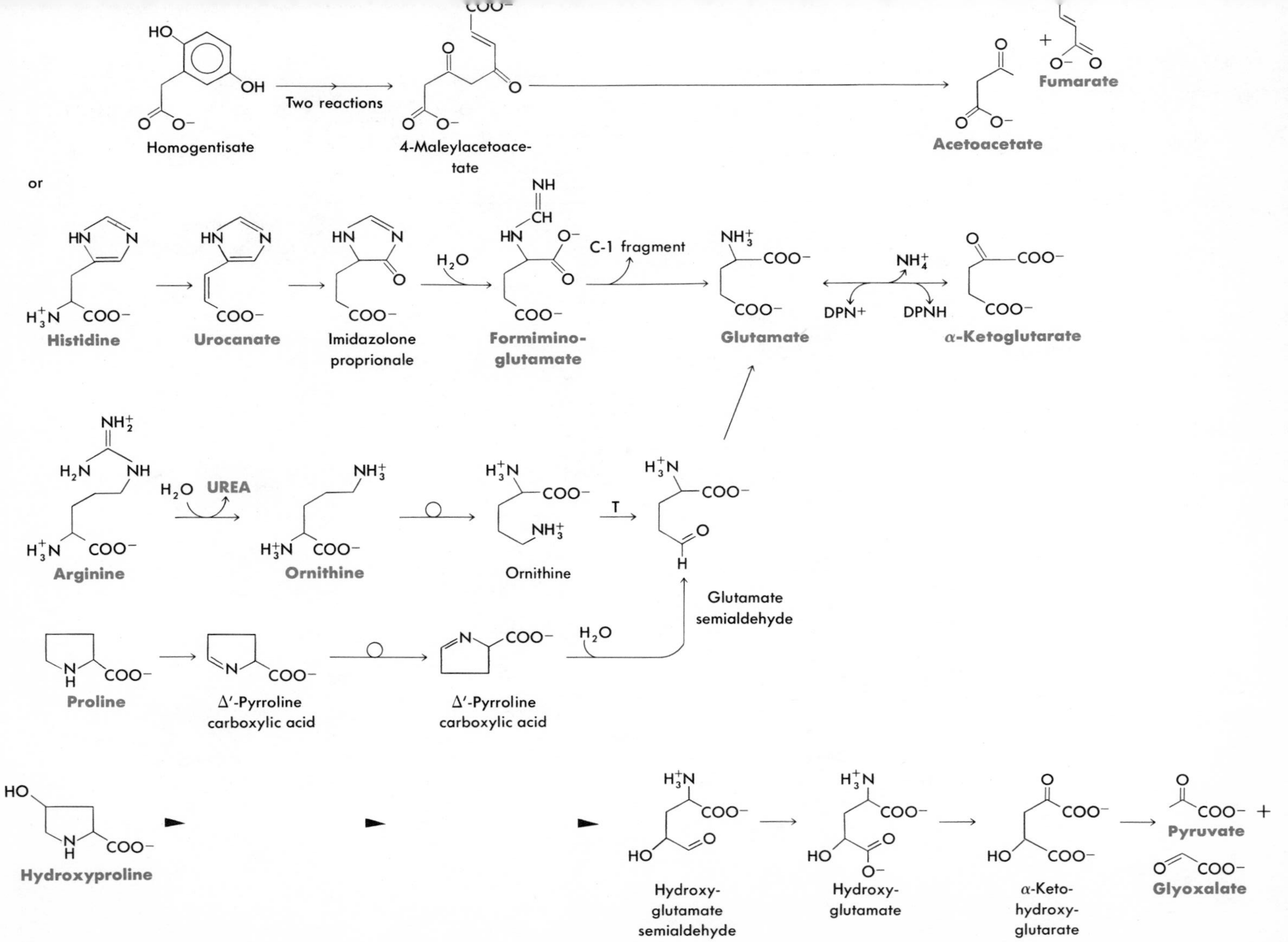

Fumarate

Acetoacetate

α-Ketoglutarate

Homogentisate

4-Maleylacetoacetate

Two reactions

NH_4^+

DPNH

DPN^+

Glutamate

C-1 fragment

Formimino-glutamate

H_2O

Imidazolone proprionale

Urocanate

Histidine

or

Arginine

UREA

H_2O

Ornithine

Ornithine

Glutamate semialdehyde

T

Δ'-Pyrroline carboxylic acid

Δ'-Pyrroline carboxylic acid

H_2O

Proline

Hydroxyproline

Hydroxy-glutamate semialdehyde

Hydroxy-glutamate

α-Keto-hydroxy-glutarate

Pyruvate

Glyoxalate

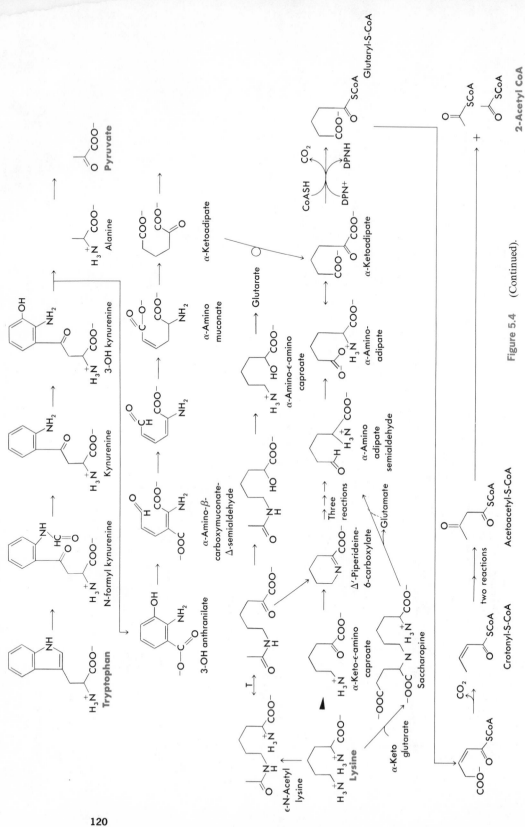

Figure 5.4 (Continued).

arginine, and proline can be converted to glutamate which undergoes de-amination (D) to α-ketoglutarate. The ammonia released in this reaction is excreted as such or converted to urea and then excreted as described in Section 5.10. The pathway from proline to glutamate involves two oxidations with DPN^+, and a hydrolytic step; these reactions are typical of similar reactions described in Chapter 4. The first step in the conversion of arginine is a novel one; it involves hydrolysis of the guanidinium group to give urea and ornithine. This reaction is the source of urea, and the synthesis of arginine using ammonia is the means of protecting many organisms from the toxic effects of accumulated ammonia. The further conversion of ornithine involves a typical transamination reaction (T). Histidine is converted by a pyridoxal phosphate-dependent enzyme to the unsaturated derivative urocanate, which in two steps is converted to formiminoglutamate. Conversion of the latter to glutamate requires the transfer of a one-carbon fragment using a folic acid derivative. The addition and removal of one-carbon pieces is accomplished in a number of different ways, and this important part of the cell's synthetic system is discussed in Section 5.9. The transfer of one-carbon fragments will be indicated by the abbreviation C-1 fragment or by a word formula. Alanine, serine, glycine, hydroxyproline, and cysteine all can be converted to pyruvate for energy production, as shown in Figure 5.4. An alternative pathway to 3-phosphoglycerate exists for glycine, also as shown in Figure 5.4. This route requires that reducing power and ATP be expended, but the product can be utilized for carbohydrate synthesis more readily than can pyruvate. The conversion of glycine to serine is readily reversible and an alternate route is thus available for glycine. Glycine can be converted by deamination (D) to glyoxalate which can in turn be oxidized to oxalic acid with the production of DPNH, H^+. The oxalic acid can be excreted or converted to carbon dioxide and a C-1 fragment, as shown in Figure 5.4. Glyoxalate can also be metabolized via the glyoxalate cycle in some plant tissues (Figure 4.17).

The degradation of hydroxyproline, which is very different from that of proline, is shown in Figure 5.4. The last step in the sequence is catalyzed by an enzyme which resembles aldolase in its action. Two moles of DPNH, H^+ are produced in the conversion.

Cysteine can be converted to pyruvate by at least three pathways (Figure 5.4). In mammals, most of the dietary sulfur is excreted as sulfate (700 mg/day in man) indicating that the major pathway is that involving sulfinate intermediates.

Aspartate, the only remaining nonessential amino acid, is readily converted to, or synthesized from, oxaloacetate by transamination.

$$
\begin{array}{ccc}
\text{COO}^- & & \text{COO}^- \\
| & & | \\
\overset{+}{\text{H}_3}\text{N}-\text{CH} & \underset{\text{T}}{\longleftrightarrow} & \text{C}{=}\text{O} \\
| & & | \\
\text{CH}_2 & & \text{CH}_2 \\
| & & | \\
\text{COO}^- & & \text{COO}^-
\end{array}
$$

aspartate   oxaloacetate

B. Essential Amino Acids

When a more than adequate diet of amino acids is supplied, man can utilize the excess of even those that are essential for the production of energy. The major pathways for the degradation of the essential amino acids are also presented without discussion in Figure 5.4, but literature references are given at the end of the chapter to provide access to detailed commentary.

Much more complex conversions are involved in converting the amino acids to metabolites that fit into the energy-producing systems than are required for the carbohydrates and lipids. The major site of amino acid degradation is the liver, and many of the enzymes required to process amino acids are produced by the liver only after a meal containing the amino acids. The requirement for synthesis of a number of enzymes on demand may seem to be a wasteful process, but it is not. It would be more wasteful to maintain a constant high level of enzymes that are called into use only occasionally.

5.8 AMINO ACID SYNTHESIS

A. Nonessential Amino Acids

Most of the nonessential amino acids can be synthesized by direct reversal of the degradative pathways. Glutamate, aspartate, alanine, glycine, serine, ornithine, and proline fall in this category, and their biosynthetic pathways are as shown in Figure 5.4. The pathway for the synthesis of arginine is discussed in Section 5.10, where its role in the formation of urea is presented. Histidine biosynthesis involves the complex sequence of reactions shown in Figure 5.5. This system has been extensively studied in *E. coli* and *Salmonella* and the control of its operation is well documented. The carbon chain of histidine is derived from 5-phosphoribosyl pyrophosphate (PRPP) which can be formed from ribose-5-phosphate of the pentose pathway described in Chapter 4. The nitrogen and carbon of the imidazole ring of histidine derives from the purine ring of ATP, a most unusual use of this metabolite.

Hydroxyproline is synthesized from proline after the latter has been incorporated into protein. The enzyme responsible utilizes molecular oxygen, Fe^{2+}, ascorbate, and α-ketoglutarate as cofactors. The role of these cofactors is not fully understood.

B. Essential Amino Acids

The pathways for the synthesis of the essential amino acids are shown in Figures 5.6 through 5.10. No further discussion of these specific pathways will be presented. It should be apparent that if a cell can obtain an amino

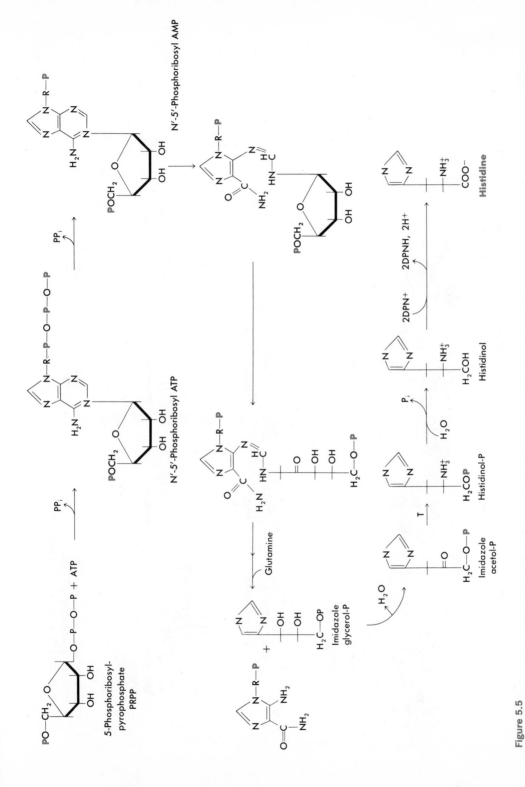

Figure 5.5

Histidine synthesis. Note the formation of N′-5-phosphoribosyl ATP, the conversion to L-histidinol and oxidation to L-histidine.

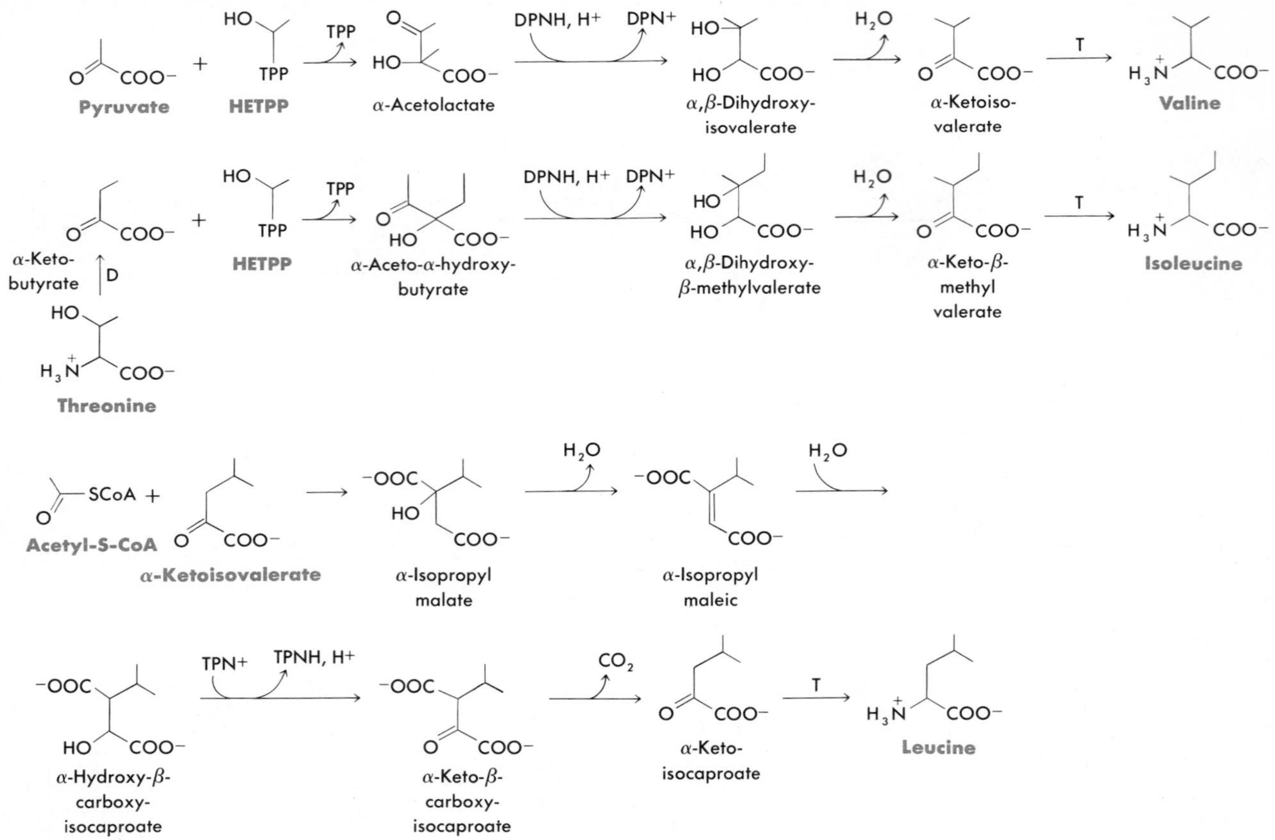

Figure 5.6

Branched chain amino acid leucine, valine, and isoleucine synthesis. Note the initial thiamine-PP dependent condensations and the final transamination reaction (T). TPP = thiamine pyrophosphate. HETPP = hydroxyethyl thiamine pyrophosphate.

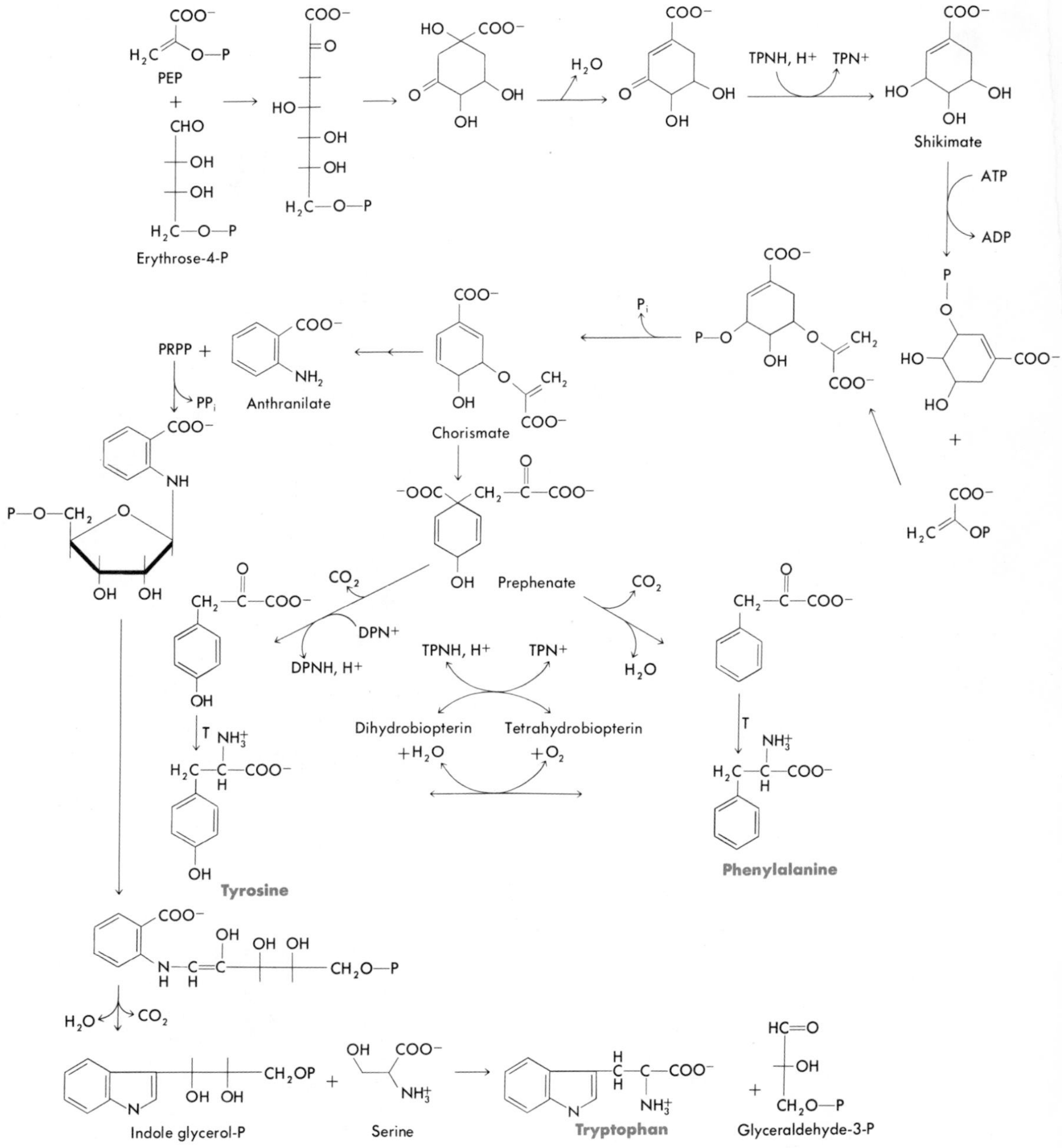

Figure 5.7   Aromatic amino acid tryptophan, tyrosine and phenylalanine synthesis. Note the intermediates shikimate, chorismate, and arthranilate. Note also the interconversion of phenylalanine and tyrosine.

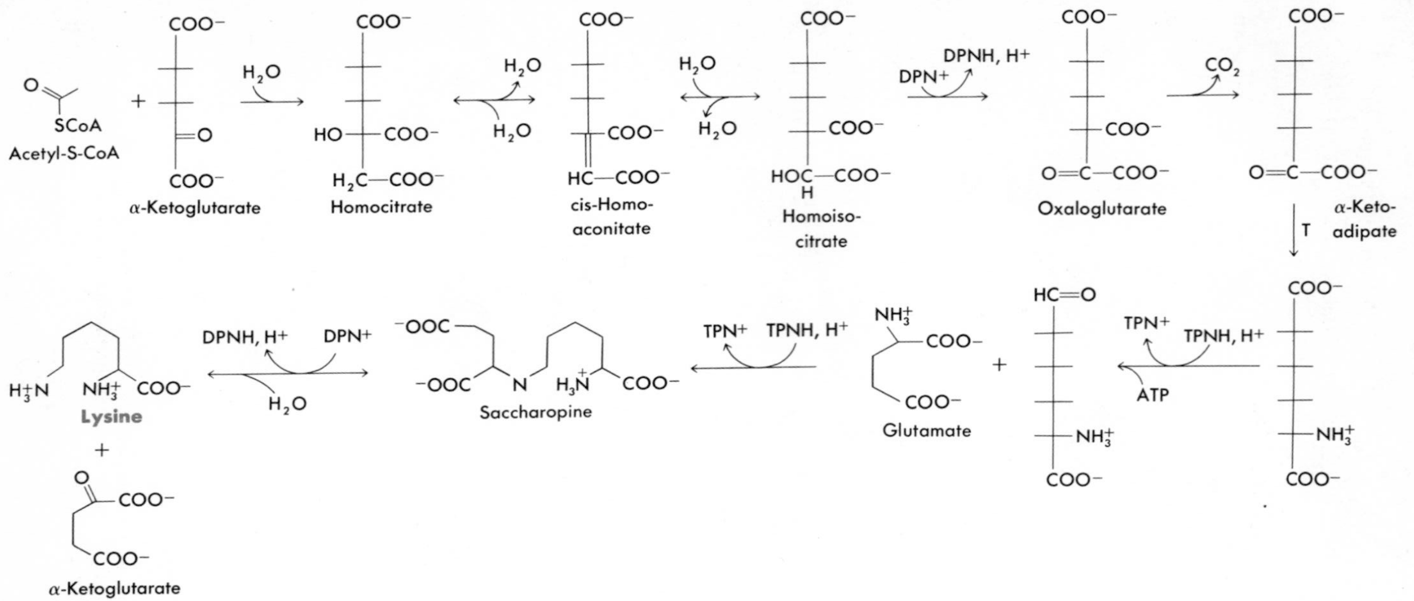

α-Keto-adipate

T

CO_2

Oxaloglutarate

TPN^+ $TPNH, H^+$

ATP

NH_3^+

$HC=O$

+

NH_3^+ Glutamate

$DPNH, H^+$

DPN^+

Homoiso-citrate

H_2O H_2O

cis-Homo-aconitate

H_2O H_2O

Homocitrate

H_2O

Acetyl-S-CoA

α-Ketoglutarate

TPN^+ $TPNH, H^+$

DPN^+ $DPNH, H^+$

H_2O

Saccharopine

Lysine

+

α-Ketoglutarate

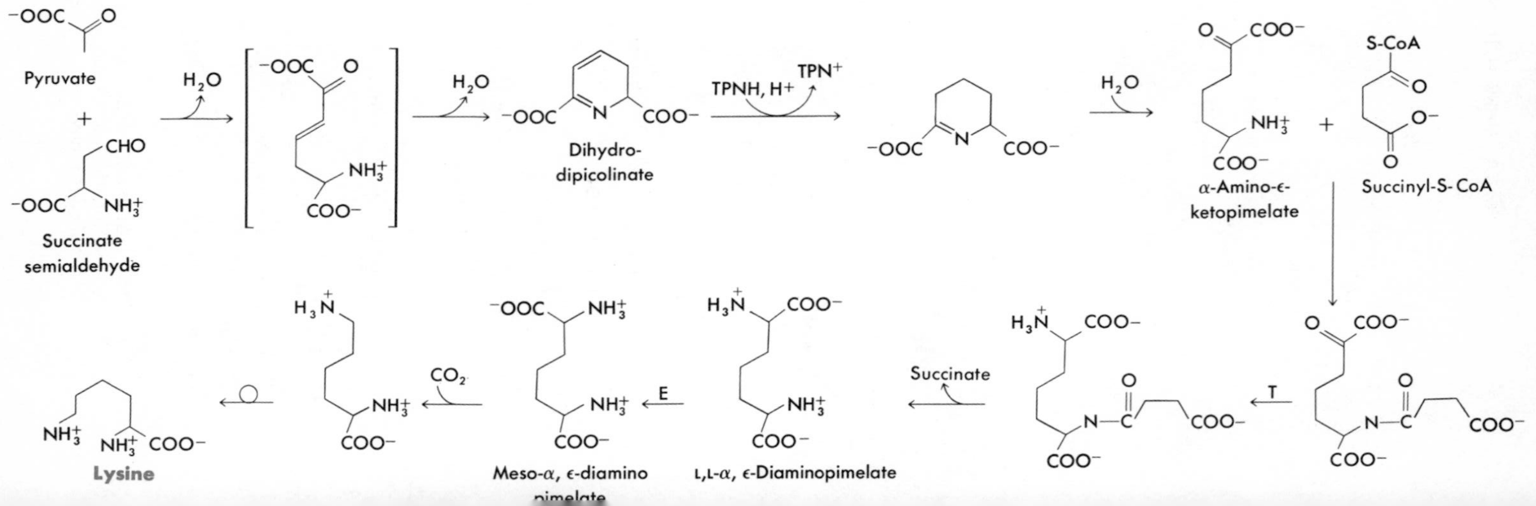

Succinyl-S-CoA

+

α-Amino-ε-ketopimelate

H_2O

T

Succinate

L,L-α,ε-Diaminopimelate

Meso-α,ε-diamino pimelate

E

CO_2

Lysine

Dihydro-dipicolinate

$TPNH, H^+$ TPN^+

H_2O

H_2O

Pyruvate

+

CHO

Succinate semialdehyde

Figure 5.8 Saccharopine and diaminopimelate pathways of lysine synthesis. Lysine is synthesized via the saccharopine pathway in yeasts and molds. Note the interesting homology with tricarboxylic acid cycle in the initial portion of the pathway. E = epimerase; $\xrightarrow{\ \_\Omega\_\ }$ = rotation of structure without changing its chemical composition; T = transaminase. Lysine is synthesized by the diaminopimelate pathway in bacteria and vascular plants. Note the succinylation of the amino group to prevent spontaneous cyclization.

Figure 5.9 Methionine synthesis. Note the intermediate cystathionine and the final methylation of homocysteine. The aspartate carboxyl group is reduced after phosphorylation with ATP.

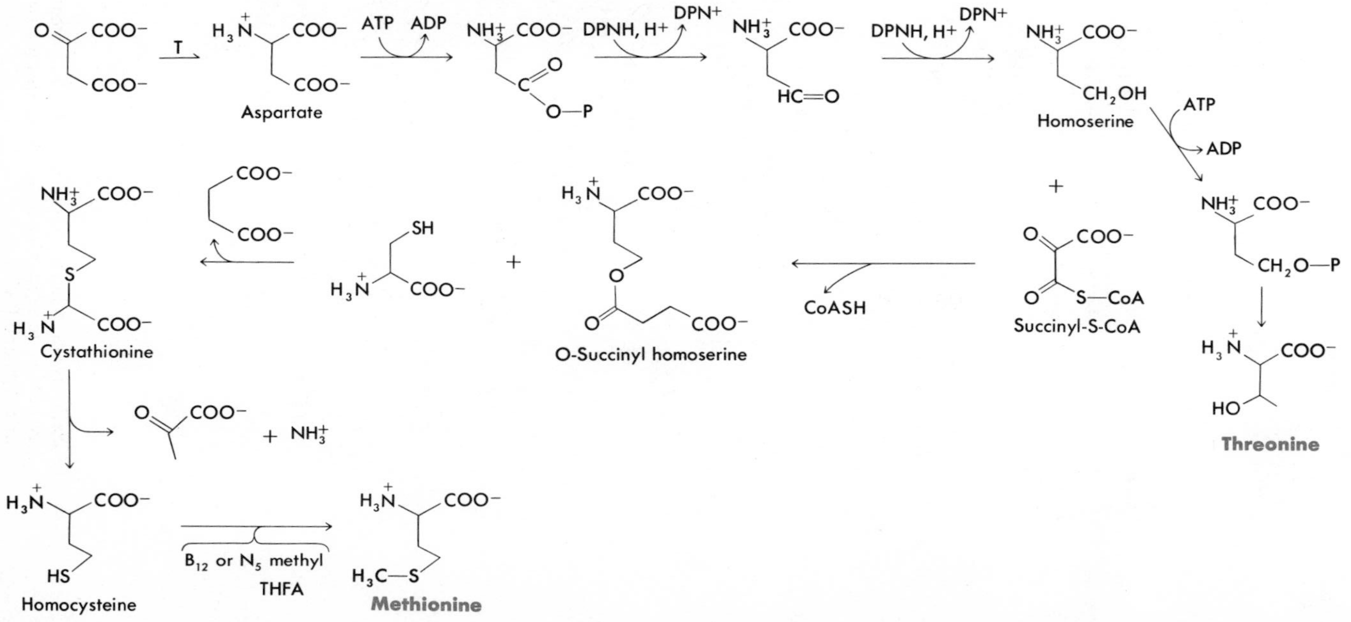

Aspartate

Cystathionine

Homocysteine

Homoserine

Threonine

Succinyl-S-CoA

O-Succinyl homoserine

Methionine

B_{12} or N_5 methyl THFA

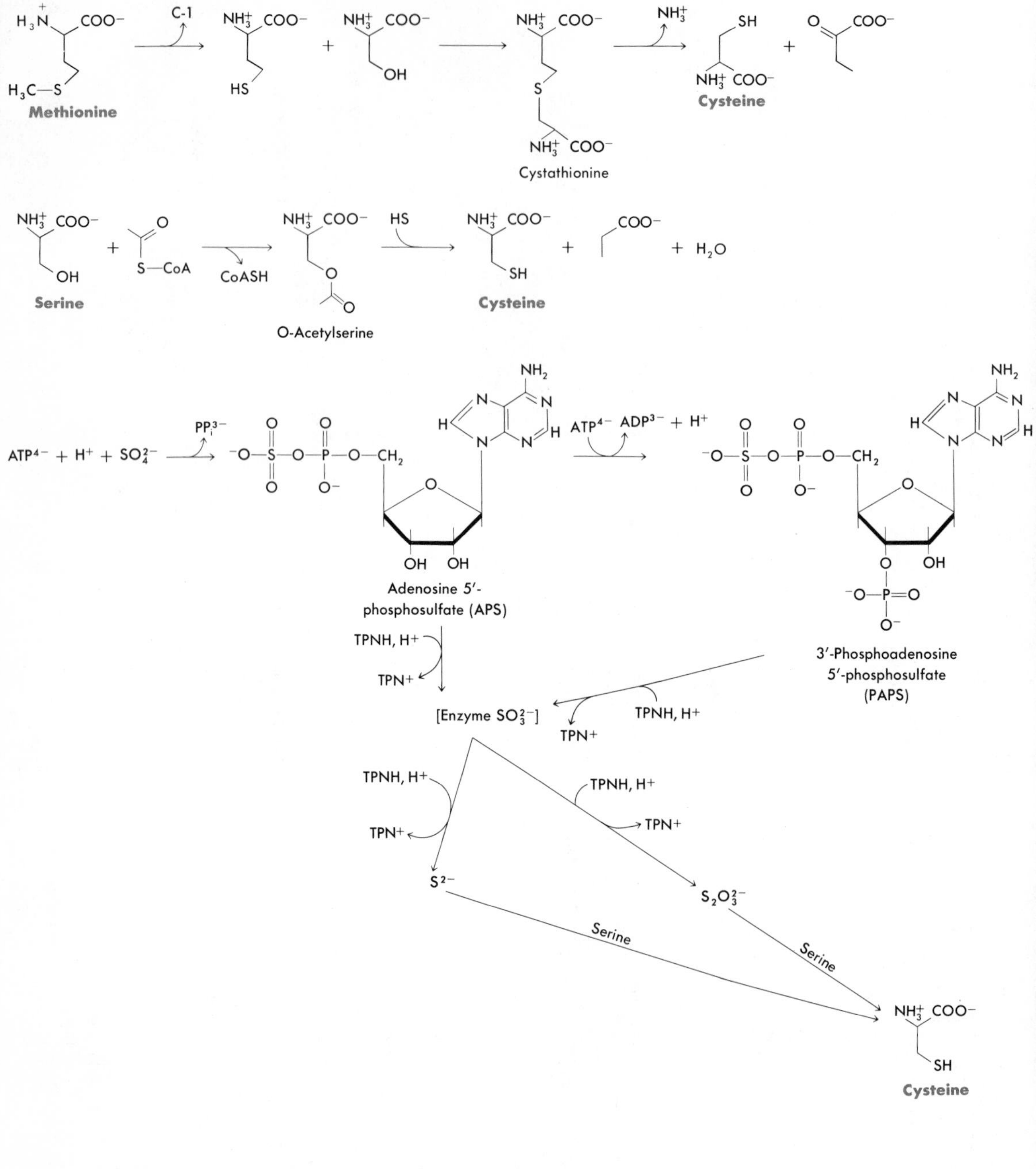

Figure 5.10 Pathways of cysteine synthesis. Note the formation of o-acetyl serine and cystathionine as intermediates. Note also the two active sulfate intermediates APS and PAPS.

acid, such as one of the essential ones, in a reliable way from its environment, it effects a considerable economy.

5.9 ONE-CARBON METABOLISM

Several of the metabolic sequences outlined above included steps in which one carbon atom was added to a structure. The carbon in some cases was added as a methyl group and in others as a formyl or hydroxymethyl group. A number of systems exist for making these transfers. They are shown in Figure 5.11. The three important cofactors in the system are S-adenosyl-

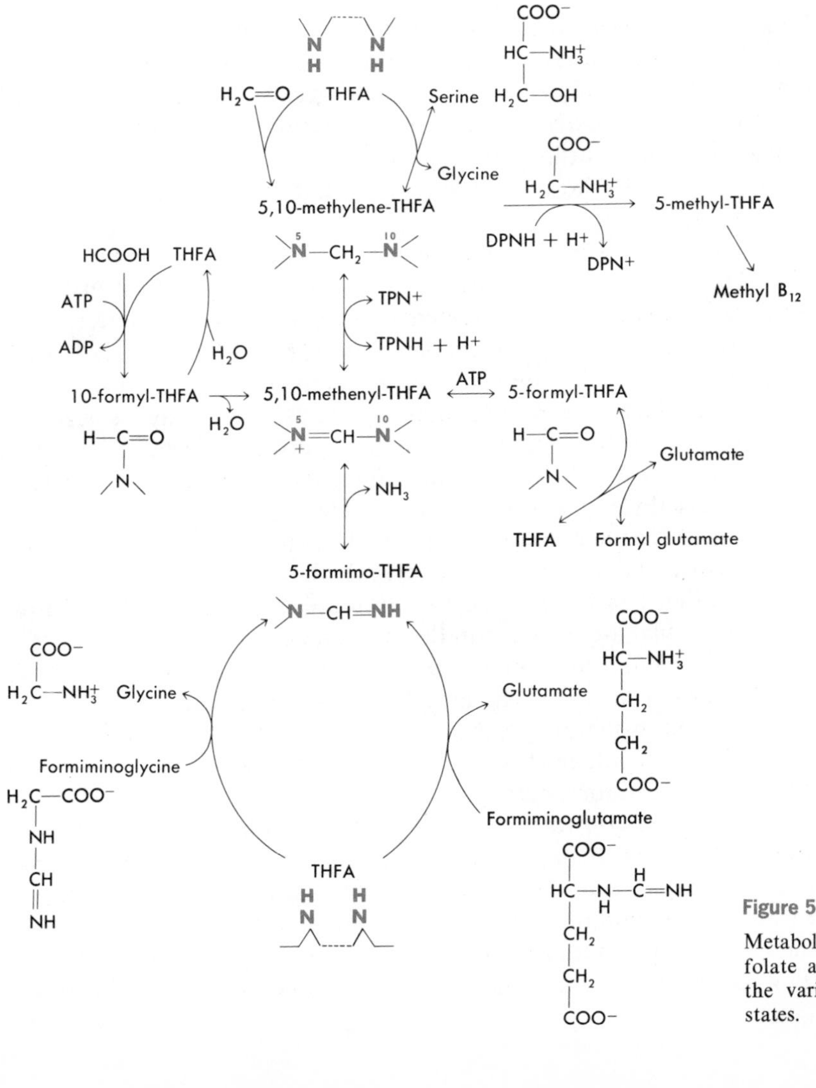

Figure 5.11

Metabolic reactions of tetrahydrofolate and its derivatives. Note the various oxidation reduction states.

methionine, methylcobalamin (derived from vitamin B_{12}), and a variety of tetrahydrofolate compounds (derived from the vitamin folic acid). The structures of these compounds are shown in the Appendix.

In Figure 5.12 are shown the interconversions that can be achieved with tetrahydrofolate derivatives and some of the reactions in which they play a role. The transfer of methyl groups is also presented in Figure 5.12. The derivatives formed by methyl group transfer, such as choline and creatine, play vital roles in metabolism.

5.10 NITROGEN EXCRETION PRODUCTS

The bulk of the nitrogen entering the animal body comes from ingested protein. The amino acids derived from the protein yield their nitrogen as ammonium ion by deamination and transamination as already described. Some ammonia derives from deamination of the purines and pyrimidines (the amino bases). There is little or no capacity to store protein or amino acids. Some nitrogen can be stored, however, as glutamine or as asparagine (see subsequent section).

Nitrogen is excreted in a variety of forms, depending upon the animal species. The elegant phylogenetic adaptability of the nitrogen excretory pattern of the animal to its environmental need is truly remarkable.

If the nitrogen excretory products of a wide variety of animals are examined, it will be seen that although several compounds are excreted by an animal, one product usually predominates. Thus, there may be small or even sizable amounts of amino acids, creatine, purines, or betaines excreted. The chief products are, however, ammonium ion, urea, and uric acid. In some cases, trimethylamine oxide is also excreted. These excretory products are rather characteristic phylogenetically and the names *ammoniotelic, ureotelic,* and *uricotelic* have, therefore, been applied. The conversion of ammonium ion to other less toxic products may represent a required adaptation to the limited availability of water in the environment.

Marine invertebrates, for example, excrete ammonia. Their surface membranes are more or less freely permeable to water and salts and, therefore, ammonia formed in the body can readily diffuse out into the surrounding sea. Since the salt content of the body is approximately that of the ocean, there may be no need for a permeability barrier.

For *fresh water invertebrates*, a different situation obtains. Here the membranes must be relatively impermeable to salt and water in order to maintain the cellular salt content. The membranes are semipermeable, permitting some water to pass into the cells because of the osmotic pressure differential. But then it is pumped out again to maintain the cellular salt content. In this situation, ammonia is excreted in a very diluted urine of low osmotic strength.

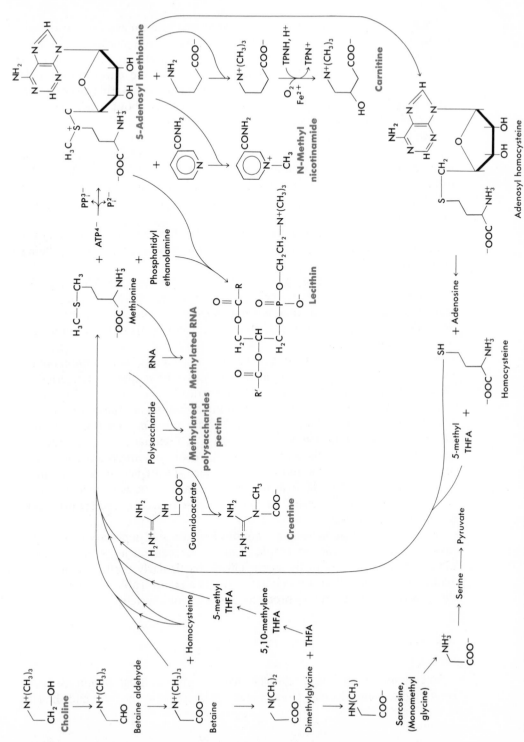

Figure 5.12 Transmethylation pathways. Note the variety of methylated products formed through methyl transfer reactions.

131

Fresh water teleost fish operate by the same mechanism and excrete ammonia in a very dilute urine. *Marine teleosts* excrete ammonia mostly by way of the gills, even though they have a relatively poor water supply. In addition to ammonia, which constitutes about two thirds of the nitrogen excreted, about one third is excreted as trimethylamine oxide. Marine teleosts are constantly losing water, because sea water contains about 3 per cent salt while their blood contains only about 1 per cent salt.

Marine elasmobranchs or cartilaginous fish are ureotelic, forming and even retaining large amounts of urea within their bodies. The concentration of urea in their blood, for example, is about 2–2.5 percent. This raises the osmotic pressure of blood to a level which is higher than that of sea water and thus prevents the water loss of the marine teleosts. They also excrete part of the nitrogen as trimethylamine oxide.

Fresh water elasmobranchs are also ureotelic, but the amount of urea retained in their bodies is less, the concentration in blood, for example, being of the order of 1 percent.

A particularly fascinating group is the *Dipnoi* or *lungfish*. When water is available in the rainy season, they, like fresh water teleosts, are ammoniotelic. During the drought, they become encased in cocoons and convert to ureotelism, the urea being stored. When the water returns, the accumulated urea is excreted en masse.

Amphibia are also fascinating. Tadpoles are aquatic and ammoniotelic, like fresh water teleosts. During metamorphosis, the tadpole is converted to an amphibian and gradually becomes ureotelic.

The two main evolutionary lines from the amphibia are the *mammals* and the *reptiles and birds*. Among the reptiles are the *Chelonia* (tortoises and turtles) and the *Sauria* (snakes and lizards). The aquatic Chelonia excrete ammonia and urea. This indicates that in evolution these aquatic forms probably derived from the terrestrial. The terrestrial Chelonia excrete urea. The desert-living or dryland forms excrete mainly uric acid together with some urea. The wholly terrestrial Sauria and the birds also excrete uric acid. Mammals excrete urea.

Uric acid excretion is a further adaptation to water deprivation. It is the major excretory product in reptiles and birds, even during early development, when it is found in the eggs. This is particularly useful because uric acid is so insoluble that it precipitates out as a solid. Table 5.3 summarizes the major nitrogen excretory products of the various vertebrates.

Urea Cycle

Since ammonium ion is relatively toxic to multicellular organisms, it is converted to neutral urea. Urea is made principally in the liver and the en-

TABLE 5.3 NITROGEN EXCRETION PRODUCTS OF VERTEBRATES[a]

Group	Environment	Water Supply	$(CH_3)_3\ N{\rightarrow}O$	NH_3	Urea	Uric Acid
Pisces (fish)	Fresh water	Abundant	−	+	−	−
Teleostei (bony)	Salt water	Poor	+	+	−	−
Elasmobranchii	Fresh water	Abundant	−	−	+	−
(cartilaginous)	Salt water	Good	+	−	+	−
Dipnoi (lung fish)	Fresh water	Abundant	−	+	−	−
	Terrestrial		−	−	+	−
Amphibia						
Urodela	Fresh water	Abundant	−	+	−	−
Anura-tadpole	Fresh water	Abundant	−	+	−	−
frog	Fresh water/ terrestrial	Good/poor	−	−	+	−
Reptilia						
Chelonia (turtles	Fresh water	Abundant	−	+	+	−
and tortoises)	Fresh water/ terrestrial	Good/poor	−	−	+	−
Sauria (snakes	Terrestrial	Poor	−	−	(+)	−
and lizards)	Terrestrial	Poor	−	−	−	+
Aves (birds)	Terrestrial	Poor	−	−	−	+
Mammalia	Terrestrial	Poor	−	−	+	−

[a] From E. Baldwin, *Dynamic Aspects of Biochemistry*, 5th Ed., Cambridge University Press, 1967.

zymatic pathway for its formation is known as the urea cycle. The overall stoichiometry is shown below.

$$2NH_3 + CO_2 + 3ATP^{4-} + 2H_2O \longrightarrow \underset{\underset{NH_2}{|}}{\overset{\overset{NH_2}{|}}{C}}{=}O + AMP^{2-} + 2ADP^{3-} + 2P_i^{2-} + PP_i^{3-} + 3H^+$$

As written, this is an ATP-requiring cycle which produces acid. The reactions which make up the cyclic pathway are shown in Figure 5.13. Ammonia is activated at the expense of two moles of ATP to form the intermediate carbamoylphosphate in a reaction which may require acetylglutamate as cofactor. Carbamoylphosphate *condenses* with ornithine to form citrulline and inorganic phosphate. Aspartate supplies the second N required for urea formation, it is formed by transamination with glutamate and oxaloacetate. The glutamate in turn arises from the combined action of the transaminase and the glutamate dehydrogenase run under reductive conditions with DPNH + H+, NH+₄, and α-ketoglutarate (Figure 5.3). For the transfer of N from aspartate to citrulline, nature has devised an unusual reac-

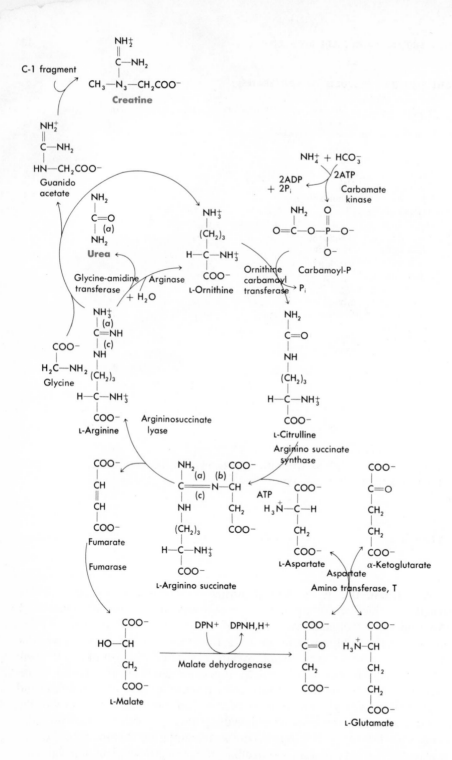

Figure 5.13   The urea cycle. Note the intermediates citrulline, argininosuccinate, and arginine. Note also the formation of creatine.

tion sequence; at the expense of one ATP, citrulline *condenses* with aspartate forming a new N—C linkage (*a*) in the bridge compound L-argininosuccinate. In the next step the transfer of N is accomplished by *breaking the N—C bond* (*b*) in argininosuccinate to form arginine and fumarate. Urea is formed *hydrolytically* by cleavage of the N—C bond (*c*) of arginine to reform ornithine, which completes the cycle. The fumarate is also *rehydrated* to malate, *oxidized* to oxaloacetate, and *transaminated* to aspartate. As can be seen from the stoichiometry of the reaction, the two N—C bonds are formed at the expense of three ATPs. Since there is an oxidation step included in the pathway between fumarate and aspartate, three ATPs are regained and the whole process within the cell becomes self-sustaining. Although liver is the major site of urea synthesis, some synthesis does occur in kidney and brain. The enzymes of the urea cycle are found in these organs.

Creatine Biosynthesis

Creatine biosynthesis is related to urea biosynthesis in that arginine is the *amidino* group donor to glycine to form guanidoacetate. In the following reaction, guanidoacetate is *methylated* with S-adenosylmethionine as methyl donor to creatine and the demethylated S-adenosylhomocysteine. These two steps are shown as an offshoot of the urea cycle in Figure 5.13.

5.11 NUCLEIC ACID METABOLISM

General

The second major class of nitrogen-containing compounds are the nucleic acids. They are polymers of nucleotides containing purine and pyrimidine bases. The five major bases have already been shown (Section 4.5). In addition, the polymers contain ribose or 2-deoxyribose and phosphate. A portion of the structure of a nucleic acid is shown in Figure 5.14. Within the cell the nucleosides derived from nucleic acids can be cleaved either hydrolytically to yield the base and sugar or phosphorolytically to yield the base plus the sugar-1-phosphate (see Section 6.1). The sugars are metabolized by the pathways described in Chapter 4. In the following section, the degradation of the purine and pyrimidine bases is considered. Although these are not usually important sources of energy, their degradation is important since they are breakdown products of normal cell processes and must be disposed of to maintain cell function. The synthesis of these bases is then considered since they are essential to the transmission and transcription of genetic information and the synthetic capability is present in virtually all cells.

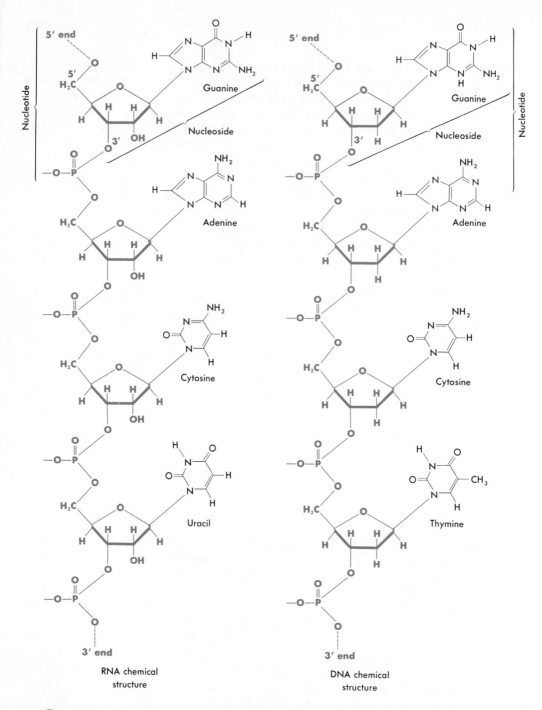

Figure 5.14 Chemical structures of the nucleic acids DNA and RNA. Note the differences between the two, including ribose (RNA) and 2-deoxyribose (DNA), and in the six-membered pyrimidine bases uracil (RNA) and thymine (DNA). The sites of linkage for the purine (nine-membered ring) and pyrimidine (six-membered ring) bases are as numbered. The phosphopentose backbones are indicated in color, and the 3' and 5' ends of the polymers (referring to pentose carbon atoms) are as labelled. Nucleoside = base + sugar; nucleotide = nucleoside + phosphate.

Purine and Pyrimidine Base Degradation

Uric acid, the major degradation product of the purine bases, adenine and guanine, is formed by *deamination* and *oxidation*. The metabolic pathways are shown in Figure 5.15.

The major pathways of pyrimidine degradation are shown in Figure 5.16. In general, the components of the ring system can be metabolized, but in some disease states β-aminoisobutyrate is excreted.

5.12 PYRIMIDINE AND PURINE NUCLEOTIDE SYNTHESIS

The purine and pyrimidine bases, like urea, arise from ammonia. Surprisingly, urea itself is not a precursor of the ureide portions of their ring systems. This was shown most conclusively with isotopic tracers when it was found that labeled urea was not incorporated into uric acid excreted in the urine of birds.

However, the ring systems are constructed from small molecules, including CO_2, NH_4^+, aspartate, glycine, and formate. Elegant tracer experiments

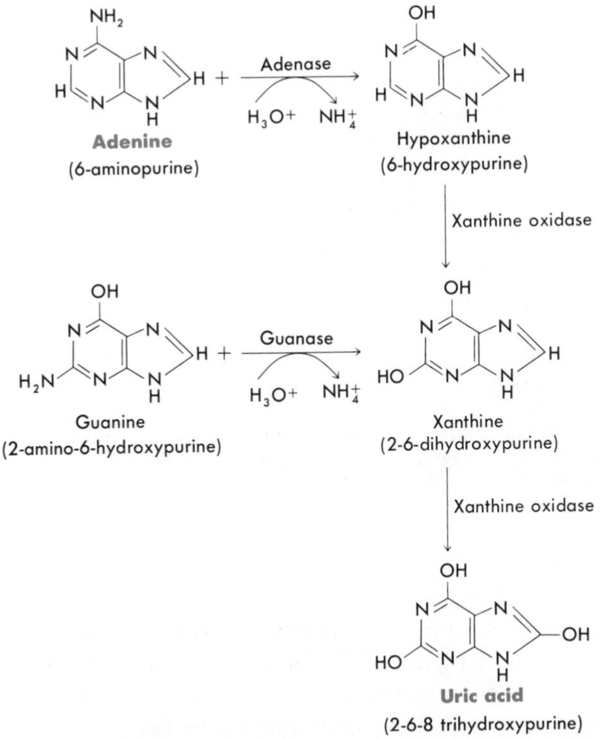

Figure 5.15

Pathways of uric acid formation. Note the hydrolytic and oxidative interconversions to uric acid.

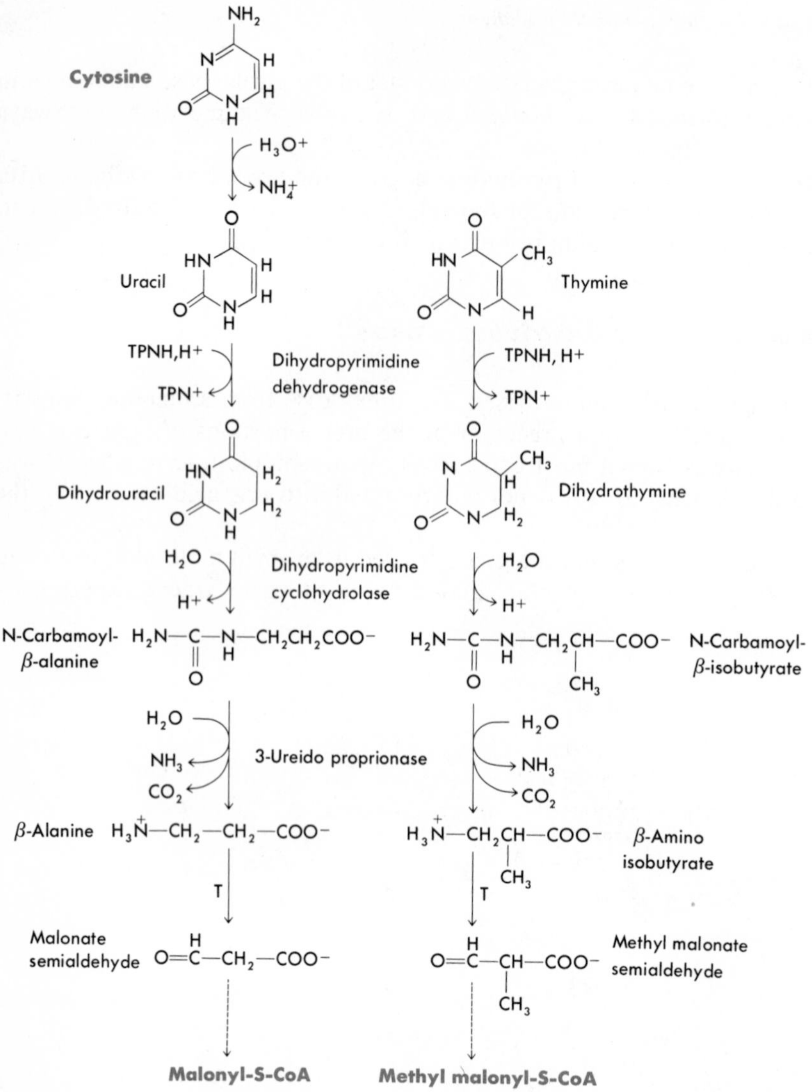

Figure 5.16   Pyrimidine degradation. Hydrolysis is followed by reduction and ring open-
ing to give the β-amino acids. These are degraded to CoASH derivatives
which can be further metabolized.

established the origin of each atom.

The origins of the two nitrogen and four carbon atoms of the six-membered pyrimidine ring is shown in Figure 5.17. As may be seen, N-l is from
ammonia, C-2 from CO_2, and the remaining four atoms from aspartate.

The pathway for the biosynthesis of the pyrimidine nucleotides is an open

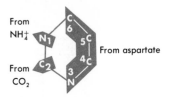

Origins of the Purine C and N Atoms

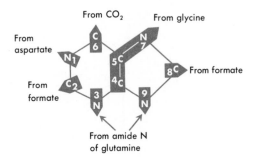

Figure 5.17

Origins of pyrimidine and purine carbon and nitrogen atoms. Origins were determined by isotopic tracer studies.

(noncyclic) series of reactions (Figure 5.18). It starts with the reaction which initiates urea formation and in which CO_2 and ammonia condense in the presence of ATP to form active carbamoylphosphate, which condenses with (carbamoylates) aspartate. A new N—C bond (*a*) is formed (25) and the new compound is carbamoylaspartate. A second N—C bond (*b*) is formed by a *dehydration* reaction, forming the six-membered ring of dihydroorotate. This ring is oxidized to the pyrimidine orotate by a DPN-linked dehydrogenase.

The ribose and phosphate are then added to the pyrimidine ring. Ribose is *phosphorylated* on the C-5 hydroxyl to form ribose-5-phosphate, which is then *pyrophosphorylated* on the C-1 hydroxyl in a pyrophosphate transfer. The product is the triply-phosphorylated 5-phospho-l-pyrophosphoryl ribose (PRPP). This *condenses* with orotate, forming the new β-N-glycoside bond with inversion of configuration of the anomeric C-atom by displacement of the pyrophosphate.

Orotidylate is then *decarboxylated* to uridylate. The uridylate is converted to UDP and UTP by two successive reversible phosphate transfer reactions with ATP. The UTP is finally *aminated* with glutamine to CTP at the expense of ATP.

The origins of the four nitrogen and five carbon atoms of the purine ring system are shown in Figure 5.17. As may be seen, N-1 is from aspartate, N-3 and N-9 are from the amide N of glutamine, while N-7 is from glycine. C-2 and C-8 are from formate, C-6 from CO_2, and C-4 and C-5 are from glycine.

The pathway for biosynthesis of purine nucleotides is again a noncyclic series of reactions shown in Figure 5.19. Initially phosphoribosyl pyrophosphate (PRPP) is *aminated* by reaction with glutamine on C-1 of the ribose

Figure 5.18

Synthesis of pyrimidine nucleotides. Note the synthesis of the two C—N bonds (*a*) and (*b*), the dehydrogenation, decarboxylation, conversion to the nucleotide via PRPP, phosphorylation, and finally amination. The aspartate transcarbamylase is end product inhibited by CTP.

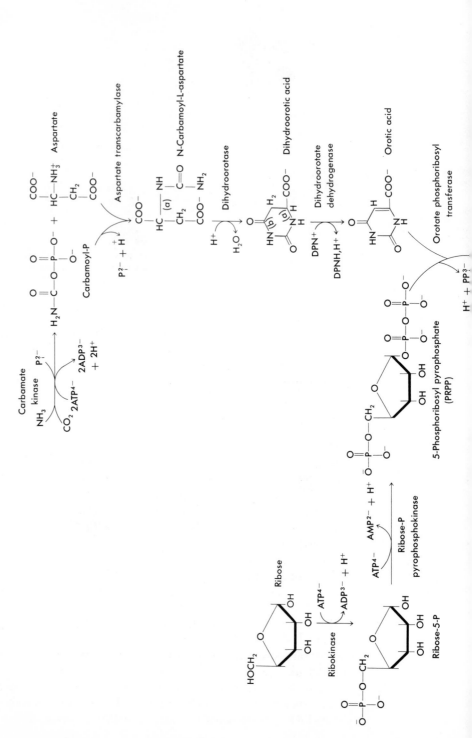

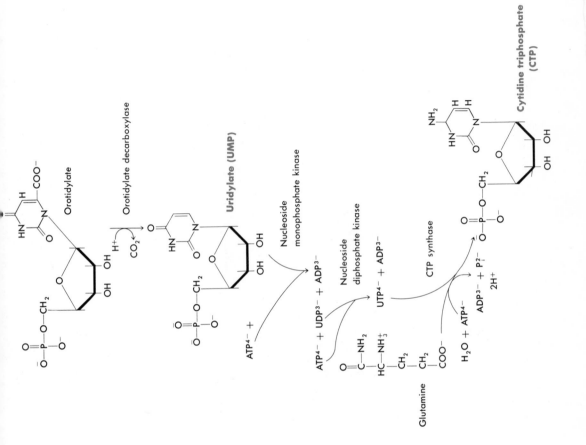

Orotidylate

Orotidylate decarboxylase

H^+ CO_2

Uridylate (UMP)

Nucleoside
monophosphate kinase

$ATP^{4-} +$ $\longrightarrow$ $ADP^{3-} + UDP^{3-} + ADP^{3-}$

Nucleoside
diphosphate kinase

$ATP^{4-} + UDP^{3-} + ADP^{3-}$ $\longrightarrow$ $UTP^{4-} + ADP^{3-}$

CTP synthase

Glutamine

$H_2O + ATP^{4-}$ $\longrightarrow$ $ADP^{3-} + P_i^{2-}$
$2H^+$

Cytidine triphosphate
(CTP)

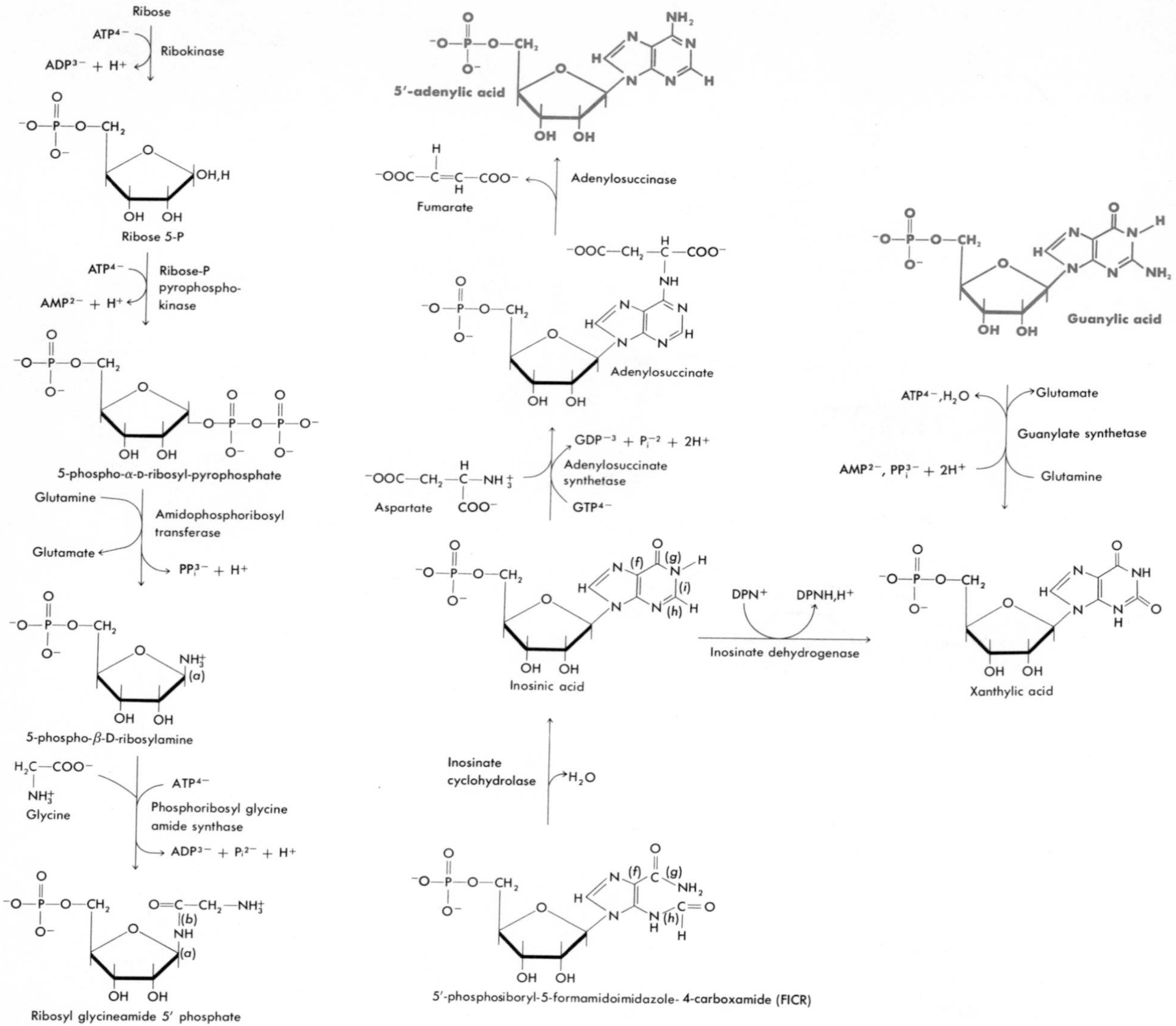

Guanylic acid

Guanylate synthetase

ATP^{4-}, H_2O → Glutamate

AMP^{2-}, PP_i^{3-} + $2H^+$ → Glutamine

Xanthylic acid

Inosinate dehydrogenase

DPN^+ $DPNH,H^+$

NH_2

5'-adenylic acid

Adenylosuccinase

$^-OOC{-}CH_2{-}C{-}COO^-$ / NH — Adenylosuccinate

$^-OOC{-}CH = CH{-}COO^-$ / Fumarate

GDP^{-3} + P_i^{-2} + $2H^+$

Adenylosuccinate synthetase

GTP^{4-}

Aspartate $^-OOC{-}CH_2{-}C{-}NH_3^+$ / COO^- H

Inosinic acid

Inosinate cyclohydrolase

$-H_2O$

$+H_2O$

5'-phosphoribosyl-5-formamidoimidazole-4-carboxamide (FICR)

Ribose

Ribokinase

ATP^{4-} → ADP^{3-} + H^+

Ribose 5-P

Ribose-P pyrophospho-kinase

ATP^{4-} → AMP^{2-} + H^+

5-phospho-α-D-ribosyl-pyrophosphate

Amidophosphoribosyl transferase

Glutamine → Glutamate

PP_i^{3-} + H^+

5-phospho-β-D-ribosylamine

$H_2C{-}COO^-$ / NH_3^+ Glycine

ATP^{4-} → Phosphoribosyl glycine amide synthase

ADP^{3-} + P_i^{2-} + H^+

Ribosyl glycineamide 5' phosphate

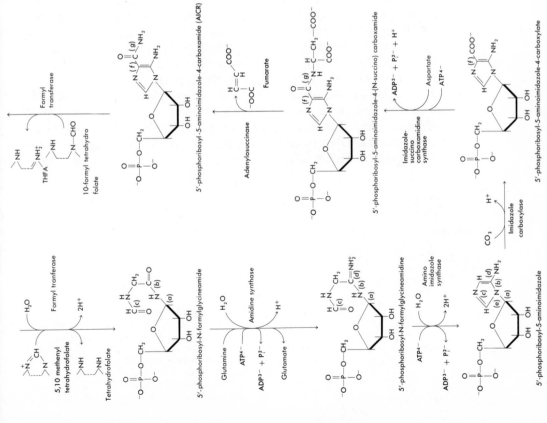

Figure 5.19

Purine nucleotide synthesis. Note the sequence of reactions for the formation of the C—N and C—C bonds denoted by the letters (a) through (i). Note the use of C-1 transfer reactions with THFA derivatives. The aspartate condensation reactions are similar to those in the urea cycle. The GTP dependent reactions are also of interest.

143

with inversion of configuration (β) and the displacement of pyrophosphate. The ring system is then built up step by step on this amino group utilizing glycine and other carbon or nitrogen additions together with cyclizing steps as shown in the figure.

5.13   THE SYNTHESIS OF NUCLEIC ACIDS

The end products of the bulk of purine and pyrimidine syntheses are not the nucleotides but the nucleic acids. The nucleotides are the precursors of these polymers and the following brief description shows how the synthesis of the polymeric materials is achieved. The structures of the nucleic acids are described in Barker's volume in this series and a detailed description of their role in the cell is given in Wold's volume in this series.

The principal nucleic acid of the nucleus, deoxyribonucleic acid (DNA), requires deoxyribose nucleoside triphosphates for its synthesis. These are synthesized by the pathways shown in Figure 5.20. The *reduction* of cytidine diphosphate (CDP) to deoxycytidine diphosphate (dCDP) is presented as a typical example of the reductive process. The other nucleotide diphosphates can be formed in an analogous reaction by the same enzyme system. The enzyme complex, ribonucleotide reductase, is subject to very precise regulation by ATP and the deoxynucleotide di- and triphosphates. The formation of thymidine triphosphate is accomplished by the methylation of deoxyuridine-5'-phosphate with N^5, N^{10}-methylenetetrahydrofolate followed by two reactions with ATP catalyzed by specific kinases.

The synthesis of the polymer DNA takes place prior to cell division in the cell nucleus. The process results in the production of a duplicate set of DNA molecules identical to those of the resting cell. The *replication* process utilizes the original DNA molecules as templates for the formation of the new set. As shown in Figure 5.21, the individual strands of parent DNA in which

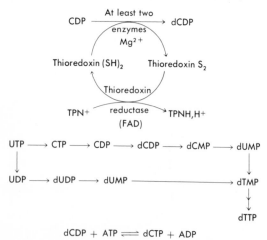

Figure 5.20

Synthesis of deoxyribose nucleoside triphosphates. The reduction of ribonucleotides to deoxyribonucleotides occurs as shown at the nucleoside diphosphate level with the example of the conversion of CDP $\longrightarrow$ dCDP. Thioredoxin is oxidized to the S-S state and subsequently reduced to the SH state by TPNH,H+. The general pathways of pyrimidine nucleotide interconversion are shown at the top and bottom.

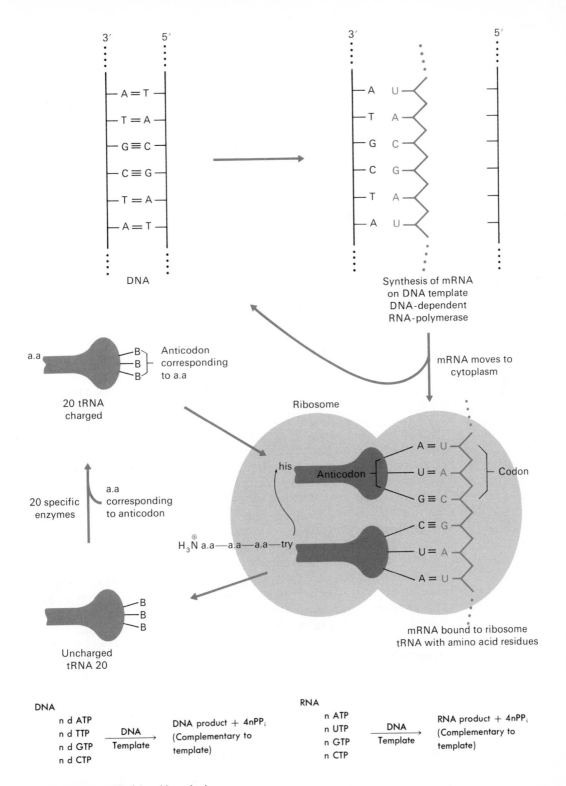

Figure 5.21 Nucleic acid synthesis.

the bases are paired, adenine with thymine and guanine with cytosine, are separated so that each can serve as a template for the synthesis of a new complementary strand. Thus, the product DNA is double-stranded with one strand inherited intact from the parent DNA molecule and the other synthesized from deoxyribonucleoside triphosphates. The enzyme DNA polymerase accomplishes this pyrophosphorylytic synthesis but requires that the DNA strands are separated for its action. It is not known how the separation of strands is achieved in the cell.

The synthesis of the various ribose nucleic acids is accomplished in a very similar fashion as also shown in Figure 5.21. The enzyme DNA-dependent RNA polymerase is capable of catalyzing the production of RNA complementary in sequence to added DNA with the exception that the RNA contains uridine rather than thymine. Synthesis occurs from the 5′ end of the molecule. In vivo only one strand of the double-stranded DNA serves as a template for RNA synthesis. Presumably all forms of RNA are synthesized in a similar fashion.

5.14 THE SYNTHESIS OF PROTEINS

The proteins are polymers of amino acids and each specific protein has a unique amino acid sequence. Thus, the problem of synthesizing a protein has at its core the requirement of a method for specifying the sequence of amino acids so that each molecule of a given protein will have the same sequence. The system is presented diagrammatically in Figure 5.22. DNA in the nucleus contains a "library" of information concerning amino acid sequences in the proteins of the cell. This information is coded in the sequence of bases in the DNA and, as pointed out above, this information can be transmitted from generation to generation with little possibility for error. When a specific protein is to be synthesized, a messenger RNA (mRNA) molecule is synthesized which contains the information to specify the amino acid sequence. Three bases are required to specify one amino acid (three-letter "words") so that the mRNA contains three times as many nucleotides as the protein will have amino acids. The mRNA moves to the cytoplasm and forms a complex with particles known as *ribosomes,* which provide a locus for the enzymes involved in protein synthesis. The message in mRNA, when bound to the ribosome, can be "read" by transfer RNA (tRNA) molecules, which are small (approximately 70 nucleotides long) and each of which contains a three-base sequence complementary to one of the three-letter words of mRNA. There are at least twenty different tRNA molecules, one for each of the amino acids. The tRNA molecules not only have recognition sites for the code words of mRNA but are recognized by specific enzymes in the cytoplasm and are charged by them with the specific amino acid for which they carry the complementary code (Figure 5.21). The process of assembling the protein

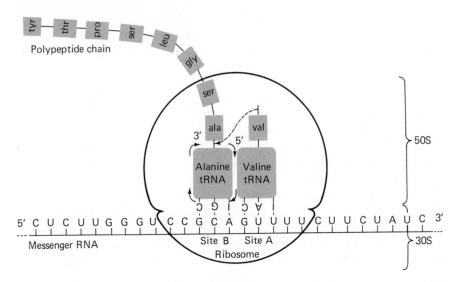

Figure 5.22 The two portions of the ribosomes, 50S and 30S, are shown together with the messenger RNA. The synthesis of the new bond is from val to ala, with peptide transferred from site B to site A. From F. Lipmann, *Science*, **164**, 1024 (1969).

takes place on the ribosome and the growing peptide chain is transferred to the amino acid attached to the most recently added tRNA. The system can produce proteins at a remarkable rate, requiring only seconds to complete a molecule having several hundred amino acid residues. A good deal of energy in the form of nucleoside triphosphate is used in this process.

The following sections deal with the synthesis of some other important nitrogen-containing compounds, heme, glutathione, and cell-wall peptido-glycan.

5.15 HEME SYNTHESIS

Isotopic studies demonstrated that glycine and acetate were precursors in heme biosynthesis. The detailed pathway was then elucidated by the enzymological approach. The reaction sequence is shown in Figure 5.23. Succinyl-S-CoA, the intermediate formed in the tricarboxylic acid cycle or formed by the reversal of the succinate thiokinase reaction (Fig. 4.5, reaction 29), *condenses* with the α-C of glycine to form a C—C bond accompanied by *decarboxylation* and the release of CoASH, forming Δ-amino levulinate. The reaction is catalyzed by the Δ-amino levulinate synthetase; a pyridoxal phosphate enzyme. Two molecules of Δ-amino levulinate *cyclize* by the removal of two molecules of H_2O, forming a C—C bond, a C—N bond, and the heterocyclic pyrrole ring of porphobilinogen. This reaction is catalyzed by the Δ-amino levulinate dehydrase. Three molecules of porphobilinogen *condense* to form a linear tripyrrole, which *condenses* with another molecule of porphobilinogen to form the cyclic tetrapyrrole, urophorphinogen III. By a series of *six decarboxylations* and *five oxidations* this compound is converted to protoporphyrin IX, the most common cyclic tetrapyrrole in nature. A specific enzyme (ferrochelatase) *inserts* ferrous ion into the tetrapyrrole to form heme. By other modifications, protoporphyrin IX is converted to chlorophyll in green plants. Heme compounds are required for photosynthesis (chlorophyll), O_2 transport and binding (hemoglobin and myoglobin), electron transport to oxygen (cytochromes), and oxidation-reduction of peroxides (catalase and peroxidase). Heme has a planar structure and the highly conjugated ring system depicted (see Appendix) is one of a number of resonance structures. Since the Δ-amino levulinate synthetase is in the microsomes and the ferrochelatase in mitochondria, this is another example of a biosynthetic pathway involving more than one subcellular compartment.

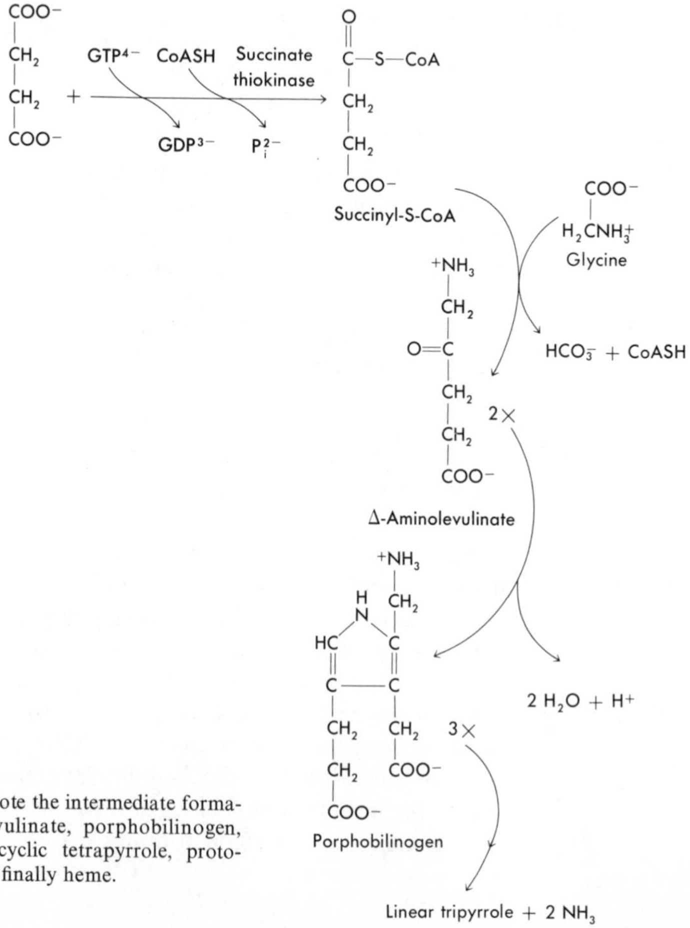

Figure 5.23

Heme synthesis. Note the intermediate formation of amino levulinate, porphobilinogen, linear tripyrrole, cyclic tetrapyrrole, protoporphyrin IX, and finally heme.

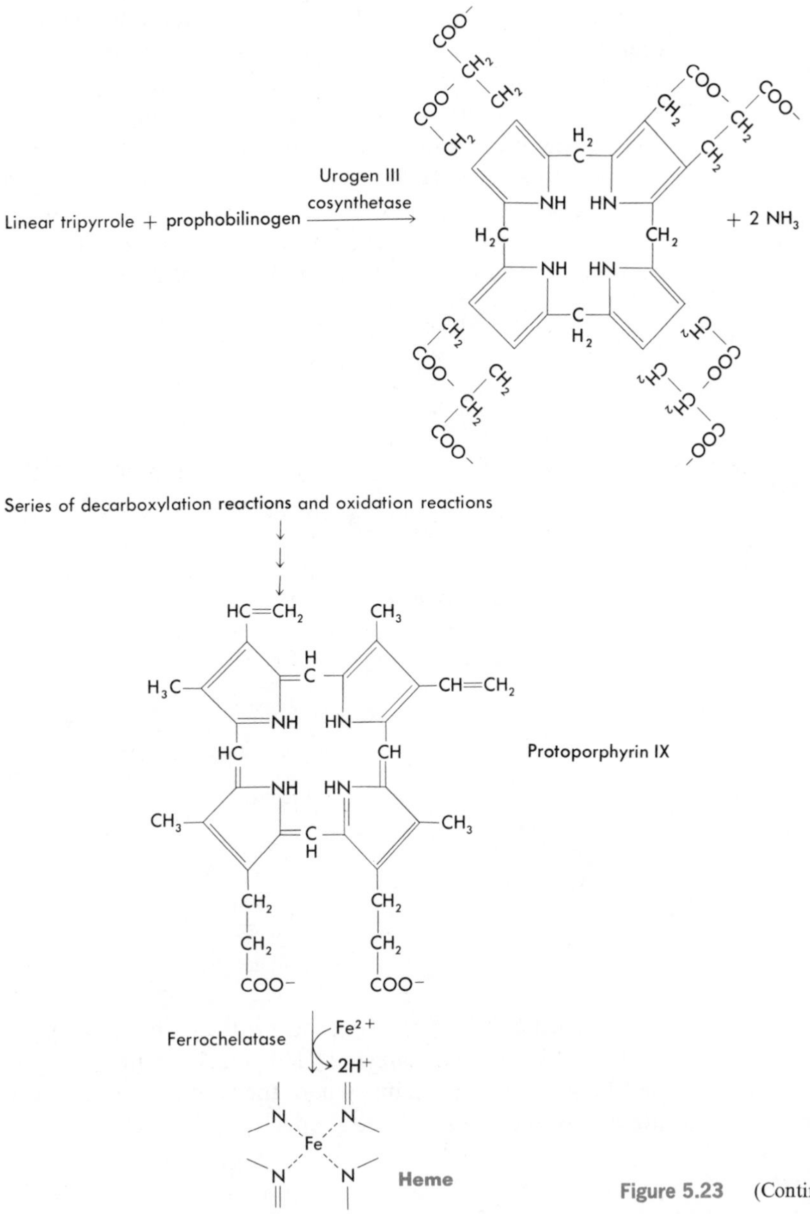

Linear tripyrrole + prophobilinogen $\xrightarrow{\text{Urogen III cosynthetase}}$ + 2 NH$_3$

Series of decarboxylation reactions and oxidation reactions

$\downarrow$
$\downarrow$
$\downarrow$

Protoporphyrin IX

Ferrochelatase

Fe^{2+}

2H$^+$

Heme

Figure 5.23   (Continued).

5.16   GLUTAMINE AND GLUTATHIONE SYNTHESIS

While there is little or no storage of protein as such, as previously mentioned nitrogen may be stored as NH$_3$, in the form of the amide linkages of glutamine and asparagine. Asparagine is especially important and abundant in plants. Glutamine is formed from glutamate via glutamine synthetase (Figure 7.12). Enzyme-bound γ-glutamylphosphate is the presumed intermediate. Asparagine may be formed by an analogous reaction, but in addition is formed by transamination from glutamine.

The tripeptide glutathione (γ-glutamylcysteinylglycine) is a rather widely distributed peptide. It serves an important intracellular role as a redox substance. For example, it is an intermediate in maintaining hemoglobin in its reduced state in the erythrocyte. The two amide linkages are formed in two reactions at the expense of two molecules of ATP.

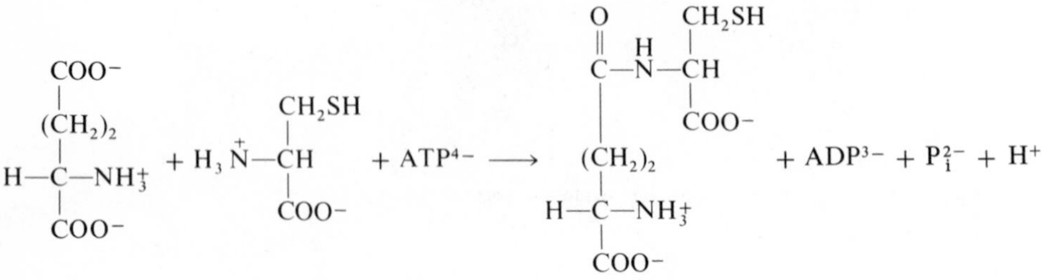

$$\gamma\text{-glutamylcysteine}$$

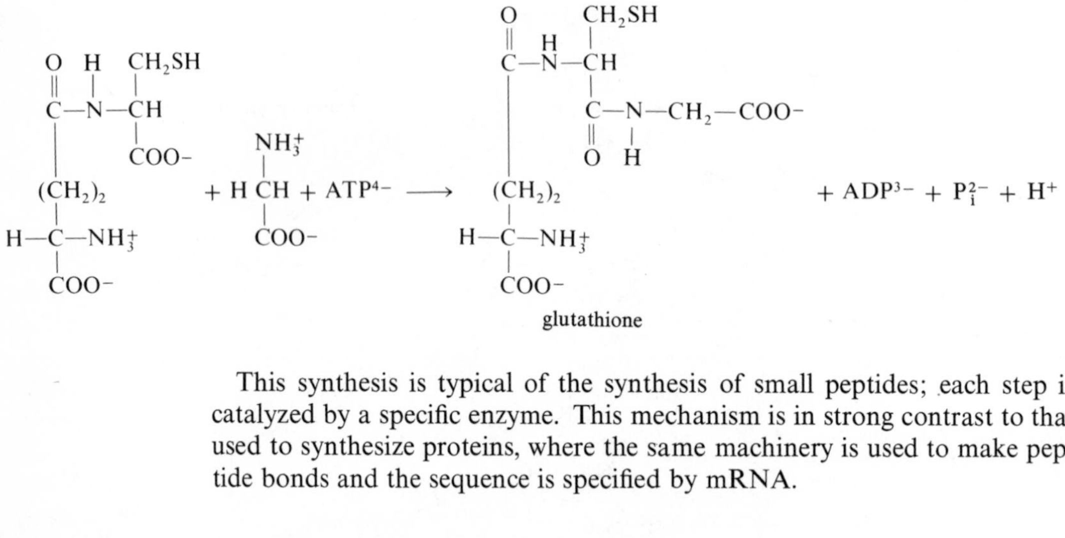

$$\text{glutathione}$$

This synthesis is typical of the synthesis of small peptides; each step is catalyzed by a specific enzyme. This mechanism is in strong contrast to that used to synthesize proteins, where the same machinery is used to make peptide bonds and the sequence is specified by mRNA.

5.17 SYNTHESIS OF PEPTIDOGLYCAN—A STRUCTURAL BIOPOLYMER

The enzymatic synthesis of the peptidoglycan of the *bacterial cell wall* of *S. aureus* is an elegant example of the principles involved in the utilization of the energy of ATP for unidirectional heteropolymer biosynthesis. Peptidoglycans from other bacterial sources are constructed on the same general pattern but have specific differences in constituents. A portion of the two-dimensional structure of peptidoglycan of *S. aureus* is shown diagrammatically in Figure 5.24.

Biosynthesis may, for convenience, be divided into three stages: (1) the synthesis of precursors, (2) synthesis of linear peptidoglycan strands from the precursors, and (3) cross-linking of the linear strands to form the two- or three-dimensional structure.

The two precursors are UDP-N-acetylglucosamine and UDP-N-acetyl-muramyl pentapeptide. The series of reactions by which these precursors are formed is shown in Figure 5.25 (I).

The second state in biosynthesis is the polymerization of the two uridine nucleotide precursors UDP-acetylmuramyl pentapeptide and UDP-acetyl-glucosamine to form the linear peptidoglycan. The overall reaction is shown below:

$$n\text{UDP-MurNAc} + n\text{UDP-GlcNAc} \longrightarrow (\text{Glc-NAc-Mur-Ac})_n + n\text{UDP}^{3-} + n\text{UMP}^{2-} + n\text{P}_i^{2-} + 3n\text{H}^+$$

<table>
<tr><td>L-ala</td><td></td><td>L-ala</td></tr>
<tr><td>|</td><td></td><td>|</td></tr>
<tr><td>D-glu</td><td></td><td>D-glu</td></tr>
<tr><td>|</td><td></td><td>|</td></tr>
<tr><td>L-lys</td><td>⟶</td><td>L-lys</td></tr>
<tr><td>|</td><td></td><td>|</td></tr>
<tr><td>D-ala</td><td></td><td>D-ala</td></tr>
<tr><td>|</td><td></td><td>|</td></tr>
<tr><td>D-ala</td><td></td><td>D-ala</td></tr>
</table>

The series of reactions which sum up to this reaction, as written, are shown in Figure 5.25 (II). First, the UDP-acetylmuramyl pentapeptide is *transferred* to a high-molecular-weight *C-55 polyisoprenoid,* splitting out UMP and forming a pyrophosphoryl bridge. In the next reaction this *condenses* with UDP-acetylglucosamine, this time splitting out UDP and forming the disaccharide (pentapeptide) P-P-isoprenoid. This disaccharide is then *transferred* as a unit to an existing acceptor in the cell wall, *lengthening* the chain in the wall by a disaccharide unit and *releasing* the pyrophosphate form of the phosphorylated isoprenoid. This pyrophosphate is then *cleaved* hydrolytically in the last reaction to inorganic phosphate and the C-55 isoprenoid.

Two additional modifications take place in this second phase: (1) the *amidation* of the *α-carboxyl* group of D-glutamate to *isoglutamine* and (2) the *attachment* of pentaglycine bridging groups. The amidation reaction takes place on the disaccharide (pentapeptide) P-P-isoprenoid and is shown in Figure 5.25 (II). The reaction is similar in principle to glutamine synthetase except that the α-carboxyl group is amidated to form an isoglutamine. It is to be noted that the Δ-*carboxyl* group is linked to the α *amino of lysine,* the adjacent amino acid in the chain. This is perhaps the only instance in which the isoglutamine is so linked.

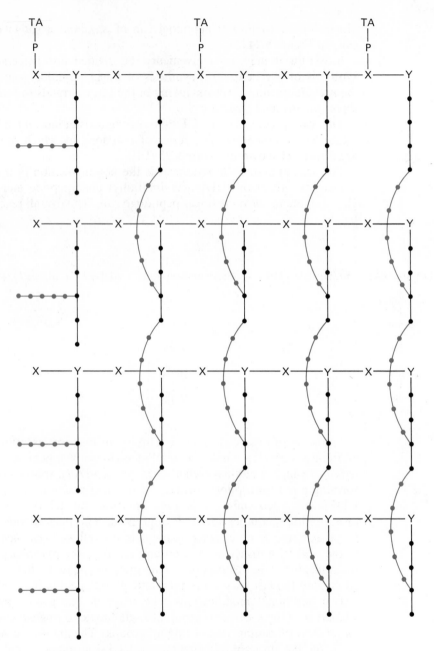

X = acetyl glucosamine

Y = acetyl muramic acid

●—●—● = L—alanyl —D—isoglutaminyl— L —lysyl —D—alanine

●—●—● = pentaglycine

TA —P = teichoic acid antigen

The biosynthesis of the pentaglycine bridges involves *activation* of glycine to glycyl-tRNA as in the first reaction of protein synthesis. Five glycyl-tRNA's are then *added sequentially* to the ε-*amino of lysine* in a novel reaction to form the decapeptide derivative of the isoprenoid. This then is the disaccharide derivative which *condenses* with the acceptor molecule to enlarge the chain and to split out the isoprenoid pyrophosphate. The pentaglycine bridge synthesis is unusual in that glycyl-tRNA is required in peptide bond synthesis in which protein is *not* made.

In the third or final phase, the peptidoglycan chains are cross-linked, again by a new reaction, through the pentaglycine bridges.

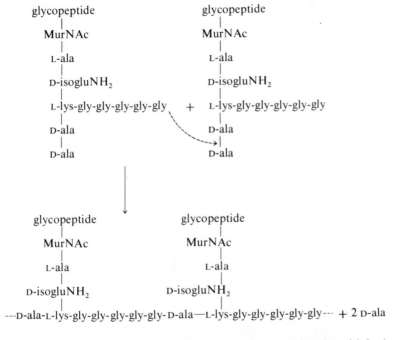

This is a transpeptidization reaction in which the new peptide bond gly-D-ala is formed at the expense of an existing peptide bond by splitting out the terminal D-ala. Thus, the resultant product has a tetrapeptide left re-

Figure 5.24

Peptidoglycan structure. A two dimensional structure for the heteropolymer is shown. Four repeating acetylglucosamine (X) and acetyl muramic acid (Y) chains are shown. The acetyl muramic residues are linked to the L-alanyl-Disoglutaminyl-ε-lysyl-D-alanine side chains O—O—O—O. These are cross-linked at the lysyl residues by the pentaglycine bridges. Four pentaglycine chains are also shown prior to cross-linking at the left. The linkage of acetyl glucosamine to teichoic acid antigen is shown at the top. From J. S. Strominger, K. Izaki, M. Matsuhashi, D. J. Tipper, *Fed. Proc.,* **26,** 9 (1967).

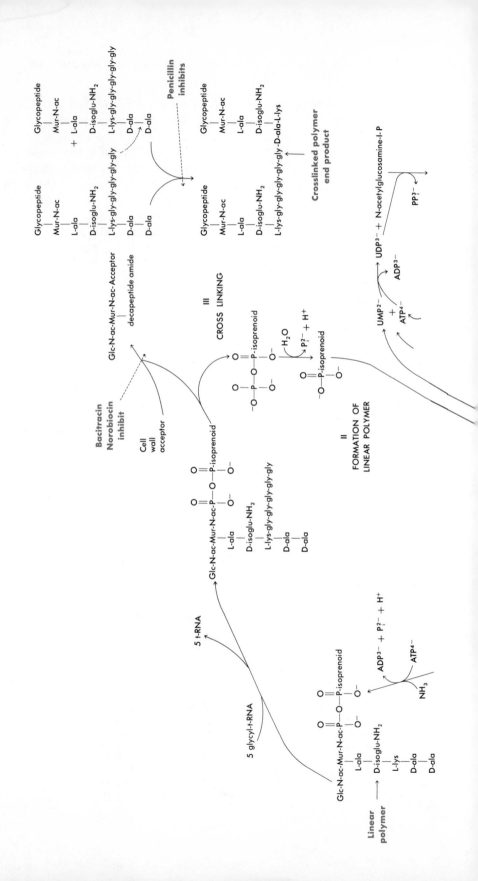

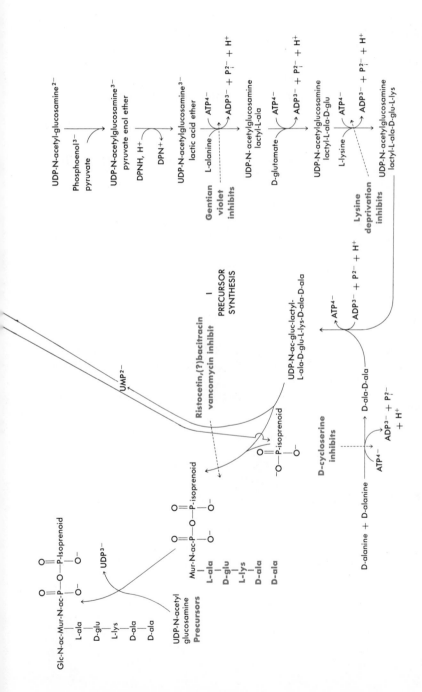

Figure 5.25 Reactions of peptidoglycan synthesis. Reactions are divided into three stages labelled 1—Precursor synthesis; 11—Formation of linear polymer; and 111—Cross linking. The individual reactions in each stage can be followed on the figure and are described in the text. The inhibitions by gentian violet, lysine deprivation, cycloserine, ristocetin, bacitracin, novobiocin, and penicillin are as shown. Note the unusual chemical features including D-amino acids, isoglutaminyl linkages, the isoprenoid lipid carrier, and the use of glycyl-t-RNA in this remarkable pathway. Adapted from J. L. Strominger, K. Izaki, M. Matsuhashi, D. J. Tipper, *Fed. Proc.*, **26,** 9 (1967).

maining L-ala-D-isogluNH$_2$-L-lys-D-ala, in place of the original pentapeptide L-ala-D-isogluNH$_2$-L-lys-D-ala-D-ala. The cross-linking is via the pentaglycine bridge from the ε-amino of lysine to the carboxyl of D-ala. This is the reaction which is specifically inhibited by the antibiotic penicillin. Figure 5.25 also shows the sites of inhibition by other substances.

In this chapter, the degradation of nitrogen-containing compounds for energy and the disposal of nitrogen wastes have been described. The synthesis of these compounds is presented and the broad outlines of energy utilization in the synthesis of nucleic acids and proteins have been drawn.

REFERENCES

Baldwin, E., *Dynamic Aspects of Biochemistry,* 5th ed., Cambridge University Press, Cambridge, Mass., 1967.

Braunstein, A. E., *The Enzymes,* (P. D. Boyer, H. Lardy, K. Myrback, eds.), Vol. 2, Chapter 6, pp. 113–181 (1960).

Cohen, P. P., and G. W. Brown, Jr., "Ammonia metabolism and urea biosynthesis," in *Comparative Biochem.,* **2,** M. Florkin and H. S. Mason eds., Academic Press, New York, 1960.

Davidson, J. N., and W. E. Cohn, *Progress in Nucleic Acid Research,* Academic Press, New York.

Greenberg, D. M., *Metabolic Pathways,* **3,** Academic Press, New York, 1969.

Meister, A., *Biochemistry of the Amino Acids,* 2nd ed., Academic Press, Inc., New York, 1965.

Strominger, J. L., Izaki, K., Matsuhashi, M., and D. J. Tipper, "Peptidoglycan Transpeptidase and D-alanine Carboxypeptidase Penicillin Sensitive Enzymatic Reactions," *Federation Proceedings,* **26,** 9 (1967).

White, A., Handler, P., and E. L. Smith, *Principles of Biochemistry,* 4th ed., McGraw-Hill Book Company, New York, 1968.

EVALUATION OF THE IN VIVO SIGNIFICANCE OF METABOLIC REACTIONS

SIX

Now that we have considered the metabolism of energy, the fuels and the nitrogen-containing compounds, we will turn to a discussion of the regulation of metabolism. In this chapter, we will deal with the question of how we can estimate the in vivo significance of metabolic reaction sequences. To a certain extent, we have touched on this question in Chapter 2, where the approaches used in ordering the reactions of metabolism and the chain of experimental biochemical systems was presented. Granted now that one has ordered a sequence of reactions into a metabolic pathway, the next question is: "What is the intracellular or in vivo significance of these reactions?" This question can be broken down into three detailed parts concerned with (1) the *quantitative assessment* of metabolic flow, (2) the *apportionment* of metabolic flow through competing systems, and (3) the *control* of the metabolic flow. The first two of these parts will be considered in this chapter, while the latter part concerning control will be discussed in a general way in Chapter 7 and will be the principal subject of Chapters 8, 9, and 10, which deal with the control of carbohydrate and lipid metabolism, the control of metabolism of the nitrogen-containing compounds, and the control of energy metabolism, respectively.

The quantitative and qualitative assessment of the in vivo significance of metabolic pathways has been approached in a number of ways. It may be useful to consider these approaches as two experimentally distinct types, depending on the sequence of steps in which the experimental evidence is collected. In the first type (*the in vitro* ⟶ *in vivo approach*), one would begin the investigation with known properties of all the appropriate purified enzymes and proceed by studying systems of increasing complexity. In essence, this would be done by building up models, and comparing their properties with the in vivo properties of the whole organ or animal. In the second type (*the in vivo* ⟶ *in vitro approach*), one starts with the known properties of the intact system and then proceeds by chemically dissecting and studying individual components in a progression of increasing simplicity. In spite of the opposite "polarity" of the approaches, the final answers and the total information should be the same. The selection of either type of approach is often simply a matter of the personal background and preference of the individual investigator, but may also be determined by sheer necessity. The history of biochemical research illustrates the latter point.

Initially, observations in biochemistry were made with the in vivo systems. The in vitro systems were developed later as a consequence of the early observations and their significance assessed according to the in vivo ⟶ in vitro approach. As more and more in vitro data accumulated, giving clues to previously undetected in vivo properties, it became feasible to seek the answers by the in vitro ⟶ in vivo approach. Another way of looking at this is to say that in vivo events predict that certain components, reactions, or phenomena should be observable in vitro. The search for the confirmation of these predictions led to some unexpected observations which, in turn, predicted that additional in vitro events be sought. This view emphasizes the complementary interaction of the two different approaches, leading to the development of a branch of natural science in ever-broadening cycles of increased refinement. Several examples of both approaches could be cited here, but the reader is left to consider the individual pathways in this book with this experimental distinction in mind. It appears that in vivo observations may have been more productive in suggesting major metabolic reactions than the in vitro ones (see Section 7.5).

6.1 SEPARATE PATHWAYS FOR SYNTHESIS AND DEGRADATION

As more and more pathways have become established, it has become clear that biosynthesis and degradation are separate reactions. This means that those sequences which utilize energy are separate from those which provide energy. The accumulated evidence on this point is impressive. In every case examined, amino acids, nucleotides, coenzymes, fatty acids, phospholipids, steroids, as well as the biopolymers, proteins, RNA, DNA, glycogen (already discussed in Chapters 3 and 4), this is the case. *This separation of pathways must be an essential feature for the efficiency of living systems.*

The presence of the two distinct pathways may mean that several intermediates are common substrates in both biosyntheses and degradations—as is the case in glycolysis, for example. Here several enzymes may also be common catalysts used in both directions. Therefore, to drive a given set of reactions one way or the other, it must be essential for the cell to separate the biosynthetic apparatus from the corresponding degradative apparatus. This is achieved either by compartmentalization or by interlinked control through a single regulatory substance, which activates ("turns on") one reaction (e.g., biosynthesis) and inhibits ("turns off") the other (e.g., degradation). The best example to illustrate and contrast biosynthetic and degradative reactions is the general pattern of reactions which interconvert monomers and polymers.

For these interconversions there are three types of reactions, hydrolysis, phosphorolysis and pyrophosphorolysis, and these are illustrated in Figure 6.1. Phosphorylases make use of P_i to cleave glycoside bonds of polysaccharides, nucleosides, and diester linkages of RNA. The glycogen phosphorolysis reaction has already been given (Figure 4.4). The reactions of

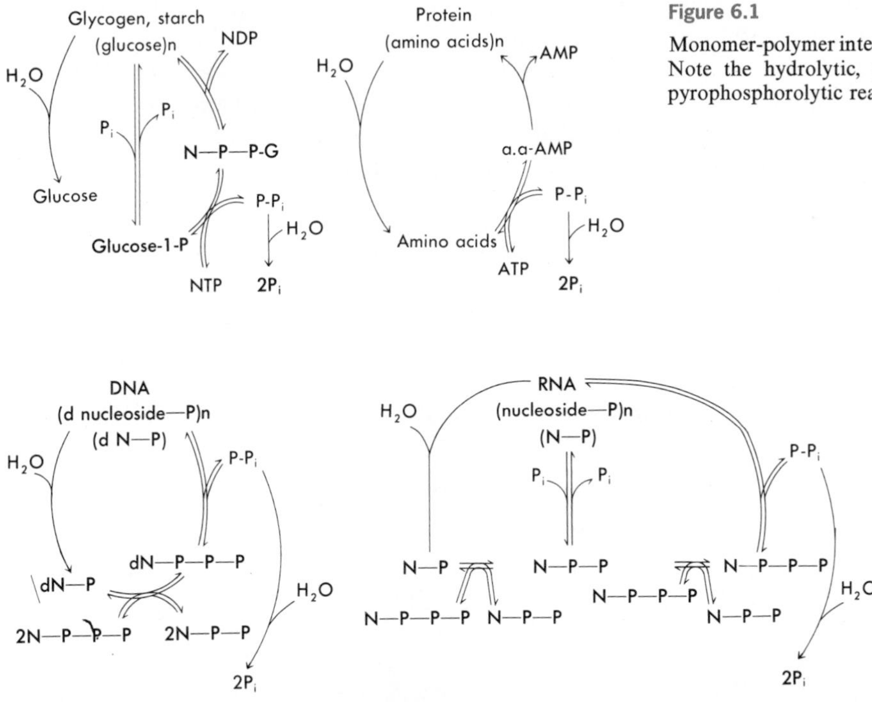

Figure 6.1

Monomer-polymer interconversion systems. Note the hydrolytic, phosphorolytic and pyrophosphorolytic reactions.

nucleoside (or deoxyribonucleoside) and RNA phosphorolysis are given in Eqs. (1) and (2). These are both readily reversible reactions.

$$\text{ribonucleoside} + P_i \rightleftharpoons \text{base} + \text{ribose-1-P} \tag{1}$$

$$\text{or} \qquad\qquad\qquad \text{or}$$

$$\text{(deoxyribonucleoside)} \qquad\qquad \text{(deoxyribose-1-P)}$$

$$\text{RNA} + P_i \rightleftharpoons \text{nucleoside diphosphate} \tag{2}$$

Pyrophosphorylases utilize pyrophosphate to cleave glycosidic and phosphate bonds in reactions which are analogous to those catalyzed by phosphorylases. Several examples have been given in Sections 4.1 and 4.5. Like the phosphorylase reactions, the pyrophosphorylase reactions are also reversible. Yet, when the pyrophosphorylase reactions are considered, their role appears to be strictly biosynthetic. When the biosyntheses of the biopolymers (Chapters 4 and 5), proteins, the nucleic acids, and glycogen, as well as the coenzymes, are considered together, these sequences are "driven toward" synthesis by the hydrolysis of the leaving pyrophosphate group to inorganic phosphate. Alternatively, phosphorolytic reactions appear to be associated with degradations "driven by" the relatively high intracellular concentrations of inorganic phosphate in order to provide for the energy requirements of the cell. The hydrolytic reactions are strictly degradative. They take place either intracellularly, for example, as catalyzed by a battery of enzymes in particles known as *lysosomes,* or extracellularly, catalyzed by a number of enzymes associated with digestion in the gastrointestinal tract.

A tabulation of the biosynthetic reactions associated with pyrophosphate release is given in Table 6.1. As can be seen, this is a general process and involves a number of the nucleoside triphosphates, including ATP, GTP, CTP, UTP, deoxythymidine triphosphate (dTTP). Table 6.2, by way of contrast,

TABLE 6.1   BIOSYNTHETIC PATHWAYS INVOLVING PYROPHOSPHATE RELEASE[a]

General Class	Specific Compounds	Reactants
Polysaccharides		
Pectins, chitins	UDP glucose	Glucose-1-P + UTP
Disaccharides	UDP-N-acetylglucosamine	N-acetylglucosamine-1-P + UTP
Bacterial cell walls	UDP xylose	Xylose-1-P + UTP
Bacterial capsules	GDP mannose	Mannose-1-P + GTP
Ascorbate, T-even phage DNA, glycolipids Gangliosides	TDP glucose	Glucose-1-P + dTTP
Glycogen	UDP glucose	Glucose-1-P + UTP
Starch	ADP glucose	Glucose-1-P + ATP
Lipids	Acyl-S-CoA	Fatty acid + CoA-SH + ATP
Phospholipid	CDP choline	P-choline + CTP
	CDP ethanolamine	P-ethanolamine + CTP
	CDP diglyceride	Phosphatidic acid + CTP

TABLE 6.1 (*Continued*)

General Class	Specific Compounds	Reactants
Steroids, terpenes	Geranyl-PP	Isopenenyl-PP + dimethyl allyl-PP
	Farnesyl-PP	Isopentenyl-PP + geranyl-PP
	Squalene-	Farnesyl-PP + farnesyl-PP
	cholyl-S-CoA	Cholic acid + CoASH + ATP
Proteins	Amino acyl RNA	Amino acid + transfer RNA + ATP
Nucleic acids	DNA	DNA primer + dATP, dCTP, dTTP, dGTP
	Acceptor RNA	RNA primer + ATP, CTP
	DNA-directed RNA	DNA primer + ATP, CTP, UTP, GTP
	RNA-directed RNA	RNA primer + ATP, CTP, UTP, GTP
Nucleotides		
De novo pathway:		
Pyrimidine	Orotidylate	Orotate + PRPP
Purine	5-Phosphoribosylamine	Glutamine + PRPP
	Guanylate	Xanthylate, glutamine + ATP (or NH_3)
Salvage pathway		
Pyrimidine	Uridylate	Uracil + PRPP
Purine	Adenylate, inosinate	Adenine
	Guanylate	Hypoxanthine, guanine + PRPP
Coenzymes	Nicotinic acid ribose-5'-P	Nicotinic acid + PRPP
DPN, TPN, FAD,	Deamido-DPN	Nicotinic acid ribose-5'-P + ATP
thiamine-PP	DPN	Deamido-DPN, glutamine + ATP
	FAD	riboflavin-5'-P + ATP
	Thiamine-P	"Thiazole"-P, "pyrimidine"-PP
CoASH	Pantothenate	pantoic acid + β-alanine + ATP
	dephospho-CoA	Phosphopantotheine + ATP
Phosphoadenylsulfate	Adenylsulfate	Sulfate + ATP
Transmethylation	S-Adenosylmethione	Methionine + ATP
Amino acids		
Histidine	Phosphoribosyl-ATP	ATP + PRPP
Tryptophan (indole	P-ribosyl anthranilic acid	Anthranilic acid + PRPP
glycerol P)	Argininosuccinate	Citrulline + aspartate + ATP
Arginine		

[a] Modified from A. Kornberg, "On the Metabolic Significance of Phosphorolytic and Pyrophosphorolytic Reactions," in *Horizons in Biochemistry,* M. Kasha and B. Pullman (eds.), Academic Press, New York, 1962.

lists the phosphorolytic reactions associated with biodegradations. The number is much smaller than the number of synthetic reactions, but taken together with the hydrolytic reactions, the total degradative capacity of the cell is obviously high.

There is an additional advantage of separation of biosynthetic and degra-

TABLE 6.2   DEGRADATIVE PATHWAYS INVOLVING PHOSPHATE[a]

Degradative Pathway	Substrate Degraded	Phosphorylated Product
Polysaccharide monosaccharide	Glycogen	α-Glucose-1-P
	Sucrose	α-Glucose-1-P
	Maltose	β-Glucose-1-P
Monosaccharide acyl-P	3-Phosphoglyceraldehyde	1,3-Diphosphoglycerate
	Xylulose 5-P	Acetyl-P
	Pyruvate	Acetyl-P
Threonine acyl-P	Aspartic β-semialdehyde	Aspartyl-P
"Acetyl" $\rightarrow$ CO$_2$ + H$_2$O	Intermediate in aerobic phosphorylation	ATP
Nucleic acid	RNA	Nucleoside diphosphate
	Ribonucleosides	Ribose-1-P
	Deoxyribonucleosides	Deoxyribose-1-P

[a] Modified from A. Kornberg, "On the Metabolic Significance of Phosphorolytic and Pyrophosphorolytic Reactions," *Horizons in Biochemistry*, M. Kasha and B. Pullman (eds.), Academic Press, New York, 1962.

dative pathways to the cell. It permits the separate *control* of these reaction pathways. Such separate control permits the direction of metabolic flow to be established. We will have more to say about this subject in subsequent chapters.

6.2   QUANTITATIVE ASSESSMENTS OF METABOLIC PATHWAYS

We can now consider the quantitative aspects of the in vivo-in vitro problem. What we would like to do first is to measure the overall rate of product formation through a pathway in vivo. The catalytic activities of the enzymes of the pathway could then be separately determined in vitro, using *both* steady-state in vivo substrate concentrations as well as saturating in vitro substrate concentrations. The rate-limiting reactions could in this way be identified and the key question asked: "Are the catalytic activities of the isolated rate-limiting enzymes measured in vitro sufficient to account for the metabolic rate (or *flux*) measured in vivo?"

Metabolic Flux in Brain

Let us examine a concrete example to help clarify some of these points. In the mouse brain, for example, glucose (and glycogen) are converted to lactate via glycolysis under anaerobic conditions, whereas in the presence of oxygen most of the glucose (and glycogen) is oxidized completely to CO$_2$. The yield of ATP in glycolysis is two per mole of glucose converted to lactate (or three per mole of glycogen-glucose converted); in complete oxidation, the ATP yield is 38 moles per mole of glucose. Under normal aerobic conditions, there is a steady-state ratio of lactate production (glycolysis) and CO_2 production (oxidation), but if the oxygen supply were to be suddenly cut off, the tissue could use only glycolysis to produce high-energy phosphate compounds and as a result, a change in the metabolic flow of different substrates would be observed. If we know the normal aerobic flow, the change will allow such an evaluation of the glycolytic flow triggered by anoxia.

Such measurements have been made in the mouse brain, the brain being one of the organs recognized as most sensitive to oxygen levels. If it is deprived of oxygen for only a few minutes, irreversible changes set in. The plan of the experiment is as follows: At varying times following the onset of anoxia effected by decapitation, the brains are rapidly stabilized by freezing at $-150°C$. From the frozen tissue, the metabolites are extracted, taking suitable precautions in order that their original concentrations within the cells are maintained. By analyzing with sensitive and specific enzymatic methods, the substrate levels are determined. We will not discuss here the micromethods which have been developed for this purpose. But the student is referred to O. H. Lowry and co-workers to make himself familiar with the precision and care possible in this type of analysis.

It is of interest to first determine aerobic glucose metabolic flow and high-energy phosphate metabolic flow prior to the onset of anoxia. In order to do so, we will make certain assumptions. First, we calculate the high-energy phosphate ($\sim P$) flow or flux by summing (Table 6.3) the creatine-P, plus ATP times two—($2 \sim P$ per ATP), plus lactate fluxes (adult, 26.7 mmoles/ kg/min; 10 days old, 5.9 mmoles/kg/min). Now we assume that:

1. The rates of $\sim P$ use during the first few seconds of anoxia are unchanged from the pre-anoxic period.
2. Glucose and glycogen are the only energy sources.

TABLE 6.3   **INITIAL FLUXES FOR MAJOR ENERGY SOURCES AFTER DECAPITATION**[a]

Group	Creatine-P	ATP	Glucose	Glycogen (as Glucose)	Lactate	$\sim P$	Maximal Pre-decapitation Glucose Flux
			mmoles/kg/min				
Adult	-11	-2.2	-6.5	-2.2	$+11.3$	26.7	0.81
10 days old	-4.8	-0.26	-1.6	-0.0	$+0.6$	5.9	0.18

[a] Modified from O. H. Lowry, J. V. Passonneau, F. X. Hasselberger, and D. W. Schulz, "Effect of Ischemia on Known Substrates and Cofactors of the Glycolytic Pathway in Brain," *J. Biol. Chem.,* **239,** 18 (1964).

3. Under aerobic conditions fifteen percent of the glucose is converted to lactate, with a yield of 2ATP per mole of glucose.

4. The remaining 85 percent is oxidized to CO_2 with a yield of 38ATP per mole oxidized (Section 4.2).

We calculate that for each mole of glucose utilized, 33 equivalents of $\sim P$ would be generated (33 is the combined 15 percent glycolysis and 85 percent oxidation). For the adult, 26.7/33 rounded off to 27/33 (Table 6.3) would be equivalent to 0.81 mmoles of glucose oxidized/kilogram/minute. (This would be the maximum predecapitation glucose flux.) This may now be compared with the sum of the glucose and glycogen fluxes (8.7 mmoles/kg/min). Thus, one can realize that anoxia has increased glucose breakdown via glycolysis from 0.81 to 8.7, or over ten-fold in the adult. A similar calculation with the 10 day old animals shows a change from 0.18 to 1.6 mmoles/kg/min. Despite the assumptions involved, these are good approximations. An experiment of this type is shown in Figure 6.2. The speed of the changes in the key metabolites measured can be appreciated from this figure. Within minutes following the onset of anoxia produced by decapitation, glycogen and glucose reserves are called upon and are broken down. Lactate begins to accumulate rapidly. In spite of the increased glycolytic flux, the demand for $\sim P$ is too great, and ATP and P-creatine levels fall. It may be seen (Table 6.3) that the lactate flux (11.3 mmoles/kg/min) is in reasonable agreement with the sum of the glucose and glycogen fluxes (8.7 mmoles/kg/min) for the

Figure 6.2   Time course of substrate changes in brain with anoxia.

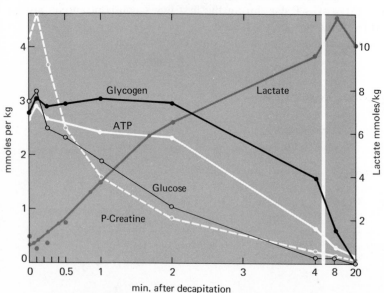

adult and that there is also reasonable agreement in the case of the 11 day old animals (0.6 as compared to 1.6 mmoles/kg/min).

In these experiments, brain levels of the intermediates in glycolysis as well as ∼P compounds were determined. Table 6.4 gives levels of the glycolytic intermediates in 10 day old mouse brain before and 25 seconds after the

TABLE 6.4   GLYCOLYTIC SUBSTRATE LEVELS IN μMOLES/KG WET WEIGHT IN MOUSE BRAIN BEFORE AND AFTER ANOXIA[a] (10 DAY MICE)

Substrate	Initial	After 25 seconds of anoxia
Glycogen	2,780	2,930
Glucose	2,560	1,930
Glucose-6-P	224	91
Fructose-6-P	50	27
Fructose-1,6-diphosphate	27	153
Dihydroxy-acetone-P	13	39
Glyceraldehyde 3-P	0.9	3.3
1,3-Diphospho-glycerate	1	1
3-Phospho-glycerate	25	85
2,3-Diphospho-glycerate	29	29
2-Phospho-glycerate	2.8	8.8
P-pyruvate	3.5	8.5
Pyruvate	39	72
Lactate	770	1,820
α-Glycero-phosphate	48	76
ATP	2,580	2,410
ADP	690	730
AMP	130	130
Phosphocreatine	3,740	2,000
P_i	3,350	4,410

[a] Modified from O. H. Lowry, J. V. Passonneau, F. X. Hasselberger, and D. W. Schulz, "Effect of Ischemia on Known Substrates and Cofactors of the Glycolytic Pathway in Brain," *J. Biol. Chem.*, **239**, 18 (1964).

onset of anoxia. Look first at the initial normal levels. Absolute tissue levels of glycogen and glucose are highest. As one goes down through the glycolytic intermediates, levels decrease progressively through glucose-6-phosphate and fructose-6-phosphate and generally remain low until one reaches pyruvate and lactate, the end products of glycolysis, where they rise again. Note that at pyruvate, the levels are beginning to rise. 1,3-Diphosphoglycerate is present at lowest concentration (in fact, too low to determine). Levels of the phosphorylated intermediates (including P_i) are high. In the adenine nucleotide series, there is a progressive decrease from ATP to ADP to AMP. Phosphocreatine $\sim$P is present in this tissue in a concentration which is approximately equivalent to that of ATP. After 25 seconds of anoxia, changes in tissue concentrations of some of these intermediates occur to affect a decrease in glucose, ATP, and phosphocreatine, an increase in all or most of the glycolytic intermediates and in the end products as well. This is consistent with an activation of glycolysis. This experiment gives us an estimate of the overall rate of glycolysis in vivo as the first prerequisite to answering the question posed at the beginning of this section.

If the catalytic activity of the enzymes of glycolysis themselves are now determined in terms of their maximal potencies or V_{max} (saturating substrate), these values may be tabulated (Table 6.5). The enzyme with the lowest potency on the main pathway of glycolysis (not including glycero-P-dehydrogenase) is *aldolase,* with hexokinase and phosphofructokinase next in line. The maximum potency of aldolase (7.6 mmoles/kg/min, 10 days old) is still several fold in excess of the maximum flux of glycolysis brought on by

TABLE 6.5   **ENZYME ACTIVITIES (10 DAY MICE)**[a]

Enzyme	Maximum Potency or V_{max} mmoles/kg/min
Hexokinase	15.2
P-glucoisomerase	154
P-fructokinase	26.7
Aldolase	7.6
Glycero-P-dehydrogenase	1.93
Glyceraldehyde-P-dehydrogenase	96
P-glycerate kinase	750
P-glycerate mutase	145
Enolase	36
Pyruvate kinase	95
Lactate dehydrogenase	129

[a] Modified from O. H. Lowry and J. V. Passonneau, "The Relationship between Substrates and Enzymes of Glycolysis in Brain." *J. Biol., Chem.* **239,** 31 (1964).

TABLE 6.6   KINETIC CONSTANTS [a]

Enzyme	K_a (Carbohydrate) μm	K_b (Nucleotide) μm	k_2 (V_{max}^b/K_a)	$(A)_{max}/K_a$ [c]
Hexokinase	40	130	380	65
P-glucoseisomerase	210		730	1.1
P-fructokinase	270	25	99	0.18
Aldolase	12		630	18
Glycero-P dehydrogenase	37	2.2	52	1.6
Glycerald-P dehydrogenase	44	22	2,180	0.08
P-glycerate kinase	9	70	83,200	<0.1
P-glycerate mutase	240		600	0.35
Enolase	33		1,090	0.37
Pyruvate kinase	55	180	1,730	0.06
Lactate dehydro-genase	140	2.8	920	0.7

[a] Modified from O. H. Lowry and J. V. Passonneau, "The Relationship between Substrates and Enzymes of Glycolysis in Brain," *J. Biol. Chem.*, **239**, 31 (1965).

[b] Values for V_{max} from Table 6.5.

[c] A_{max} is peak value of substrate level found in tissues.

anoxia (1.6 mmoles/kg/min). Thus under conditions of saturating amounts of substrate, the maximum potency of the enzyme is of sufficient magnitude to account for the rates of glycolysis. Do these conditions of saturating substrate actually occur in the cell? If one compares the tissue levels of substrate (Table 6.4) with the K_m* (K_a and K_b used in Table 6.6 for that substrate), it is clear that the answer is no. In fact, for the six enzymes in the lower portion of glycolysis, tissue substrate levels (A_{max}) are below K_a values ($A_{max}/K_a < 1$) (Table 6.6, last column). At low substrate concentrations (under these circumstances) it can be shown that

$$\frac{V_{max}}{K_m} = k_a \tag{3}$$

which has the dimensions and properties of a first order rate constant, and that the tissue substrate concentration (A) can be estimated from Eq. (4).

$$(A) = \text{flux}/k_a. \tag{4}$$

* For a discussion and definition of K_m and V_{max}, see Chapter 3.8 and Glossary.

In the case of the lower six enzymes of glycolysis, the velocity of the reaction is thus related to the substrate concentration in a first order (linear) manner.

In the upper portion of glycolysis, including the low potency aldolase and excluding the case of phosphofructokinase (which is an exception and will be discussed separately in Chapter 7), the tissue substrate levels may be equal to or greater than the K_m values $[(A)_{max}/K_a > 1)]$. In this set of circumstances, the velocity (flux) is primarily a function of enzyme concentration, and the estimate of rate under saturated conditions is an acceptable approximation.†

Thus, from these experiments, it can be appreciated that the metabolic flux measured in vivo can be adequately accounted for by the activities of the enzymes measured in vitro.

6.3 QUANTITATIVE APPORTIONMENT OF FLOW THROUGH COEXISTING METABOLIC PATHWAYS

The importance of isotopes in metabolic studies has already been discussed (Section 2.2). Evaluation of specific labeling patterns produced when small precursors are converted to products serves to validate metabolic pathways in vivo. In addition, where than one convergent or divergent pathway exists, some estimate can be made of the potential of each pathway under a specific set of conditions, provided the two pathways give different labeling patterns.

An example with isotopic tracers can first be used to illustrate the type of data that suggests that a specific pathway exists in an organism rather than an alternative pathway. ^{14}C carboxyl-labeled acetate was first injected *intravenously* into the jugular vein of the goat. The lactose was isolated from the milk of the udder, hydrolyzed into its constituent glucose and galactose residues, and then each sugar degraded into each of its separate C atoms. The data shown in Table 6.7 (Experiment 1) were obtained. Almost equal amounts of radioactivity were present in the glucose and galactose moieties (46 percent and 51 percent respectively). The labeling pattern in galactose was also similar to glucose, with the exception that relatively more radioactivity was observed in C-1 and C-2 of the galactose.

On the other hand, when the same labeled compound was injected directly into the perfusing fluid of the udder, the data shown in Table 6.7 (Experiment 2) was obtained. Only a minimal amount of radioactivity was observed in the glucose (6.0 percent). The galactose which had almost the total of the radioactivity (96 percent) had an unusual labeling pattern. Most of the radioactivity was in C-3 and C-4, but C-3 had in this instance less than half

---

† Having determined the tissue metabolite levels, it may be of interest to see if they agree or disagree with the equilibrium constants determined for the individual isolated reactions. This has been done in a number of instances and both answers have been found.

TABLE 6.7[a]   **RELATIVE DISTRIBUTION OF RADIOACTIVITY IN GLUCOSE AND GALACTOSE FROM LACTOSE**

	C-1	C-2	C-3	C-4[b]	C-5	C-6
			Experiment 1 (Intravenous Injection)			
Glucose	3	4	78	100	2	2
Galactose	13	23	66	100	3	2
Glucose	46 percent					
Galactose	51 percent					
Lactose	100 percent					
			Experiment 2 (Udder Perfusion)			
Galactose	4	4	41	100	1	2
Glucose	6 percent					
Galactose	96 percent					
Lactose	100 percent					

[a] Modified from H. G. Wood, "Polysaccharides in Biology," Transactions of 3rd Conference of the J. Macy Foundation, G. Springer (ed.), 1958.

[b] Values relative to C-4 set at 100.

the radioactivity of C-4. What was the explanation of the different distributions of radioactivity in the two experiments?

The redistribution of isotope along the carbon chains of precursors and products in the pentose phosphate pathway is shown in Table 6.8. By the nonoxidative reactions of the pentose pathway (Section 4.3) isotope is shifted from the original C-3 position of hexose into the C-2 and C-1 of the pentose (pentose *c*). If labeled pentose is then converted back into hexose through the nonoxidative transaldolase-transketolase pathway, label is shifted into the C-2 and C-1 of hexose, thus diminishing radioactivity in the C-3 position. In these reactions C-4, C-5, and C-6 are not affected. Thus, one can conclude that galactose (Table 6.7, Experiment 1) had undergone more extensive pentose pathway metabolism than had glucose.

The fact that glucose was relatively free of radioactivity when galactose had most of the radioactivity (Table 6.7, Experiment 2) indicated that the two sugars were not arising from a common origin. Two reaction sequences had been proposed for the biosynthesis of lactose.

Sequence A

$$H^+ + \text{glucose-l-P}^{2-} + UTP^{4-} \xrightleftharpoons{\overset{\text{UTP uridyl}}{\text{transferase}}} UDPG^{2-} + PP_i^{3-} \quad \text{(Chapter 4, Equation 20)}$$

$$UDPG^{2-} \rightleftharpoons UDP\,Gal^{2-} \tag{5}$$

TABLE 6.8   TRANSALDOLASE-TRANSKETOLASE MECHANISM OF PENTOSE PATHWAY[a]

Non-Oxidative Mechanism

```
                     1
 1   1          1    2
 2   2      1   2    3           1    3
 3   3      2 3 3    3           2    3
 4 + 4 + 4 → 4+4 +4 → 4 + 4 →    4  + 4
 5   5   5  5 5 5    5   5       5    5
 6   6   6  6 6 6    6   6       6    6
        pentose         pentose pentose
          a                b       c
```

```
        1  1  3   ⅓(1 + 1 + 3)
        2  2  3   ⅓(2 + 2 + 3)
        4  4  4 = 4
        5  5  5   5
        6  6  6   6
        pentose
         a  b  c
```

Oxidative Mechanism

```
               1 CO₂
        1       +
        2       2
        3       3
        4 hexose → 4 pentose
        5       5
        6       6
```

[a] Modified from H. Z. Sable, "Biosynthesis of Ribose and Deoxyribose," *Adv. Enzymol,* **28,** 391 (1966), Interscience Publishers.

$$\text{UDP Gal}^{2-} + \text{G-l-P}^{2-} \longrightarrow \text{lactose 1-P}^{2-} + \text{UDP}^{3-} + \text{H}^+ \tag{6}$$

$$\text{lactose l-P}^{2-} \longrightarrow \text{lactose} + \text{P}_i^{2-} \tag{7}$$

Sequence B

$$\text{H}^+ + \text{glucose-l-P}^{2-} + \text{UTP}^{4-} \rightleftharpoons \text{UDPG}^{2-} + \text{PP}_i^{3-} \quad \text{(Chapter 4, Equation 20)}$$

$$\text{UDPG}^{2-} \rightleftharpoons \text{UDP Gal}^{2-} \tag{5}$$

$$\text{UDP Gal}^{2-} + \text{glucose} \longrightarrow \text{lactose} + \text{UDP}^{3-} + \text{H}^+ \tag{8}$$

These two sequences differ in that in sequence A both glucose and galactose residues come from the same hexose monophosphate source, namely, glucose-l-P. In sequence B, on the other hand, glucose arises not from the hexose monophosphate pool but from free glucose itself (Eq. 8). The differential labeling of the glucose and galactose in the two experiments of Table 6.7 is compatible with two different metabolic sources for the two hexoses, therefore favoring sequence B and not sequence A. The fact that galactose rather than glucose (Experiment 1) had undergone more extensive metabolism through the pentose pathway is also in keeping with this conclusion. The same conclusion can also be drawn from Table 6.7 (Experiment 2) where the amount of radioactivity in the two sugars is also clearly different. The small amount of radioactivity in the glucose as compared with galactose indicates that when glucose enters the mammary gland cell from the udder it is converted directly into lactose without entering into the general metabolism. Subsequent verification of sequence B was obtained when the enzyme catalyzing reaction (8) (UDP galactose: D-glucose-l-galactosyltransferase) was isolated from mammary gland and the reaction established in vitro.*

Next let us consider the apportionment of metabolic flow through coexisting pathways. It is possible to estimate directly the relative contribution of the pentose cycle and glycolysis in any tissue or organism by the following type of experiment. Glucose-1-^{14}C and glucose-6-^{14}C give ^{14}C-CO_2 at the same rate if glycolysis alone operates (coupled to pyruvate oxidation). In the pentose pathway, however, C-1 only is converted to CO_2, C-6 being completely inert (Table 6.8, oxidative mechanism). Thus, if one compares the rate of ^{14}C-CO_2 production from C-1-^{14}C glucose in one experiment, and from C-6-^{14}C glucose in a parallel experiment, the latter gives an estimate of the sum of glycolysis and pentose pathway. The difference between the two rates thus gives the rate of pentose oxidation directly. (Rate of C-6 $\longrightarrow$ CO_2 = rate of glycolysis, rate of C-1 $\longrightarrow$ CO_2 minus rate of C-6 $\longrightarrow$ CO_2 = rate of pentose oxidation.) Obviously this can only be a rough estimate, but under specified conditions the results are quite reproducible and are probably significant. In this way, it has been estimated that in liver the glucose metabolic flow through the two pathways is about equal, while in muscle and yeast, glycolysis accounts for at least 95 percent of the glucose breakdown.

In this chapter we have discussed the in vitro-in vivo problem in terms of the quantitative assessment and the apportionment of metabolic flow. We have seen that in terms of directionality, synthetic energy requiring reactions are usually irreversible. Pyrophosphate release may be a generally occurring biochemical hallmark. The phosphorolytic reactions tend to be generally reversible and degradative, while the hydrolytic reactions are irreversible and degradative.

The quantitative aspects of the problem have also been considered. The relationship of enzyme velocity and substrate levels have led to an evaluation

---

* Thus the elegant interpretation of a specific labeling pattern in an in vivo experiment led the way in establishing a metabolic pathway at the enzymatic level.

of the rate-limiting steps in a reaction sequence. Other quantitative aspects concerned with multiple coexisting pathways were also discussed. It was concluded that one could evaluate and relate metabolic pathways in vivo to in vitro systems.

REFERENCES

Kornberg, A., "On the Metabolic Significance of Phosphorolytic and Pyrophosphorolytic Reactions," *Horizons in Biochemistry*, (M. Kasha and B. Pullman, eds.), Academic Press Inc., New York, 1962.

Lowry, O. H., J. V. Passonneau, F. X. Hasselberger, and D. W. Schulz, "Effect of Ischemia on Known Substrates and Cofactors of the Glycolytic Pathway in Brain," *J. Biol. Chem.*, **239**, 18 (1964).

Lowry, O. H., and J. V. Passonneau, "The Relationship between Substrates and Enzymes of Glycolysis in Brain," *J. Biol. Chem.*, **239**, 31 (1964).

Sable, H. Z., "Biosynthesis of ribose and deoxyribose," *Adv. Enzymol.*, **28**, 391 (1966), Interscience Publishers.

"Studies on Purified Citrate Enzymes—Metabolic Interpretations," in *P. Srere in Metabolic Roles of Citrate*, (T. W. Goodwin, ed.), 1968, p. 11.

Wood, H. G., *Polysaccharides in Biology, Transactions of 3rd Conf.* (G. Springer, ed.), J. Macy Found., Madison Printing Co., Madison, N. J., 1958.

GENERAL ASPECTS OF METABOLIC CONTROL

SEVEN

In Chapter 6 we discussed the *in vitro-in vivo* problem in terms of quantitative assessment and the apportionment of metabolic flow through competing systems. In the present chapter we will discuss this problem from the point of view of the control of metabolic flow. Recall that the process of metabolic control was first introduced in Chapter 1. Here the importance of the so-called intrinsic or nonhormonal controls, as well as the extrinsic or hormonal controls was pointed out. Control mechanisms are necessary for life to proceed within well-defined limits.

As in the case of the ordering of the metabolic pathways (Chapter 2), a number of independent approaches were also employed to study the control of metabolism. These include measurements both of substrate levels *in vivo* and of enzyme activities *in vitro,* under a variety of perturbing conditions, to stress the capacity of the systems under study. *Hormonal perturbations* have proved extremely important in this connection. Whenever possible, specific genetic metabolic blocks are studied since they provide a completely independent approach. Appendix Table A.5 lists the endocrine glands of the mammal and the various hormones secreted by these glands.

The fundamental questions are: "How do we recognize control points in metabolism in vivo?" "How do the control characteristics of the pure enzyme or enzyme system catalyzing the reaction at the control point as determined in vitro relate to the metabolic control in vivo?" Finally, "By what criteria can we determine whether the perturbed metabolic flow in vivo is related to the in vitro effects of the same perturbing agents?"

Metabolic control is affected by certain *regulatory metabolites* (also termed effectors, modifiers, or modulators) which modify enzyme activity. Appendix Table A.6 lists some of the most common regulatory metabolites which act at several sites. Note that they are small, charged, and chemically diverse. They are active in more or less 2 concentration ranges—macro and micro. The words "stimulation" and "inhibition," frequently used to describe altered enzyme activity, are not adequate in the present context. The effector usually *modifies the affinity of the enzyme* for its substrate and/or other reaction components. The terms *positive* or *negative effector* indicate whether the effector has decreased or increased the affinity of the enzyme for its substrate.

Different *regulatory enzymes* have different kinetic regulatory patterns, but a fairly representative pattern for a regulatory enzyme is shown in Figure 7.1. The plot of velocity against substrate concentration is typically S shaped or sigmoid. At low substrate concentration, the slope is increasing. In ordinary Michaelis-Menten kinetics, which is first order, there is a hyperbolic curve with a slope that is decreasing. The sigmoid kinetics requires that more than one molecule of substrate interact in a rate-limiting way with

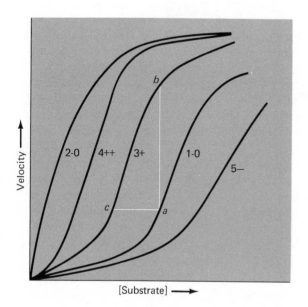

Figure 7.1

Kinetics of a regulatory enzyme. Curve 1-0, an S shaped or sigmoid curve representing a regulated enzyme without effectors; curve 2-0, a hyperbolic curve representing an unregulated enzyme; curves 3+ and 4++, addition of two concentrations of a positive effector; curve 5−, addition of a negative effector. Redrawn from D. E. Atkinson, *Science*, **150**, 851 (1965).

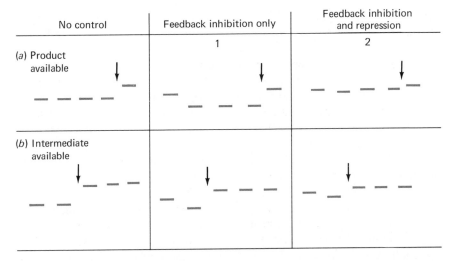

Figure 7.2   Substrate levels in regulated and unregulated enzyme systems. Note the much "tighter" control with both feedback and repression as compared with feedback alone. With product available (a) antecedent substrate levels tend to fall by feedback alone, and are normalized by feedback and repression. A similar situation holds with an intermediate made more available (b), except that the final regulation by feedback and repression is not as normal as in (a). ↓ indicates point of control. Redrawn from D. E. Atkinson, *Science,* **150,** 851 (1965).

each molecule of enzyme. The addition of a positive or negative effector does not typically alter maximum velocity but shifts the whole curve either to the right (negative) or to the left (positive). At intermediate substrate concentrations, the slope remains steep and virtually constant. In Figure 7.1, let the starting point be "a." If a positive effector is added and the substrate concentration is maintained, the velocity is increased to point "b." However, if the velocity were held constant by decreasing the substrate concentration in the presence of the same positive effector, the velocity would be that represented by point "c." In intermediate cases, the new position may be located anywhere in the area "abc." In general, the metabolic controls operate to modify the control exerted by *mass action* (substrate concentration alone). When excess end product accumulates, it inhibits the first or any early enzymatic step in the metabolic pathway [Figure 7.2 (a)] and thus restores metabolite levels *toward* normal. The nature of this negative control may be either an enzyme *inhibition* (a1) and/or an enzyme *repression,* the latter occurring by a decrease in the number of enzyme molecules. If many or all of the enzymes of a sequence are repressed simultaneously, this is known as *coordinate repression.* If this slower control (repression) is applied *in addition* to inhibition, an even closer approximation of metabolite levels toward normal is achieved [Figure 7.2 (a2)]. The same general situation obtains when the tissue level of an intermediate metabolite increases because of increased availability from external reactions, as shown in Figure 7.2 (b).

The opposite type of control is that in which an early metabolite *accelerates* its own metabolism. This represents a positive rather than negative signal. Examples of the stimulation of glycogen synthase by glucose-6-P and of lipogenesis by citrate will be discussed in Chapter 8. In the initiation of glycogenesis and lipogenesis, this mechanism is of obvious importance.

The more finely controlled the regulation of the metabolite levels, the greater the sensitivity of the control that is required. High sensitivity is, therefore, of advantage to the cell. Most regulatory enzymes give sigmoid curves when velocity is plotted against effector concentration as well as against substrate concentration. However, there is a threshold effector concentration below which no control is obtained. Above this threshold, there is a continuously variable, finely controlled response. The sensitivity of the control is usually further enhanced when the enzyme is affected by *both* positive and negative effectors. In this case, the ratio of (both) positive and negative effector concentrations can be varied even more delicately to obtain a heightened sensitivity.

In addition to these "rheostat" controls, there are on-off or "switch" type controls. These occur when a single effector is effective in an almost absolute sense, that is, when there is an absolute requirement for a regulatory metabolite. Several examples are known, including the requirement of pyruvate carboxylase for acetyl-S-CoA, phosphorylase *b* for AMP, and UDPG glycogen synthase *D* form for glucose-6-P (see Section 8.1). In these cases the effector usually increases the *maximum velocity* of the enzyme.

To complete the picture, other factors must also be considered. Many of the regulatory properties are sensitive to small fluctuations in pH which can occur locally at specific intracellular sites where the enzymes are located. It is also possible that regulatory enzymes are attached to structural elements within the cell and thus bear a spatial relationship to other related enzymes. If effectors or other factors affect the conformation of the enzyme molecules, then these changes may also alter the relationship to neighboring enzymes and thus affect the metabolic sequence. These factors related to the supramolecular specificity will undoubtedly become better studied and understood in the future.

7.1 SUBSTRATE MEASUREMENTS AND CROSSOVER POINTS

In Chapter 6 we discussed the determinations of levels of the chain of substrates of glycolysis (Table 6.4), pointing out that the absolute levels of the starting precursors and final products were higher than levels of intermediates in the central portion of the pathway. It is now of interest to reconsider the central portion of the pathway and to examine the changes induced by anoxia. The decrease in glucose levels already discussed is carried forward into the hexose monophosphates, where decreases in glucose-6-P and fructose-6-P levels are also observed. However, with fructose-1,6-diphosphate, in direct contrast to the preceding metabolites, marked increases in tissue concentrations are observed with anoxia. This is an abrupt change, and its effect may be detected along with the remainder of the glycolytic pathway.

For easy visualization, the level of each substrate is plotted (Figure 7.3) as percent of the initial value. This point of change between hexose monophosphate and hexose diphosphate can be easily seen in Figure 7.3 and it becomes progressively greater as the duration of anoxia increases from 4 to 25 seconds. This change indicates that anoxia brings about an *activation or a facilitation* of phosphofructokinase since the level of the substrate fructose-6-P is below normal and the level of the product fructose-1,6-diphosphate is above normal. This point of change (Figure 7.3) is termed a *positive crossover point.*

With substrate measurements one can also observe the opposite type of crossover, a *negative crossover point.* In this instance the effect is to *decelerate* a reaction or reactions, because of an inhibitory influence. An example is provided in recent work where the intermediates in gluconeogenesis starting with alanine as substrate were determined (see also Section 3.5). If tryp-

Figure 7.3   An example of a positive crossover point between glucose-6-P and fructose-1,6-diphosphate. Note that this is heightened by increasing the time of anoxia from four to 25 seconds. From O. H. Lowry, J. V. Passonneau, F. X. Hasselberger and D. W. Schulz, *J. Biol. Chem.,* **239,** 18 (1964).

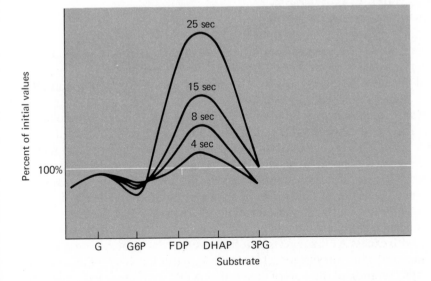

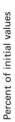

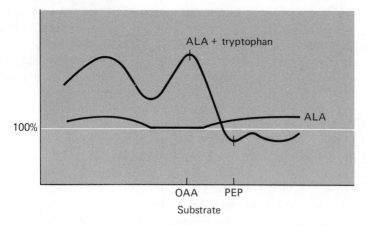

Figure 7.4

An example of a negative crossover point between oxaloacetate and phosphoenolpyruvate in gluconeogenesis brought on by the administration of tryptophan. The control curve was obtained with alanine in the absence of tryptophan. From C. M. Veneziale, P. Walter, N. Kneer, and H. A. Lardy, *Biochemistry,* **6**, 2129 (1967).

tophan is administered, gluconeogenesis was found to be blocked. Figure 7.4 shows that the negative crossover point occurs between oxaloacetate and phosphoenol-pyruvate. Substrates immediately behind oxaloacetate in the pathway are elevated and substrates immediately preceding phosphoenol-pyruvate are slightly depressed from their normal levels. It thus appears that simply measuring substrate levels can point out enzyme sites of control along metabolic pathways. It must be emphasized that while crossover points indicate sites of control, the converse does not necessarily hold; namely, sites of control do not always give crossover points.

7.2 ENZYME ACTIVITY MEASUREMENTS— THE PHOSPHOFRUCTOKINASE MODEL

When substrate measurements indicate a *site* of control, it is of great interest to determine the *mode* of control by *direct enzyme measurements.* There are several instances of this type of correlation, and one of these, phosphofructokinase, will be discussed.

It was demonstrated a number of years ago that phosphofructokinase (PFK) (Figure 4.2, reaction 3) was inhibited by an excess of one of its substrates, ATP. This type of inhibition of a number of kinases by excess ATP is now recognized as a general phenomenon. The interesting point is that the inhibition by excess ATP can be counteracted by the other substrate, fructose-6-P. This kinetic behavior of the enzyme is shown in Figure 7.5. The fact that the velocity with low and high concentrations of fructose-6-P is the same at low ATP concentrations, and only differs after the maximum velocity has been obtained with excess ATP, suggests that fructose-6-P does not influence the K_m (see Glossary) of the enzyme for ATP nor the V_{max} (see Glossary) of the enzyme. One interpretation of this sort of data is that ATP is inhibitory by virtue of its

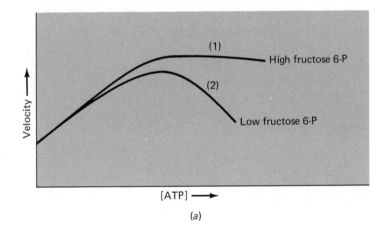

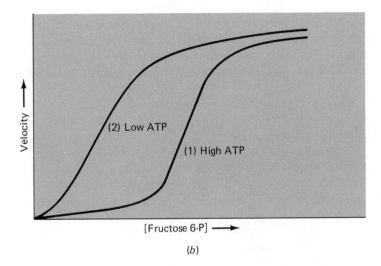

Figure 7.5
Phosphofructokinase kinetics-effects of increasing ATP concentration at low and high fructose-6-P concentrations (Experiment *a*); and of increasing fructose-6-P concentrations at low and high ATP concentrations (Experiment *b*). Redrawn from E. R. Stadtman, *Adv. Enzymol.,* **28,** 41 (1966).

binding to a second or regulatory site which is present and distinct from the substrate site. Fructose-6-P could thus influence the binding constant (K_I) of the enzyme for ATP at this regulatory site. A number of other P-compounds also reverse or "deinhibit" the inhibitory action of excess ATP at this regulatory site. Interestingly, these include just those compounds which would be expected to accumulate in cells in vivo when ATP breaks down (e.g., during anoxia), for example, ADP, AMP, P_i, fructose-1,6-diphosphate, and even NH_4^+ from the breakdown of nitrogen-containing compounds. Thus, it is possible to essentially "turn off" PFK under conditions of high ATP and low fructose-6-P (generally aerobic conditions), or to "turn on" PFK under conditions of decreased ATP and high fructose-6-P together with increased ADP, AMP, P_i, and fructose-1,6-diphosphate (generally anaerobic conditions). This is shown kinetically in Figure 7.5 (*b*). In the presence of high ATP concentrations, the velocity of the reaction is almost zero at low fructose-6-P concentrations. As the concentration of fructose-6-P increases, the enzyme becomes active and finally attains full activity.

PFK has also been shown to be inhibited in a specific way by citrate, one of the early products of the tricarboxylic acid cycle. This is an example of a type of *end product inhibition* (see Glossary) and like the inhibition by ATP, is of great physiological significance.

7.3   HORMONAL PERTURBATIONS—THE PHOSPHORYLASE AND GLYCOGEN SYNTHASE MODELS

Phosphorylase

Other examples in which the elucidation of the *site* of control by crossover points determined from substrate measurements led to the elucidation of the *mode* of control at the enzymatic level is that of the enzymes catalyzing glycogen breakdown and synthesis. In these cases hormonal perturbations were employed.

When the levels of glycogen, glucose-1-P, glucose-6-P and glucose were measured in liver slices in response to treatment with the hormones epinephrine and glucagon, a positive crossover point was present between glycogen and glucose-1-P, indicating control of phosphorylase. Consequently, direct measurements of phosphorylase activity (Figure 4.2, reaction 12) were undertaken by Sutherland. The plan was simple. Slices were incubated in the presence or absence of the hormone under conditions as close to physiological as possible, and at different times of incubation, the slices were removed from the incubation media and frozen. The frozen slices were then homogenized in the cold and the total enzyme activity was determined, always in a *comparative* way, relating the control samples to the hormone-treated samples. In this way, what was emphasized was not the enzyme activity in an *absolute* sense, but rather the *change* which occurred as a result of the hormone treatment.

The results of two such experiments are shown in Figure 7.6. In the presence of the hormones, the activity of phosphorylase was *altered*.

It is interesting to note that the hormones did not *increase* the enzyme activity originally present, but rather *prevented or retarded the decrease* of enzyme activity of the control (Figure 7.6, Experiment 1). If the hormone were added after a 20 minute incubation, it acted to restore the enzyme activity almost back to control levels (Figure 7.6, Experiment 2).

It was soon discovered by a series of elegant experiments with the purified enzymes from both liver and muscle that the inactivation of active phosphorylase occurred with the release of P_i from the enzyme, and that the activa-

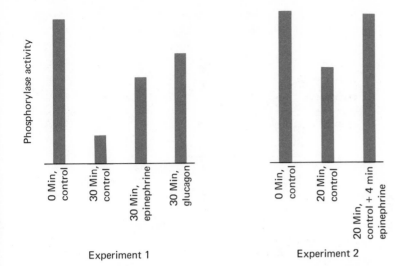

Experiment 1   Experiment 2

Figure 7.6   Phosphorylase activation in liver slices by hormones. Note that phospho-rylase was either reactivated after prior inactivation (Experiment 2) or maintained, i.e., prevented from becoming inactivated (Experiment 1). In this experiment the hormones were incubated with liver slices which were then homogenized and phosphorylase assayed directly in the homogenates or in extracts of the slices. Height of bar represents activity of the enzyme. Redrawn from E. W. Sutherland, Proc. of 3rd Intern. Cong. of Biochem., Academic Press, Inc., New York, 1956.

tion of inactive phosphorylase was a phosphorylation reaction requiring ATP. The reactions are shown in Eqs. 1 and 2.

$$\text{inactive phosphorylase (E)} + n\text{ATP} \longrightarrow \text{active phosphorylase-P (E-P)} + n\text{ADP} \qquad (1)$$

$$\text{active phosphorylase-P (E-P)} + n\text{H}_2\text{O} \longrightarrow \text{inactive phosphorylase (E)} + n\text{P}_i \qquad (2)$$

With these two pieces of information, the hormone effects on phospho-rylase activity, and the recognition of the two distinct forms of the enzyme, inactive E and active E-P, it was possible to test the hormone action as directly involved in the phosphorylation-dephosphorylation reactions. To this end, slices were incubated in $^{32}\text{P}_i$ with and without hormone. After an experimental period tissue was again fixed by freezing and homogenized, phosphorylase was purified, and its radioactivity was determined. As shown in Figure 7.7 the two hormones caused an increase in bound $^{32}\text{P}_i$ (Experiment 1) in the enzyme itself. Most of this $^{32}\text{P}_i$ was released by a liver phosphatase (Experiment 2) which is known to catalyze the reaction of Eq. (2) above. (In all likelihood, the remaining radioactivity was $^{32}\text{P}_i$ which was bound to the enzyme nonspecifically and probably noncovalently. This system will be further discussed in Chapter 8.)

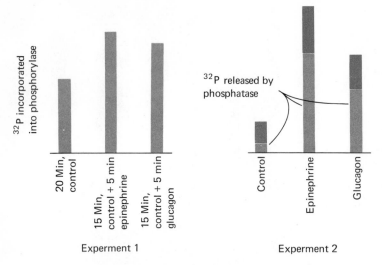

Figure 7.7   Hormonal control of the phosphorylation of the enzyme phosphorylase. Experiment 1. ^{32}P incorporated into phosphorylase without and with hormones. Experiment 2. ^{32}P released from phosphorylase by hydrolysis of seryl-P residues with a phosphoprotein phosphatase. Note that with hormone treatment, larger amounts of ^{32}P were incorporated into the enzyme, which could then be released by phosphatase action. The ^{32}P remaining (not released by phosphatase action) probably represents ^{32}P bound to the enzyme non-specifically, and probably not covalently. Height of bars represents amount of ^{32}P incorporated into the enzyme. Redrawn from E. W. Sutherland, *Proc. of 3rd Intern. Cong. of Biochem.,* Academic Press, Inc., New York, 1956.

Glycogen Synthase

The opposite type of control, namely the stimulation of the synthesis of glycogen from glucose, has been recognized for some time as a prime action of another hormone, insulin. A second hormonally perturbed enzyme system has been identified in which direct enzyme measurements were made at a site indicated as a site of facilitation by *prior* substrate measurements. From studies of the levels of the intermediates glucose-6-P and glucose-1-P in diaphragm muscle following insulin treatment, it became apparent that glucose-1-P levels were relatively decreased in comparison to increased levels of glucose-6-P and glycogen. It was known that glucose-6-P under certain conditions stimulated the enzyme UDPG glycogen synthase in vitro. To design an assay for insulin effects on the synthase, the possible effects of glucose-6-P had to be evaluated. This was done by assaying synthase in parallel (1) directly without added glucose-6-P (minus) and (2) with saturating levels of glucose-6-P added (plus). In this way it was possible to distinguish between direct effects of insulin on synthase and effects of increased glucose-6-P levels (induced by insulin) on synthase. The results in Figure 7.8 show that with normal tissue levels of glucose-6-P (Experiment 1) the insulin

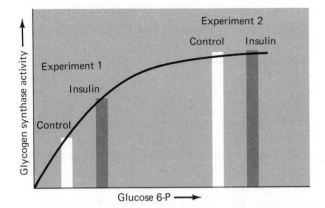

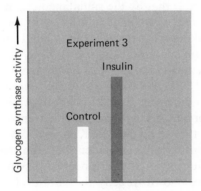

Figure 7.8

Control-insulin glycogen synthase activity difference based on the hypothesis of enzyme activation by glucose-6-P. At low glucose-6-P levels (1) the influence of insulin to stimulate the enzyme is seen. At high glucose 6-P levels when the enzyme is maximally stimulated the difference between the control and the insulin treated enzyme activities disappear (2). When the experiment is done in the complete absence of added glucose and with the tissue levels of glucose-6-P markedly reduced (Experiment 3), the difference between the control and the insulin-treated is maintained indicating that insulin has acted to stimulate the enzyme directly and not via glucose-6-P.

stimulation of synthase could be explained in terms of the difference in glucose-6-P levels. Experiment 2, in which high levels of glucose-6-P had been added, are also consistent with this explanation. However, in Experiment 3, done under conditions in which any excess carbohydrate was removed from the tissue so that the levels of glucose-6-P were extremely low and did not differ significantly in the insulin-treated samples and the control, it is clearly shown that insulin causes an increased activity of synthase which cannot be explained by glucose-6-P effects.

Investigation of the biochemical mechanism of the insulin-induced glycogen synthase activation revealed that this enzyme also exists in an active and an inactive form, and that these forms can be distinguished by their dependence on the presence of glucose-6-P for enzyme activity. These two forms were termed synthase I (independent of glucose 6-P) and synthase D (dependent on glucose 6-P. The I form is, therefore, the "*active*" (or more active) form of the enzyme, and the D form is the "inactive" (or less active) form. An interconversion mechanism similar to that of phosphorylase was then discovered, in which the I form was converted to the D form by an

ATP-dependent phosphorylation of the enzyme, and in the reverse direction, the D form converted to the I form with the release of P_i [Eqs. (3) and (4)].

$$\text{glycogen synthase } I \text{ (E)} + n\text{ATP} \longrightarrow \text{glycogen synthase } D\text{-P (E-P)} + n\text{ADP} \tag{3}$$

$$\text{glycogen synthase } D\text{-P (E-P)} + n\text{H}_2\text{O} \longrightarrow \text{glycogen synthase } I \text{ (E)} + n\text{P}_i \tag{4}$$

Note that although the biochemical mechanisms of Eqs. (3) and (4) are identical to Eqs. (1) and (2), the biological polarity or "sense" is inverted. The control potentiality of this *dual reciprocal* system is such that in the case of phosphorylase, phosphorylation with ATP activates and dephosphorylation inactivates; in the case of glycogen synthase phosphorylation inactivates and dephosphorylation activates the enzyme. This aspect and the relation to hormonal control will be further discussed in Chapter 8. The important principle to be illustrated here is that by the simultaneous control of two opposing enzyme systems, the *direction* of metabolic flow is dramatically influenced. Another point worth making is the special experimental conditions needed to detect the insulin effect on synthase. The special assay ($\pm$ glucose-6-P) was required to detect the change in enzyme activity brought on by the hormonal perturbation. Had the activity of the fully stimulated enzyme (+ glucose-6-P) been measured alone, no difference would have been detected. The interrelationships of the phosphorylase and synthase interconversions are summarized in Figure 7.9. With all three enzymes, PFK, phosphorylase, and glycogen synthase, there is a "comfortable" agreement between the crossover points which indicate metabolic control at the respective enzyme sites and the enzyme studies which have shown directly the nature of the control of the enzyme catalysts themselves.

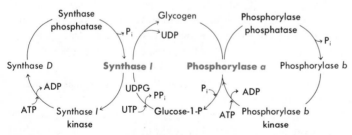

Figure 7.9   Interconversion of phosphorylase and glycogen synthase. Both enzymes are interconverted by a phosphorylation-dephosphorylation reaction sequence involving separate phosphoprotein kinases and phosphatases. Note that the biological polarity is reversed in the two enzyme systems; i.e., phosphorylation activates phosphorylase and inactivates synthase, whereas dephosphorylation inactivates phosphorylase and activates synthase. (See also Fig. 8.2 and 8.3).

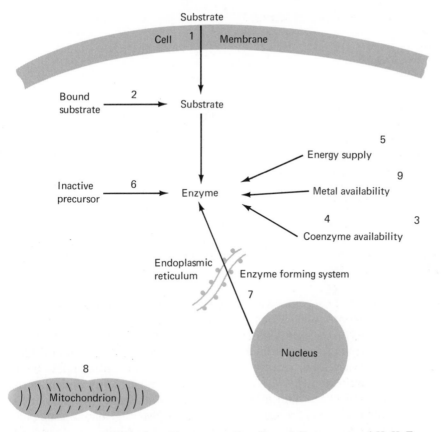

Figure 7.10   Cellular sites of hormone action. From J. Tepperman and H. H. Tepperman, *Pharm. Rev.,* **12,** 301 (1960).

7.4   CELLULAR SITES OF HORMONAL CONTROL MECHANISMS— A LISTING

Hormonal or externally imposed controls appear to be "superimposed" on metabolic controls at all levels. With hormonal controls, we must be concerned with mechanisms of action at the cellular level as well as with loci of action in a biochemical sense. This may come about because "supramolecular" arrangements within the cell and within cellular organelles may be intimately related to hormone actions.

The potential cellular sites of hormone action are illustrated in Figure 7.10. The figure schematically shows the cell membrane, the nucleus, the mitochondrion, and the endoplasmic reticulum. Nine potential mechanisms of hormone action are numbered in relation to the cellular organelles and are listed in Table 7.1.

TABLE 7.1   CELLULAR HORMONE MECHANISMS OF ACTION[a]

1. Control of membrane permeability
2. Release of bound substrate intracellularly
3. Control of coenzyme availability
4. The hormone itself functioning as a coenzyme
5. Control of the availability of energy as $\sim$P
6. Control of inactive-active enzyme interconversions
7. Control of enzyme formation and degradation
8. Control of mitochondrial structure and function
9. Control of ion, especially metal ion, availability

[a] From J. Tepperman and H. M. Tepperman, *Pharm. Rev.*, **12**, 301 (1960).

7.5 CRITERIA FOR JUDGING THE IN VIVO SIGNIFICANCE OF IN VITRO HORMONE EFFECTS

In discussing the *in vitro-in vivo* problem in Chapter 6, we outlined the two experimental approaches which have been used to study this question, namely, (1) in vitro ⟶ in vivo and (2) the in vivo ⟶ in vitro. Some of the reasons for the success of method (1) were pointed out. Method (2) has been rather unsuccessful because of the failure to meaningfully relate the in vitro to in vivo effects. This lack of success has been singularly evident in the case of biochemical mechanisms of hormone action, where the landscape is literally strewn with the "parched bones of dead theories" based principally on in vitro experiments. Hunter and Lowry have thoughtfully reviewed this question in terms of the action of drugs on enzymes. The following list of five criteria is modified from their review:

1. that the enzyme concerned is affected by the hormone or drug in the living cell in the same way (manner) as it is in vitro;
2. that the effect of the hormone or drug on the enzyme explains quantitatively the overall metabolic effects of the hormone or drug;
3. that the in vitro enzyme effect occurs with a concentration of hormone or drug no greater than that necessary to produce the in vivo effect;
4. that the in vitro effect has the same pattern of organ specificity as the in vivo effect. That is to say, that organs which respond in vivo respond in vitro, and organs which are unresponsive in vivo are likewise unresponsive in vitro.
5. that the structure activity relationship of a series of chemically related compounds with a gradation of biological activity (for example, a series of steroids) is similar in its action pattern in vitro and in vivo.

These criteria should constantly be kept in mind in judging the biological significance of a hormone or drug effect observed in vitro.

7.6   FEEDBACK CONTROLS IN BACTERIAL SYSTEMS

The influence of *feedback control* as well as *directionality* in metabolism has been elegantly studied in bacterial systems. Here four different examples of feedback control mechanisms have been elucidated and these will be briefly discussed as illustrations of how the cell meets the requirements for specific regulation.

Enzyme Multiplicity

This is illustrated diagrammatically in Figure 7.11. In *E. coli*, the phosphorylation of aspartate to aspartyl-P is the first reaction (1) in the biosynthesis of lysine, methionine, threonine, and isoleucine (in color). To regulate this highly branched pathway, three separate aspartokinases are present which are regulated by different effector substances. One of these (*a*) is specifically and completely inhibited by lysine. The synthesis of this enzyme is also *repressed* by lysine (for a discussion of repression, see Section 7.7). The second (*b*) is present in small amounts and is specifically inhibited by homoserine. The third (*c*) is specifically and completely inhibited by threonine. Thus synthesis of aspartyl-P is insured even in the presence of an excess of one of the amino acid end products, but the overall rate of aspartyl-P synthesis depends on the extent to which each or all of the three pathways are turned "on" or "off." In order to further direct the diminished aspartyl-P along the desired pathway, further controls are obviously required. These are also present and shown in the figure by the selective inhibition of the first

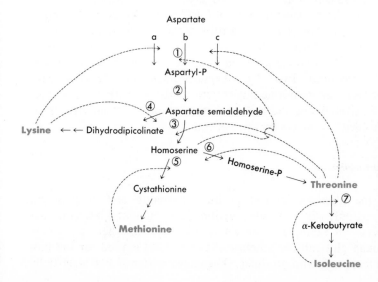

Figure 7.11

Metabolic control of lysine, methionine, and isoleucine synthesis by enzyme multiplicity feedback inhibition. Catalytic reactions ⟶. Allosteric inhibitions ---→. The three aspartokinases (1) *a*, *b*, and *c*, are separately inhibited by lysine, homoserine, and threonine. Directionality is imposed by further inhibitions at the branch points beyond lysine (4), methionine (5), and threonine (6). From E. R. Stadtman, *Adv. Enzymol.,* **28,** 41 (1966).

step diverging from the common pathway (branching step) by the amino
acid end product, e.g., methionine inhibition of reaction (5); lysine inhibition
of reaction (4); and threonine inhibition of reaction (6). In this way, directionality is controlled.

Concerted Feedback Inhibition

Here two or more end products must be present *simultaneously* and in excess amounts to give inhibition of the key enzyme. An example of this type
of feedback regulation is the aspartokinase of *Rps. capsulatus* and *B. poly-
myxa* which in these organisms exists as a single enzyme. As expected, the
single enzyme form is not inhibited by lysine, threonine, methionine, or
isoleucine alone. When excess lysine and threonine are present together,
however, the enzyme is inhibited. This mechanism does not permit as fine a
regulation as does enzyme multiplicity but does permit the metabolic flow
to continue in the presence of an excess of only one end product.

Cooperative Feedback Inhibition

Here each end product does cause *partial* inhibition of the key enzyme,
but the simultaneous presence of two or more end products result in a cooperative inhibition in such a way that the total inhibition is greater than the
simple sum of the individual effects. To illustrate, consider that amidophosphoribosyl transferase (Figure 5.19), the enzyme catalyzing the first specific
reaction of purine biosynthesis, is inhibited by various nucleotide end products. We will consider that a given concentration of GMP gives 10 percent
inhibition and a given concentration of AMP also gives 10 percent inhibition.
The combination of these concentrations of GMP and AMP does not simply
give the algebraic sum (10 percent + 10 percent of the remaining 90 percent =
19 percent), but a much higher value, such as 50 percent inhibition. It is of
considerable interest that cooperative inhibition is not observed with every
combination of nucleotides. Two 6-hydroxypurine nucleotides (GMP + IMP,
for example) or two 6-aminopurine nucleotides (AMP + ADP, for example)
show simple additive effects, and a combination of one representative from
each series is needed for the cooperative effect.

Cumulative Product Inhibition

In this type the inhibition by each product is separate and independent,
and it appears to apply when a single reaction is common for a large number
of end products. An example is shown in Figure 7.12, where glutamine
generated through glutamine synthetase (Section 5.16) is used for the biosynthesis of at least eight end products. The enzyme from *E. coli* is partially

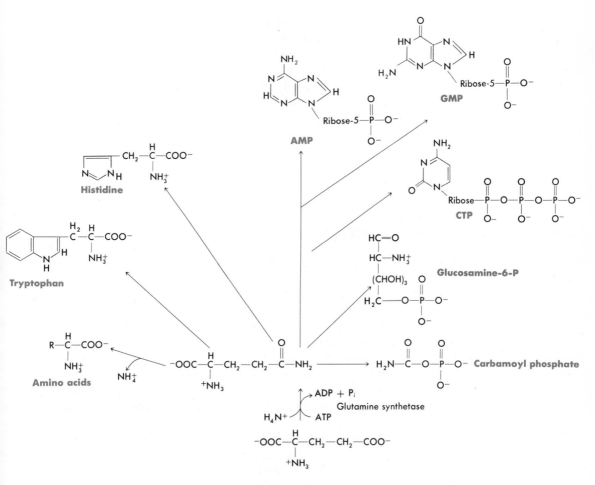

Figure 7.12 Cumulative feedback in glutamine metabolic pathways. All eight products inhibit glutamine synthetase in a cumulative manner. From E. R. Stadtman, *Adv. Enzymol.,* **28**, 41 (1966).

inhibited by saturating concentrations of each of the end products, tryptophan, AMP, GMP, glucosamine-6-P, histidine, carbamoylphosphate, glycine, and alanine, added separately. Other nitrogen compounds not products of amide nitrogen transfer from glutamine are not inhibitory. Various combinations of end products inhibit independently. For example, consider that separately tryptophan inhibits 16 percent, CTP, 14 percent, carbamoyl-P, 13 percent, and AMP, 41 percent. What would be the total inhibition by all four together? This can be calculated as follows: tryptophan inhibits 16 percent, therefore the remaining activity would be 84 percent; CTP inhibits 14 percent, therefore the inhibition would be 14 percent of 84, and the remaining activity 84 − 11.8 or 72.2 percent; the inhibition by carbamoyl-P would be 13 percent of 72.2 or 9.4 percent, the remaining activity would be 72.2 − 9.4 or 62.8 percent; the inhibition by AMP would be 41 percent of 62.8 or 25.8 percent, the remaining activity would be 62.8−25.8 or 37 percent of the original activity. Thus, in the presence of all eight inhibitors, the enzyme can be totally "turned off." With each inhibitor alone, only a partial inhibition is obtained. The elucidation of these mechanisms of control in bacterial systems constitutes a major advance in our knowledge of control mechanisms in general.

7.7 GENETIC BLOCKS OF METABOLIC CONTROLS*

In Chapter 2, the importance of genetic blocks, both bacterial and human, in delineating metabolic pathways was pointed out. In studying metabolic control, genetic mutants, especially bacterial, have been equally important.

It is a remarkable fact that in some bacteria the structural genes governing the biosynthesis of the enzymes of a given metabolic pathway are grouped in the exact order of the sequence of reactions in that pathway. For example, in *Salmonella* the structural genes for histidine biosynthesis are so arranged. This means that the chromosome contains the information *both* for the structures of the various enzymes and for the metabolic pathway catalyzed by these enzymes. In other words, the ordering of the reactions into the metabolic pathway, a remarkably impressive amount of information, is also dictated by the chromosome. A group of such consecutive genes forming an operational unit has been termed an *operon* by Jacob and Monod.

Enzymes whose structural genes are located in an operon are all *induced* or *repressed* by low-molecular-weight substances to the *same* extent. Enzymes whose structural genes are *not* located on the same operon are *induced* or *repressed* to *different* extents. This is termed *coordinate* or *noncoordinate repression,* respectively. For a schematic representation of the β-galactosidase operon see Figure 7.13.

It is worthwhile at this point to define induction and repression. In order to synthesize a given enzyme, the structural gene is an absolute requirement. In many cases, it alone is not sufficient. In addition, some low-molecular-weight compound somewhat related to the substrate of the enzyme-catalyzed reaction is required to be present for enzyme synthesis to occur. The process is termed *induction.* Other low-molecular-weight substances which may be products or somehow related to products of the enzyme-catalyzed reaction act as *corepressors* (see Glossary) by preventing the formation of enzyme in the presence of the structural gene. This is termed *repression.*

What coordinate induction or repression suggests is that when the DNA of an operon is copied as messenger RNA (see Section 5.13), the copying

* See also the book by Wold in this series, Chapter 8.

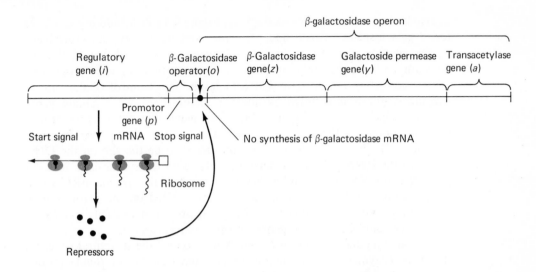

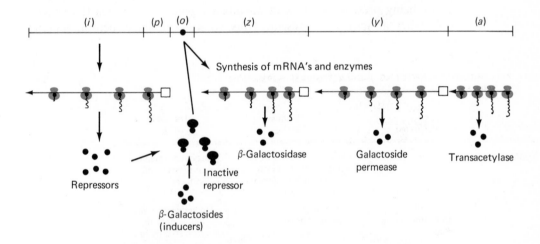

Figure 7.13   Schematic representation of the interaction of repressor, inducer, and operator to control synthesis of β galactosidase operon in E. coli. The three structural genes Z, Y, and a, code for the synthesis of the proteins galactosidase, galactose permease, and transacetylase respectively. The control or regulator genes, regulator i, promotor P and operator 0 are as shown. From J. D. Watson, *Molecular Biology of the Gene*, W. A. Benjamin, 1965.

starts at one end of the segment of the DNA molecule and proceeds in a linear fashion through to the other end.

Structural genes specify the structures of enzymes in terms of amino acid sequences. They have no direct control over the *rate* at which the

enzymes are produced. For example in Figure 7.13 Z, Y, and a genes code
for β galactosidase, galactoside permease, and transacetylase respectively.
In the absence of control, the rate of enzyme production would thus be
constant and depend only on the number of structural genes, the ribosomes, activating enzymes, amino acid levels, etc. Control of the rate of
enzyme synthesis is dictated by another set of genes, the *regulator* genes
designated as i, p, and o (Figure 7.13). The i gene codes for a repressor protein which binds to the DNA of the operator (o) gene thus preventing transcription. The promotor gene (p) is considered to be the site on the DNA
at which the RNA polymerase enzyme, catalyzing the synthesis of messenger RNA (mRNA) binds, and is thus the site where the specific mRNA synthesis begins. In contrast to operator genes, located on the chromosomes
which they control, the other regulator genes are not necessarily so located.
They may control structural genes on other chromosomes.

The three regulator genes in *E. coli*, which control the structural genes for
the three enzymes involved in the uptake and cleavage of β-galactosides,
can mutate (Table 7.2). Thus an inactive i gene (i⁻), gives rise to cells which
produce enzyme (e.g., β-galactosidase) *constitutively*, that is, without an inducer being present. Cells with an intact i gene (i⁺) produce the enzyme
only when an inducer is present. Thus, where (z) is the structural gene for

**TABLE 7.2   MUTATIONS AFFECTING β-GALACTOSIDASE FORMATION
IN E. COLI** [a]

Mutation	Gene Affected	Transcription Effect	Translation Effect
None		Operator blocked by repressor; repressor removed by combination with inducer	Enzyme formed only in presence of inducer
z⁻	Part of structural gene forming active enzyme	Structure of active center altered	No active enzyme; inactive protein formed only in presence of inducer
Oᶜ	Operator part of structural gene	Operator active, unable to combine with repressor	Enzyme formed, even in absence of inducer
i⁻	Regulator gene	No repressor formed	Enzyme formed, even in absence of inducer
iˢ	Regulator gene	Modified repressor formed, unable to combine with inducer	No enzyme formed, even in presence of inducer
p⁻	Promotor gene	RNA polymerase unable to transcribe	Make only a few percent of enzyme(s)

[a] Adopted from M. Dixon and E. C. Webb, *The Enzymes,* 2nd Edition, Academic Press, N.Y., 1964.

the galactosidase enzyme, (z−) will produce no enzyme, whereas (z+) will produce enzyme. Now, (i− z+) will produce enzyme constitutively, whereas (i+ z+) will produce enzyme only by induction. If two chromosomes (i+ z−) and (i− z+) are present together in a cell, the enzyme is formed only by induction, indicating that (i+) is dominant and (i−) is recessive.

Thus, (i+) in the absence of an inducer *prevents* the formation of the enzyme, whereas (i−) *allows* the formation of the enzyme. If an inducer is present, the negative influence of (i+) is overcome. This indicates that (i+) produces a material which normally inhibits enzyme formation, whereas (i−) does not. This material has been termed *repressor* and identified as a protein. The repressor acts by combining at the o gene and preventing transcription. This is borne out by the fact that the operator itself can mutate so that it becomes constitutive, the mutation termed (O^c). In this instance, the operator no longer is able to combine with the cytoplasmic repressor. In other words, the (O^c) and the (i−) mutations have much the same effect but for different reasons.

One reasonable effect of the inducer could, therefore, be to combine with the repressor and thus prevent it from combining with the operator. Induction (considered as +) is seen to consist of a derepression (the sum of two −'s), thus allowing the bringing together of the concepts of induction and repression. In both, enzyme production is blocked by combination of the cytoplasmic repressor with the operator. The difference is that in induction the free cytoplasmic repressor combines with the operator, while its inducer bound form does not. In repression, the free cytoplasmic repressor does not combine with the operator (considered as +), while its inducer (or in this case termed corepressor) bound form does (considered as −). These relationships are shown diagrammatically in Figure 7.14, which illustrates the uncombined active repressor acting to prevent mRNA synthesis (a) and the uncombined inactive repressor permitting mRNA synthesis (b).

An additional mutant of the regulator gene (i^s) has been discovered. With this gene, none of the enzymes of the metabolic pathway are formed in the presence of the inducer and with normal structural genes. Even an (i+) gene in another chromosome has no effect. Thus, (i^s) is dominant over (i+). The interpretation is that (i^s) forms a cytoplasmic repressor which can no longer combine, or combines very poorly with inducer but still can combine with operator. Promotor mutants (p− in Table 7.2) respond to inducer, but even when fully induced, make only a few percent of the adoptive enzyme(s) as compared with wild-type strains.

7.8 LEVELS OF METABOLIC CONTROL—A CLASSIFICATION

From the foregoing discussion, it is evident that controls may be exercised at differing levels in responsive systems. Here we will list these levels cate-

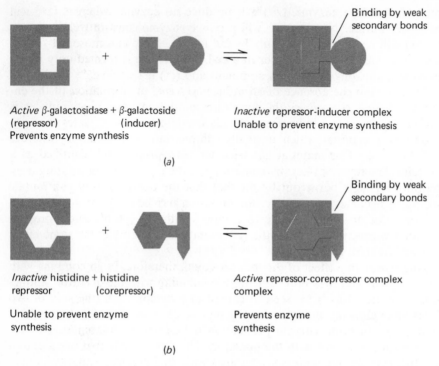

Active β-galactosidase + β-galactoside
(repressor)   (inducer)
Prevents enzyme synthesis

Inactive repressor-inducer complex
Unable to prevent enzyme synthesis

(*a*)

Inactive histidine + histidine
repressor   (corepressor)

Unable to prevent enzyme
synthesis

Active repressor-corepressor complex
complex

Prevents enzyme
synthesis

(*b*)

Figure 7.14   Schematic representation of inducer and corepressor action to control synthesis of β galactosidase operon. (*a*) uncombined repressor is active—induction; (*b*) combined repressor is active—repression. From J. D. Watson,
Molecular Biology of the Gene, W. A. Benjamin, 1965.

gorically. It is to be emphasized that this type of classification, like most, is
arbitrary.

The classification is given in Table 7.3. There are two principal categories, A and B. In A, control is exerted by an alteration of enzyme activity
with no change in the number of enzyme molecules. In B, there is an increase or decrease in the number of enzyme molecules. In the latter B group
are the induction and repression mechanisms discussed in the preceding
section, where control is exerted at the transcription level, that is, at the level
involving the transfer of information from DNA into RNA (B1). Control is
also possible at the translational level, that is, the conversion of the RNA
message into the protein amino acid sequence (B2). Control of enzyme
degradation is also possible. It is to be noted that this is obviously a gross
oversimplication for purposes of classification. Control at one level may
markedly affect another level, since the levels are so closely interrelated.

In the A group, we are concerned with two principal subgroups. In A1,
control is exerted by low-molecular-weight substances—substrates or allo-

TABLE 7.3 BIOCHEMICAL CONTROLS—A CLASSIFICATION

A. ALTERATION OF ENZYME ACTIVITY
  1. Control by low-molecular-weight substances
     (a) Substrate control
     (b) Allosteric effector control

  2. Control by enzyme or protein modification
     (a) Covalent modification—another enzyme may be required
        1) Control by irreversible covalent modification
        2) Control by reversible covalent modification
     (b) Noncovalent modification—protein-protein interactions

B. ALTERATION OF NUMBER OF ENZYME MOLECULES
  1. Control at transcription level
  2. Control at translation level
  3. Control of enzyme degradation

steric modifiers. In subgroup A2, on the other hand, control is brought about by altering the protein enzymes themselves.

In subgroup A1, probably the simplest level of control is exerted by the substrate concentration itself [A1 (a)]. If the tissue substrate level is about or below the K_m of the enzyme, the velocity will be related to the substrate concentration by the Michaelis-Menten relationship, Eq. (5).

$$v = \frac{V_{\max}S}{K_m + S} \tag{5}$$

As was shown in Section 6.2, this is the case for the six enzymes of the lower portion of glycolysis, where

$$k_a = \frac{V_{\max}}{K_m} \tag{6}$$

k_a has the properties of a first order velocity constant. Under these conditions, the tissue substrate concentration A controls flux as per (7)

$$A = \frac{\text{flux}}{k_a} \tag{7}$$

In the next class, A1 (b), the control is by allosteric low-molecular-weight activators or inhibitors. In the present chapter, we have discussed several such substances and given examples, including AMP, which activates phosphorylase, glucose-6-P, which activates glycogen synthase, and the various other end products involved in feedback inhibition.

The examples of control by single allosteric substances are probably oversimplified from the biological point of view and only reflect the limitations in our knowledge. In the cell, a number of modifiers are present at the same time which are in contact with the enzyme and *multiple* or *coordinated* substrate and allosteric control is probably of greater biological significance.

In category A2, regulation is achieved by alteration of the protein enzymes. This category is subdivided into several subgroups. In subgroup A2 (a), there is covalent alteration of the enzyme. This frequently means that an additional enzyme or "second order" catalyst is required to catalyze the structural alteration, setting up a hierarchical system. In the A2 (b) subgroup, there is no covalent alteration, rather, regulation is achieved by noncovalent protein interactions.

The covalent change may be irreversible [A2 (a), (1)], usually a hydrolytic modification. Examples are the well-known conversions of the pancreatic zymogens into their active enzyme forms (Section 5.1). The covalent modifications may also be reversible [A2 (a) (2)]. Two examples, phosphorylase and glycogen synthase, were just discussed in Section 7.3. Another fascinating case is the recently discovered bacterial glutamine synthetase system (Chapter 9) where the enzyme may be present either in an adenylated or nonadenylated form. Further details of the different classes will be discussed in subsequent chapters.

These then are the chief types of control. Undoubtedly, additional types exist and will be discovered in the future. What is already clear is that control exists at apparently all levels. Nature leaves little or nothing to chance.

In this chapter, we have discussed the in vitro-in vivo problem in terms of the question of the control of metabolism. The varied approaches and techniques used to work out the control mechanisms were presented, followed by the classification of the hormonal controls in cellular terms and of the control mechanisms in biochemical terms. In the remaining chapters, we will consider the control of carbohydrate and lipid metabolism, N-metabolism, and energy metabolism.

REFERENCES

Atkinson, D. E., "Biological Feedback Control at the Molecular Level," *Science,* **150,** 851 (1965).

Dixon, M., and E. C. Webb, *Enzymes,* 2nd ed., Academic Press, Inc., New York, 1964.

Hunter, F. E., Jr. and O. H. Lowry, "The Effects of Drugs on Enzyme Systems," *Pharm. Rev.,* **8,** 89 (1956).

Larner, J., C. Villar-Palasi, and D. J. Richman, "Insulin-Stimulated Glycogen Formation in Rat Diaphragm," *Ann. N. Y. Acad. Sci.,* **82,** 345 (1959).

Lowry, H. Pannonneau, J. V., Hasselberger, F. X., and D. W. Schulz, *J. Biol. Chem.,* **239,** 18 (1964).

Stadtman, E. R., "Allosteric Regulation of Enzyme Activity," *Adv. Enzymol.,* **28,** 41 (1966).

Sutherland, E. W., *Hormonal Regulatory Mechanisms,* Proc. of 3rd Intern. Cong. of Biochem., Acad. Press, Inc., New York, 1956.

Tepperman J., and H. M. Tepperman, "Some Effects of Hormones on Cells and Cell Constituents," *Pharm. Rev.,* **12,** 301 (1960).

Veneziale, C. M., Walter, P., Kneer, N., and H. A. Lardy, "Influence of L-Tryptophan and Its Metabolites on Gluconeogenesis in the Isolated, Perfused Liver," *Biochemistry,* **6,** 2129 (1967).

Watson, J. D., *Molecular Biology of the Gene,* W. A. Benjamin, 1965.

EIGHT

INTEGRATION AND CONTROL OF CARBOHYDRATE AND LIPID METABOLISM

In Chapters 6 and 7, we discussed the in vivo-in vitro problem in terms of quantitative aspects and control. In the next three chapters, we will discuss separately the control of the metabolism of the fuels (carbohydrates and lipids), the nitrogen compounds, and energy. This approach has the advantage of making the presentation easier to follow. The disadvantage is that it fragments metabolism. For this reason, the control of energy metabolism follows the other two, since the integrative aspects can best be developed in this order. Several control sites in carbohydrate and lipid metabolism will be considered in this chapter. These are shown in Figure 8.1. They are glycogen α-1,4 bond synthesis and degradation (labeled I); fructose-6-P phosphorylation and dephosphorylation (labeled II); glucose phosphorylation and dephosphorylation (labeled III); and pyruvate phosphorylation and dephosphorylation (labeled IV). In the tricarboxylic acid cycle, the isocitrate dehydrogenase and citrate synthase control sites will be discussed; and in fatty acid synthesis, the acetyl-S-CoA carboxylation reaction to malo-

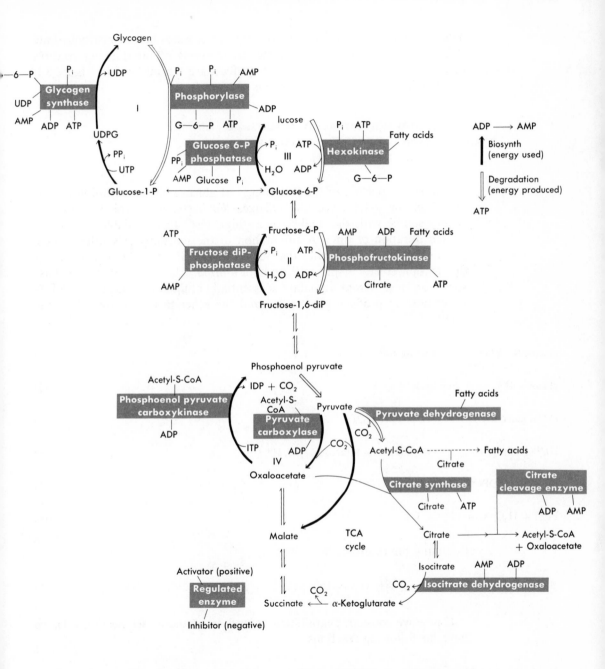

Figure 8.1   Overall regulation of carbohydrate and lipid metabolism. Sites I, II, III, and IV are glycogen synthesis and degradation (I), fructose-6-P phosphorylation and dephosphorylation (II), glucose phosphorylation and dephosphorylation (III), and pyruvate phosphorylation and dephosphorylation (IV). Modified from E. R. Stadtman, *Advances in Enzymology,* **28,** 41 (1966). D. E. Atkinson, *Science,* **150,** 851 (1965).

nate will be considered. Finally, the interrelationships between carbohydrate and lipid metabolism will be reviewed in terms of interlocking controls through metabolites. The regulatory effects are summarized in Figure 8.1, which will serve as an outline for this chapter.

8.1 COVALENT AND NON-COVALENT, HORMONAL AND NON-HORMONAL CONTROL OF GLYCOGEN 1,4 BOND SYNTHESIS AND DEGRADATION

In glycogen a portion of the free energy of glucose phosphorylation is conserved in the α-1,4 glycosidic linkages. Glycogen is a rapidly mobilized energy source with the quality of a "high test" fuel available for only a limited duration of time. A summation of the reactions of synthesis, Eqs. (1) through (6), demonstrates that the cost is 2ATP's, sum Eq. (7), assuming that pyrophosphate is split to P_i and not utilized. This is probably a good assumption since pyrophosphatase is essentially ubiquitous. One of the ATP's is required to produce glucose-1-P and the other to regenerate UTP from UDP.

$$\text{glucose} + \text{ATP}^{4-} \longrightarrow \text{glucose-6-P}^{2-} + \text{ADP}^{3-} + \text{H}^+ \tag{1}$$

$$\text{glucose-6-P}^{2-} \rightleftharpoons \text{glucose-1-P}^{2-} \tag{2}$$

$$\text{H}^+ + \text{glucose-1-P}^{2-} + \text{UTP}^{4-} \rightleftharpoons \text{UDPG}^{2-} + \text{PP}_i^{3-} \tag{3}$$

$$\text{UDPG}^{2-} + (\text{glucose})_n \longrightarrow \text{UDP}^{3-} + (\text{glucose})_{n+1} + \text{H}^+ \tag{4}$$

$$\text{ATP}^{4-} + \text{UDP}^{3-} \rightleftharpoons \text{ADP}^{3-} + \text{UTP}^{4-} \tag{5}$$

$$\text{PP}_i^{3-} + \text{H}_2\text{O} \longrightarrow 2\text{P}_i^{2-} + \text{H}^+ \tag{6}$$

Summing the reactions, we obtain

$$\text{glucose} + 2\text{ATP}^{4-} + (\text{glucose})_n + \text{H}_2\text{O} \longrightarrow (\text{glucose})_{n+1} + 2\text{ADP}^{3-} + 2\text{P}_i^{2-} + 2\text{H}^+ \tag{7}$$

If now we consider degradation as well as synthesis (see Section 4.1), we have the following reactions:

$$\text{H}^+ + \text{glucose-1-P}^{2-} + \text{UTP}^{4-} \rightleftharpoons \text{UDPG}^{2-} + \text{PP}_i^{3-} \tag{3}$$

$$\text{UDPG}^{2-} + (\text{glucose})_n \longrightarrow \text{UDP}^{3-} + (\text{glucose})_{n+1} + \text{H}^+ \tag{4}$$

$$(\text{glucose})_{n+1} + \text{P}_i^{2-} \longrightarrow (\text{glucose})_n + \text{glucose-1-P}^{2-} \tag{8}$$

$$PP_i^{3-} + H_2O \longrightarrow 2P_i^{2-} + H^+ \tag{6}$$

Summing, we obtain

$$UTP^{4-} + H_2O \longrightarrow UDP^{3-} + P_i^{2-} + H^+ \tag{9}$$

Thus, recycling glucosyl residues in glycogen synthesis and breakdown (recall Figure 4.4), in essence, amounts to a glycogen-dependent hydrolysis of UTP into UDP and P_i. If these reactions proceeded uncontrolled, it would obviously be a costly process for the cells. Control mechanisms must, therefore, exist for synthesis as well as for degradation, such that glycogen can be produced under conditions of energy excess and subsequently used when energy is needed. These control processes are extremely rapid, occurring within seconds, highly efficient, and of a complex nature. The important feature is the interdependent and complementary manner in which glycogen synthesis and glycogen breakdown are regulated, with the net result that when one is turned on, the other is turned off and vice versa.

Let us consider first the degradation in terms of the reversible activation of the key enzyme phosphorylase (see Section 7.3). These reactions arranged in a hierarchical manner are shown in Figure 8.2 with the phosphorylase-catalyzed reaction labeled (1) and the enzyme interconversions involved in the activation of phosphorylase ordered above labeled (2), (3). The important hormonal controls are labeled (4), (5). Note that the product in each step is *activator* of the subsequent step (not a substrate as in the usual arrangement of a sequence of steps). This leads to an amplification effect and is, therefore, termed a *cascade* of reactions [see Wold in this series and Figure 1.3(e)].

As the first step in the energy mobilization, this series of events (5) through (1) constitutes the turning on of the phosphorylase system. The concentration of 3′,5′-cyclic adenylate required for half maximum activation of the phosphorylase kinase kinase (4) is of the order of $10^{-8}\,M$. The concentrations of ATP required to achieve half maximum initial velocity of reactions (2) and (3) are of the order of $10^{-5}\,M$. When compared with the concentration of ATP usually present in cells ($10^{-3}\,M$), this suggests that this cascade of reactions requires only a low ATP concentration for initiation. The amplification feature of this cascade of reactions becomes very obvious in conducting experiments in the laboratory. In order to assay the various steps, the reaction to be determined is run, and then after a time period, stopped, a dilution made, the next reaction is run, stopped, another dilution made, etc. These serial dilutions demonstrate directly the increasing enzyme potency in the cascade and illustrate the extensive amplification of the initially small input signal (hormone action) to a large output effect (phosphorolysis of glycogen). In the reverse direction, the enzyme is turned off by the 2 phosphatases, stages (2) and (3), phosphorylase phosphatase "turning off" the enzyme itself and phosphorylase kinase phosphatase "turning off"

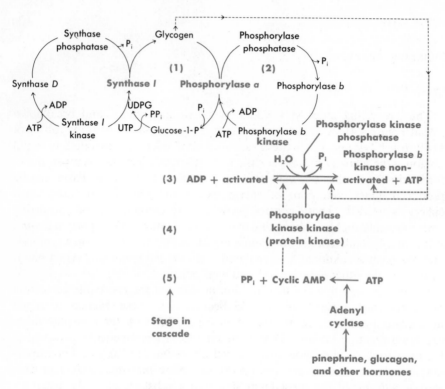

Figure 8.2   The phosphorylase cascade. Catalytic reactions ——→. Positive allosteric regulations indicated by – – –→. (1) The degradation of glycogen; (2) conversion of phosphorylase b to a; (3) conversion of non-activated to activated kinase; (4) the phosphorylase kinase kinase enzyme-site of control by 3′5′ cyclic adenylate; (5) the adenyl cyclase reaction in which ATP is converted to 3′5′-cyclic AMP. Note that glycogen is a positive effector in step (3) both by activating the non-activated phosphorylase b kinase as well as by promoting its conversion to the activated kinase by phosphorylation. Also shown are the two back reactions catalyzed by two phosphatases, phosphorylase phosphatase (2) and phosphorylase kinase phosphatase (3). As a result of an initial signal generated by such hormones as epinephrine (muscle) or glucagon (liver, heart) the adenyl cyclase is activated and the entire cascade is set into motion. See Figure 7.9.

the activation process. Also shown in Figure 8.2 is the important control by glycogen itself, which has been shown to accelerate the phosphorylase kinase reaction (3) in vitro specifically by lowering the K_m of the enzyme for its substrate. Glycogen thus participates in the stimulation of nonactivated phosphorylase kinase, as well as in the promotion of the conversion of nonactivated phosphorylase kinase to activated phosphorylase kinase by phosphorylation with ATP. It must be noted here that the terms "active" and "inactive" with reference to these enzymes is misleading. Nonactivated phosphorylase b kinase is active but with a different pH activity profile than the activated form of the enzyme. Similarly, phosphorylase b is also active but is sensitive to other regulatory processes. Nonactivated phosphorylase *b* kinase is distinguished from activated phosphorylase *b* kinase by a technique involving assay at two different pH's, 6.8 and 8.2. For the nonactivated form of the enzyme, the pH 6.8/8.2 activity ratio is 10 percent of the activity ratio for the activated enzyme.

Inactive phosphorylase (*b*) is distinguished from active phosphorylase (*a*) by its strong dependence on 5'-AMP. Thus, the ratio of activities

$$\frac{\text{activity without AMP}}{\text{activity with AMP}} \times 100$$

gives the percent of phosphorylase (*a*) in an unknown sample. AMP decreases the K_m of phosphorylase *b* for P_i and for glycogen. In turn, each of these substrates influences the enzyme affinity (K_a) for AMP. As in the case of phosphofructokinase (PFK) (Chapter 7), ATP also inhibits phosphorylase. With phosphorylase, however, ATP is not a substrate. It inhibits (as does glucose-6-P) by competing with AMP for its activating site on the enzyme. Phosphorylase *b* control is therefore similar in some aspects to PFK control (see Section 7.2). Substrates which accumulate anaerobically, such as AMP and P_i, act to deinhibit the ATP-inhibited enzyme. Aerobically, with high ATP and glucose-6-P and low AMP, ADP, and P_i, the *b* form of the enzyme may be completely inactive. Similar types of controls have been noted with phosphorylase *a*, but this form of the enzyme is markedly *less sensitive* than is the *b* form.

The importance of these coordinated substrate controls lies in their interrelationship with the phosphorylase *b* to *a* interconversions. Anaerobically, when most of the enzyme is in the *b* form, glycogenolysis can be triggered by the substrate (non-covalent) controls, that is, the AMP and P_i activation in the face of low ATP levels. This, then, is an energetically less costly method of initiating glycogenolysis than is the previously discussed ATP-dependent method triggered by the hormones. In this latter instance, the enzyme is converted to the *a* form, which is relatively insensitive to the substrate controls. The *b* form, which is present under these anaerobic conditions, is inhibited by the ATP and glucose-6-P present, and can, therefore, be "turned off." The anaerobic activation of phosphorylase *b* by AMP and P_i explains how a genetic strain of mice which lacks phosphorylase *b* kinase is able to carry on glycogenolysis, although probably somewhat less efficiently than normally.

Let us next consider the glycogen-synthesizing system, UDPG gycogen synthase, in terms of the enzyme interconversions which lead to the activation of that enzyme (Figure 8.3). In Section 7.3 it was shown that the synthase can exist in two forms, an active *I* form and an inactive *D* form, interconverted by phosphorylation and dephosphorylation. With these interconversions, as with phosphorylase, we have a cascade of reactions with many similar features to the phosphorylase system. By phosphorylation with ATP and Mg^{2+}, the active *I* form is converted to the inactive *D* form (2). This is

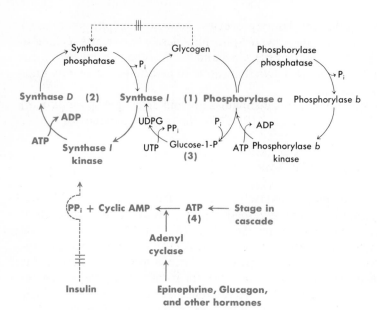

Figure 8.3

UDPG glycogen synthase cascade. Symbols as in Figure 8.2. Negative regulations indicated by $-\!+\!\!\mid\!\!+\!\!\rightarrow$. (1) synthesis of glycogen from UDPG; (2) conversion of active *I* form to inactive *D* form of synthase; (3) synthase *I* kinase which is probably identical with phosphorylase kinase kinase (4) in Figure 8.2. The control by epinephrine and glucagon is via adenyl cyclase and 3'5'-cyclic adenylate as in Figure 8.2. Note that there is no reaction between synthase conversion (2) and synthase *I* kinase (3), making this cascade one reaction less than phosphorylase. Insulin has been shown to inactivate kinase by rendering it 3'5' cyclic adenylate dependent. See Figure 7.9.

catalyzed by a phosphoprotein kinase, termed synthase *I* kinase (3). This kinase (3) responds to 3',5'-cyclic adenylate (4) just as does phosphorylase kinase kinase and with equal sensitivity to low concentrations. In fact, there is now good evidence that phosphorylase kinase kinase and synthase *I* kinase are the same enzyme. The system in muscle and liver, therefore, responds to the hormones epinephrine and glucagon with a resultant conversion of the *I* to the *D* form. The system also responds to insulin, which causes a conversion of the *D* to the *I* form. The site of action of insulin appears to be an inhibition exerted at the level of synthase *I* kinase (3), but the mechanism is as yet unknown. In the opposite direction, a phosphatase, synthase phosphatase, converts the *D* form to the *I* form by dephosphorylation.

There are a number of important nonhormonal regulators. One is glycogen itself (Figure 8.3), which acts to inhibit the synthase phosphatase. With glycogen accumulation, the phosphatase would be progressively inhibited, and as a result the synthase would be present to a greater extent in the *D* or inactive form. This relationship is seen in vivo as an inverse relationship between percent synthase in the *I* form and tissue glycogen concentration (Figure 8.4) as well as in vitro. The similarity between the two curves suggests that this in vitro effect may play an important role in the in vivo relationship.

Nucleotides including mono-, di-, and triphosphates, of which the most important are the adenine and uridine nucleotides, inhibit the enzyme. UDP, a product of the reaction, is a competitive inhibitor of UDPG utilization. Its inhibition is not completely reversed by glucose-6-P, and thus, UDP may bind to the UDPG site. The inhibition by ATP as well as by ADP and

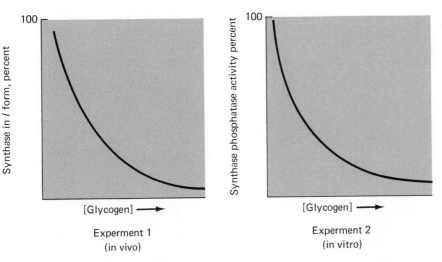

Figure 8.4 Glycogen—UDPG glycogen synthase feedback control. Experiment 1—*"in vivo"* measurements made with a number of hearts or skeletal muscles of both glycogen content and % synthase in the active or *I* form. Plotting all points gives the resultant curve, indicating that as the glycogen concentration in muscle increases the synthase is converted to the *D* form and thus inactivated. Experiment 2—*"in vitro"* as the glycogen concentration is increased the synthase phosphatase is inhibited and less *D* form of the enzyme is converted to the *I* form. The similarity between the two curves is one argument suggesting that the *in vitro* effect is physiologically significant. Modified from C. Villar-Palasi, *N.Y. Acad. Sci.*, **166**, 719 (1969).

AMP is reversed by glucose-6-P and is thus probably at a separate nonsubstrate site. Of utmost importance is the differential sensitivity of the *I* and *D* forms. The *D* form is much more sensitive to nucleotide inhibition than is the *I* form. A "physiological" mixture of nucleotides and phosphorylated compounds can "turn off" the *D* form completely at low glucose-6-P concentrations (Figure 8.5, Exp. 1) under conditions where the *I* form is active (Exp. 2). With increasing concentrations of glucose-6-P, the inhibition is overcome, the *D* form requiring a much larger concentration of glucose-6-P to restore activity than does the *I* form. Thus, the conversion of the *I* to *D* form under aerobic conditions in the presence of maintained intracellular levels of ATP can again "turn off" the enzyme by two mechanisms, the interconversion as well as the metabolite inhibition. When the *D* form is converted to the *I* form anaerobically, the enzyme would be activated again by the double mechanism of interconversion and metabolite control. It is possible that the interconversion system may be more directly related to the hormonal controls per se, since in all cases known the hormonal controls are concerned with either increasing or decreasing total enzyme activity or total physiologically effective enzyme activity.

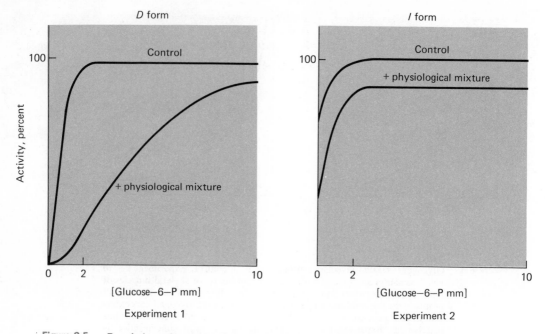

Figure 8.5   Regulation of activity of *I* and *D* forms of UDPG glycogen synthase by metabolites; effect of increasing glucose 6-P concentration. Experiment 1: *D* form. Experiment 2: *I* form. Note the marked sensitivity of the *D* form to inhibition by a physiological mixture of nucleotides at low glucose-6-P concentrations when compared with the *I* form. Modified from R. Piras, L. B. Rothman and E. Cabib, *Biochemistry*, **7**, 56 (1968).

8.2   PHOSPHOFRUCTOKINASE—FRUCTOSE-1, 6-PHOSPHATASE SITE

As with the preceding regulatory site (Figure 8.1, I), the PFK-fructose diphosphate phosphatase (FDPase) reactions (Figure 8.1, II), if summed, would result in ATP hydrolysis,

$$\text{fructose-6-P}^{2-} + \text{ATP}^{4-} \longrightarrow \text{fructose-1,6-P}^{4-} + \text{ADP}^{3-} + \text{H}^+ \tag{10}$$

$$\text{fructose-1,6-P}^{4-} + \text{H}_2\text{O} \longrightarrow \text{fructose-1-P}^{2-} + \text{P}_i^{2-} \tag{11}$$

Sum $\text{ATP}^{4-} + \text{H}_2\text{O} \longrightarrow \text{ADP}^{3-} + \text{P}^{2-} + \text{H}^+$ \tag{12}

and a wasteful energy expenditure. The control of PFK has already been discussed (Section 7.2) and was characterized by ATP inhibition and AMP and P_i stimulation. Here we will consider the control of fructose diphosphatase. This enzyme, when isolated from cells where gluconeogenesis takes place (liver, kidney and yeast), is found to be under metabolite control. It is inhibited by excess substrate (fructose-1,6-P_2), suggesting that the enzyme has a separate control site in addition to the substrate site for fructose-1,6-P_2. Nucleotides AMP as well as ADP and ATP all inhibit noncompetitively with substrate. Of significance is the fact that AMP which inhibits this phosphatase, activates PFK, thus establishing a directional control (see Figure 8.1) by simultaneously inhibiting gluconeogenesis and stimulating glycolysis.

8.3   HEXOKINASE—GLUCOSE-6-PHOSPHATASE SITE

The reactions at this site (Figure 8.1, III), if summed, would also constitute ATP hydrolysis.

$$ATP^{4-} + glucose \longrightarrow glucose\text{-}6\text{-}P^{2-} + ADP^{3-} + H^+ \tag{13}$$

$$glucose\text{-}6\text{-}P^{2-} + H_2O \longrightarrow glucose + P_i^{2-} + H^+ \tag{14}$$

Sum $$ATP^{4-} + H_2O \longrightarrow ADP^{3-} + P_i^{2-} + H^+ \tag{15}$$

Recently a novel phosphorylation of glucose to glucose-6-P has been discovered. This reaction catalyzed by glucose-6-phosphatase results in an economical reutilization of pyrophosphate for synthesis of glucose-6-P (16), rather than merely the hydrolysis of pyrophosphate to $2P_i$ (Figure 8.1, III).

$$glucose + PP_i^{3-} \longrightarrow glucose\text{-}6\text{-}P^{2-} + P_i^{2-} + H^+ \tag{16}$$

Glucose-6-phosphatase is an enzyme like fructose diphosphatase, present in those tissues carrying out gluconeogenesis (liver and kidney). It is now considered to be a multifunctional catalyst capable of phosphorylation (16) as well as dephosphorylation (14). The enzyme is subject to end product inhibition by both glucose and P_i, which probably serve to regulate the enzyme activity. The interaction with pyrophosphate is of particular interest inasmuch as it is a product in glycogen synthesis. Pyrophosphate inhibits the enzymatic hydrolysis of glucose-6-P by competing with it as a substrate for the enzyme. It also maintains glucose-6-P levels by acting as a phosphorylating agent. In these two ways, glucose-6-P is made available for glycogen synthesis.

Hexokinase is also subject to regulation by the end product, glucose-6-P (Figure 8.1). Glucose-6-P is a strong inhibitor which is noncompetitive with substrates and thus serves to control activity. P_i and ATP serve to counteract the inhibitory action of glucose-6-P on the enzyme. Both of these enzymes are subject to control by mechanisms of a more long-term adaptive nature to be discussed in Chapter 9.

8.4 PYRUVATE-PHOSPHOPYRUVATE SITES

The sum of the reactions at this site (Figure 8.1, IV), as indicated in Eqs. (17 through 20), constitute a hydrolysis of guanosine triphosphate (GTP) to guanosine diphosphate (GDP) + P_i.

$$\text{pyruvate}^{1-} + \text{HCO}_3^- + \text{ATP}^{4-} \longrightarrow \text{oxaloacetate}^{2-} + \text{ADP}^{3-} + P_i^{2-} + H^+ \tag{17}$$

$$\text{oxaloacetate}^{2-} + \text{GTP}^{4-} \longrightarrow \text{phosphoenolpyruvate}^{3-} + \text{HCO}_3^- + \text{GDP}^{3-} + H^+ \tag{18}$$

$$\text{phosphoenolpyruvate}^{3-} + \text{ADP}^{3-} + H^+ + H_2O \longrightarrow \text{pyruvate}^{1-} + \text{ATP}^{4-} \tag{19}$$

Sum $\text{GTP}^{4-} + H_2O \longrightarrow \text{GDP}^{3-} + P_i^{2-} + H^+$ \hfill (20)

In reactions (17) and (18), pyruvate is converted to phosphopyruvate by carboxylation (pyruvate carboxylase) and by decarboxylation [phosphoenol-pyruvate (PEP) carboxykinase] at the expense of an ATP and a GTP. One ATP can be recovered by the phosphorylation of ADP (pyruvate kinase) with phosphoenolpyruvate (19). The close interrelationships of this site with the tricarboxylic acid (TCA) cycle is shown in Figure 8.1. There is now ample evidence that this is the pathway of pyruvate conversion to phospho-pyruvate in gluconeogenesis. Both pyruvate carboxylase and PEP-carboxy-kinase are present in liver and kidney, organs which carry out gluconeo-genesis, as well as in other cells, including microorganisms. Pyruvate car-boxylase is low or absent from tissues which do not carry out gluconeogene-sis. On the other hand, pyruvate kinase is not found in the tissues and sub-cellular fractions where pyruvate carboxylase is present. This differential distribution acts to prevent the energy waste which would result from recy-cling of pyruvate.

Pyruvate carboxylase is subject to metabolite control of a very interesting kind. The enzyme itself contains biotin and catalyzes a two-step reaction. In the first step (21),

$$\text{HCO}_3^- + \text{ATP}^{4-} + \text{biotin-enzyme} \longrightarrow \text{-OOC-biotin-enzyme} + \text{ADP}^{3-} + P_i^{2-} + H^+ \tag{21}$$

the enzyme-biotin is carboxylated at the expense of ATP. In the second step (22), the activated CO_2 is transferred to pyruvate to form oxaloacetate (see also Section 4.10).

$$\text{-OOC-biotin-enzyme} + \text{pyruvate} \longrightarrow \text{oxaloacetate} + \text{biotin-enzyme} \tag{22}$$

For the first reaction, in addition to the substrate, ATP and Mg^{2+}, acetyl-S-coenzyme A is an *absolute* allosteric requirement (Figure 8.1). (In what pre-vious reactions have metabolite controls been of an absolute nature?) This unusual activator binds strongly enough to the carboxylase to effect a significant stabilization of the enzyme. In addition, the enzyme is inhibited by the end product ADP, which serves as a further method of regulation. Pyruvate carboxylase and acetyl-S-CoA carboxylase (another regulatory enzyme to be discussed in a subsequent section) share in common a property which has become recognized as a characteristic of many regulatory enzymes, namely, *a susceptibility to inactivation by cold.* Acetyl-S-CoA protects pyruvate carboxylase from dissociation into subunits by binding to the enzyme and by preventing this disaggregation. The important physiological implication of the acetyl-S-CoA activation is that acetyl-S-CoA, a product of fat metabolism, is an absolute requirement for the enzyme and thus promotes gluconeogenesis.

Oxaloacetate is a key intermediate required to initiate the tricarboxylic acid cycle by condensing with acetyl-S-CoA. When the supply of oxaloacetate is low, acetyl-S-CoA would tend to accumulate. Higher steady-state levels of acetyl-S-CoA would stimulate the synthesis of oxaloacetate from pyruvate and CO_2 by the pyruvate carboxylase reaction, which would then permit the tricarboxylic acid cycle to resume activity (see Figure 8.6). The functions of the cycle, both in respiration and in supplying key intermediates for transamination and other reactions, would be promoted.

The inhibition by ADP suggests that the enzyme is regulated in vivo by the ADP/ATP ratio. An increased ratio would "turn off" while a decreased ratio would "turn on" the enzyme.

The activity of pyruvate kinase has been estimated as exceeding the sum of the activities of pyruvate carboxylase and PEP carboxykinase by a factor of about 25 to 1. Since the biosynthetic enzymes (carboxylase and carboxykinase) and the degradation enzyme (pyruvate kinase) are found in different parts of the cell, this may not be a serious problem, but control mechanisms for the kinase still have been sought. End product inhibition by ATP (gly-

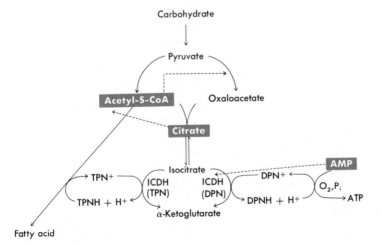

Figure 8.6

Isocitrate dehydrogenase—site of regulation of respiration and fatty acid synthesis. Catalytic reactions ——→; allosteric controls – – –→, all allosteric controls shown are positive; allosteric agents ICDH(TPN) the TPN specific form of the enzyme; ICDH(DPN) the DPN specific form. Note the control of fatty acid synthesis by citrate without control of ICDH-(TPN), and the control of ICDH-(DPN) by AMP. Note also the control of pyruvate carboxylase by acetyl-S-CoA. Modified from E. R. Stadtman, *Advances in Enzymology,* **28,** 41 (1966).

colytic direction) has been demonstrated. This is partially but not completely overcome by ADP, indicating that the enzyme is probably sensitive to the ATP/ADP ratio in vivo. Other controls have been suggested by studying metabolites which increase or promote gluconeogenesis. Two which have been found are (1) DPNH (increased DPNH/DPN$^+$ ratios in gluconeogenesis are favored by the oxidation of lactate to pyruvate) and (2) free fatty acids. Not only have free fatty acids been shown to promote gluconeogenesis, but conditions under which free fatty acids accumulate are recognized to be associated with increased gluconeogenesis (e.g., starvation, the diabetic state, high fat diets). In vitro experiments demonstrate that both DPNH and free fatty acids inhibit pyruvate kinase, suggesting that these controls may be of physiological significance. Thus, the control is of a complex nature, suggesting a number of control sites on the enzyme.

All three enzymes are also under control by hormones via mechanisms which are slower than metabolite controls and presumably involve adaptations through protein biosynthesis.

8.5 TRICARBOXYLIC ACID CYCLE CONTROLS

In this section, we will discuss the control of two key reactions, the isocitrate dehydrogenase (ICDH) and the citrate synthase. The isocitrate dehydrogenase reaction (Figure 4.5, reaction 26) represents an important control site in the TCA cycle. Two types of enzymes, one specific for DPN and another specific for TPN, have been detected and studied. Studies of the DPN-specific dehydrogenase have demonstrated an important regulatory role for AMP which stimulates the enzyme by reducing the K_m for isocitrate. The enzyme is also activated (especially at low isocitrate concentration) by ADP and deoxy-ADP, which also act by decreasing the apparent K_m of the enzyme for isocitrate. This stimulation is counteracted by ATP, adenosine diphosphate ribose, and DPNH, all of which compete with DPN$^+$. Citrate, which is inactive as a substrate, activates at low concentrations, while at high concentration, it inhibits competitively with isocitrate. The reaction has been shown to be fourth order with respect to isocitrate, indicating a high degree of cooperativity.

A plausible interlocking metabolic control model for the two ICDH enzymes is shown in Figure 8.6. The TPN-specific enzyme is not stimulated by AMP. It would appear to be concerned more with electron transfer in the biosynthesis of fatty acids where TPNH is required. On the other hand, the DPN-specific enzyme which is stimulated by AMP would appear to be concerned with the electron transport of respiration. With stimulation of respiration, AMP would be converted to ATP, constituting a self-regulating system. Electron transport through the TPN-linked enzyme would appear to be linked to the stimulation of fatty acid synthesis by means of citrate, which, as will subsequently be shown, stimulates the acetyl-S-CoA carboxylase reaction (see Figure 8.6).

Citrate synthase (Figure 4.5, reaction 23), the enzyme catalyzing the first reaction of the TCA cycle, has been shown to be inhibited by ATP. This inhibition would tend to decrease the activity of the TCA cycle and thus govern the role of ATP production by a feedback inhibition via the product ATP. The enzyme is also inhibited by CoA-S-esters of long-chain fatty acids. The type and extent of this inhibition varies with the enzyme source and specific conditions used in the assay. The possible physiological significance of this inhibition lies in the fact that acetyl-S-CoA fragments would be diverted from the TCA cycle and respiration and be used instead for other purposes, including ketone body production.

8.6 FATTY ACID SYNTHESIS

Recall that acetyl-S-CoA carboxylase (see Section 4.10) catalyzes a two-step reaction analogous to pyruvate carboxylase, Eqs. (21) and (23). The enzyme activity which has been estimated (in liver) to be present to the extent of 10 percent of the subsequent catalytic activities is, therefore, rate-limiting.

$$HCO_3^- + ATP^{4-} + \text{biotin-enzyme} \longrightarrow {}^-OOC\text{-biotin-enzyme} + ADP^{3-} + P_i^{2-} + H^+ \tag{21}$$

$$^-OOC\text{-biotin-enzyme} + \text{acetyl-S-CoA} \longrightarrow \text{biotin-enzyme} + \text{malonyl-S-CoA} \tag{23}$$

It had been known for some time that the synthesis of fatty acids is stimulated by citrate. It was assumed that citrate as a substrate acted to supply TPNH. Studies with the isolated carboxylase enzyme showed, however, that citrate is a specific allosteric activator. With citrate activation, the enzyme became altered structurally with an increase in molecular size as indicated by an increase in the sedimentation coefficient from about 18 S to about 43 S (see Glossary). The interlocking relationship of this activation with the TPN-specific ICDH reaction has been discussed (see Figure 8.6). At this time, it may be recalled that citrate specifically inhibits PFK, thus also acting as an end product inhibitor of glycolysis (Figure 8.1).

Another property of the acetyl-S-CoA carboxylase is its end product inhibition by fatty acyl-S-CoA esters. This inhibition is competitive with regard to the activator citrate and noncompetitive with regard to the substrates acetyl-S-CoA, HCO_3^-, or ATP.

In Figure 8.1, the citrate controls and additional metabolic controls by the adenine nucleotides are shown. The inhibition of PFK and of citrate synthase by citrate and the stimulation of PFK by AMP and ADP is pictured. The stimulation of ICDH by AMP and ADP and the inhibition of the citrate cleavage reaction catalyzed by ATP citrate lyase by AMP and ADP is also shown. This extramitochondrial enzyme (24)

$$\text{citrate}^{3-} + \text{CoA-SH} + \text{ATP}^{4-} \rightleftharpoons \text{acetyl-S-CoA} + \text{oxaloacetate}^{2-} + \text{ADP}^{3-} + \text{P}^{2-} \qquad (24)$$

plays the very important role of producing extramitochondrial acetyl-S-CoA for fatty acid synthesis.

8.7 CHOLESTEROL SYNTHESIS CONTROL

The principal control step of cholesterol biosynthesis is considered to be the reduction of β-hydroxy-β-methylglutaryl-S-CoA to mevalonate (Figure 4.16). There is also evidence for control sites at later stages in cholesterol synthesis. The exact mechanisms of control of sterol synthesis remain to be elucidated. A number of agents (Table 8.1) block specific enzymatic steps of cholesterol synthesis and are useful tools in studying synthetic pathways, intermediates, and reaction mechanisms. Most compounds that inhibit cholesterol biosynthesis are toxic in vivo; an exception is chlorophenoxyiso-butyrate, used clinically to lower blood cholesterol levels.

8.8 CONTROL OF GLUCONEOGENESIS BY METABOLITES DURING LIPOLYSIS

The pathway of gluconeogenesis has been detailed (Figure 4.3). This process is of extreme importance to animals which require adequate glucose to support brain metabolism. Conditions which call forth gluconeogenesis, as already mentioned, are starvation or high fat diets where adequate carbo-

TABLE 8.1   SELECTED INHIBITORS OF CHOLESTEROL BIOSYNTHESIS AND THEIR SITES OF ACTION [c]

Compound	Enzymatic Step Blocked
Chlorophenoxyisobutyrate	β-Hydroxy-β-methylglutaryl-CoA reductase
Farnesol analogs	Squalene synthetase
MER-29[a], azasteroids, benzylamines	$\Delta^{5,7}$-Sterol-Δ^7-reductase, Δ^{24}-sterol reductase
AY-9944[b], biguanides	$\Delta^{5,7}$-Sterol-Δ^7-reductase
Chelators, KCN	Δ^7-Sterol-Δ^5-dehydrogenase

[a] 1-(P-[β-diethylaminoethoxy]phenyl)-1-(P-tosyl)-2-(P-chlorophenyl)ethanol or triparanol.

[b] trans-1,4-bis-(2-chlorobenzylaminomethyl)cyclohexane.

[c] Modified from M. E. Dempsey, Ann. N. Y. Acad. Sci., **148**, 631 (1968).

hydrate supplies are not utilized and various hormonal imbalances including growth hormone excess, and epinephrine and glucagon administration. Under all of these conditions, fat reserves are called upon, triglycerides are hydrolyzed to fatty acids (lipolysis) and fatty acids accumulate in plasma.

As already discussed (Section 8.4) free fatty acids control gluconeogenesis. Following preincubation of tissue extracts in vitro, a pattern of inhibition by free fatty acids of several irreversible enzymatic steps of glycolysis has been shown. These enzymes are the kinases, and include hexokinase, PFK, as well as pyruvate kinase. Also inhibited are oxidative reactions of the pentose pathway, including glucose-6-P and 6-phosphogluconate dehydrogenases. The key bypass enzymes of gluconeogenesis, pyruvate carboxylase, PEP carboxy-kinase, FDPase, and glucose-6-phosphatase, are not affected. Thus one can begin to appreciate the pattern of control by fatty acids.

Also, as discussed, a further mechanism of control is the DPNH,H$^+$/DPN ratio, which is increased under conditions of gluconeogenesis. DPNH inhibits pyruvate kinase and also PFK. Through these coordinated controls, including the acetyl-S-CoA activation of pyruvate carboxylase, the gluconeogenesis pathway is favored.

8.9 SOME HORMONAL CONTROLS OF LIPOLYSIS INVOLVING 3′, 5′-CYCLIC ADENYLATE

The hormonal control of glycogen degradation and synthesis via 3′,5′-cyclic adenylate has already been detailed. It is appropriate to point out here that lipolysis, the hydrolysis of triglycerides to free fatty acids, is also under hormonal control by a variety of hormones and chemical agents. Some of these are shown in Figure 8.7. The catecholamines (epinephrine and norepinephrine), adrenocorticotrophic hormone (ACTH), thyroid stimulating hormone (TSH), glucagon, and other hormones act by stimulating adenyl cyclase (in vivo as well as in vitro). The concentration of cyclic adenylate in the fat cell triggers the process of lipolysis, via a protein kinase which converts the nonactivated lipase to an activated enzyme by phosphorylation with ATP, very much analogous to triggering glycogenolysis. Thyroxin also acts to increase cyclic adenylate by a mechanism in which adenyl cyclase may possibly be increased by protein synthesis.

Several other substances, including insulin, several prostaglandins and nicotinic acid act anti-lipolytically, that is, they *depress* cyclic adenylate levels once they have been elevated by the hormones which promote lipolysis. Another mechanism of regulating lipolysis is illustrated by the methylated purines (caffeine, theophylline, etc.). These agents inhibit the specific phosphodiesterase enzyme which inactivates cyclic adenylate by hydrolyzing it to 5′-AMP. Thus, the methylated purines act to increase cyclic adenylate

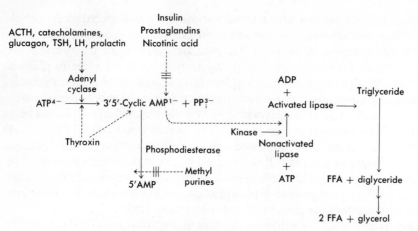

Figure 8.7   Control of lipolysis by 3'5'-cyclic adenylate. Catalytic reactions $\longrightarrow$; posi-
tive allosteric control reactions $--\rightarrow$; negative controls $-\||\!|\!|-\rightarrow$. Note
that the process is activated by a wide variety of hormones, and inhibited
by a smaller number. The similarity here to the control of glycogen metabolism is apparent with 3'5'-cyclic adenylate acting to convert an inactive to
an active form of lipase thus triggering the process. From E. W. Sutherland Jr., G. A. Robinson, R. W. Butcher, *Circulation,* **37,** 279–306 (1968).

levels in fat cells and promote lipolysis. By this coordinated control, free
fatty acids are able to favor glucose production through gluconeogenesis.

8.10   INTEGRATED CONTROL OF FUEL METABOLISM AT THE ORGAN LEVEL—STARVATION IN THE HUMAN

In order to bring together some aspects of the control of the metabolism of
the fuels and integrate to the organ level, let us examine as a model, the
perturbed state of starvation in the human being.

The "average man" (70 kg) has fuel reserves which consist of fat protein
and carbohydrate (Table 8.2) The largest reserve is fat as triglyceride

TABLE 8.2   FUEL RESERVES OF AN "AVERAGE MAN" (70 kg)[a]

Fuel	Organ or Tissue	Caloric Equivalence (kcal)
Triglyceride	Adipose tissue	100,000
Protein	Mainly muscle	25,000
Glycogen	Muscle	400
	Liver	200
Glucose	Body fluids	40

[a] From G. F. Cahill, Jr. and O. E. Owen, *Carbohydrate Metabolism and its Disorders,*
Academic Press, New York, 1968.

(100,000 kcal). The protein reserve is also large (25,000 kcal) but is *not* immediately available. It becomes available through gluconeogenesis under the destructive circumstances of tissue breakdown. Carbohydrate, readily available, is a small contributor.

Food intake and its partition and use by the organs are shown in Tables 8.3 and 8.4. Of the 1710 kcal ingested, over half (glucose and fat) is utilized by the carcass, a quarter by the brain (glucose), and the remainder by the liver (amino acids).

Man can undergo starvation for prolonged periods of time (many months) provided water is supplied. How is this stress met by the body which draws upon its fuel resources for energy production? What are the adaptive changes which permit the maintenance of organ and cell function under these conditions?

In Table 8.5 data are presented on total body fuel stores after short (overnight), intermediate (8 day) and prolonged (40 day) fasts. As can be seen, total fuel stores after 40 days of fast (60,880 kcal) are decreased to about half of those present after one day of fast (125,680 kcal). In terms of the three major fuel classes, the largest decrease occurs in lipid stores, with protein next, and carbohydrate least.

TABLE 8.3   COMPOSITION OF DIET OF "AVERAGE MAN" (70 kg) IN TERMS OF CALORIES AND GAS EXCHANGE PER 24 HOURS

Fuel	Weight (grams)	O_2 Consumed (moles)	CO_2 Produced (moles)	R.Q.	kcal
Carbohydrate (starch)	200	7.5	7.5	1.0	836
Protein	70	3.0	2.4	0.801	306
Fat	60	5.5	3.8	0.707	578
		16.0	13.7	0.864	1710

TABLE 8.4   PARTITION OF THE FUELS AMONG THE ORGANS PER 24 HOURS[a]

Organ	Fuel	Weight (grams)	kcal	O_2 Consumed (moles)
Brain	Glucose	120	423	4
Liver	Amino acid	70	300	3
Carcass	Glucose	80		
	Fat	60	987	9
			1,710	16

[a] From G. F. Cahill, Jr. and O. E. Owen, *Carbohydrate Metabolism and Its Disorders,* Academic Press, New York, 1968.

TABLE 8.5 BODY STORES AT END OF PERIOD OF FAST (kcal)^a

	Lipid	CHO	Protein
Overnight fast	100,000	680	25,000
8 day fast	88,000	380	23,000
40 day fast	42,000	380	18,500
Daily loss (*last day of period*)			
Overnight fast	1,200	200	300
8 day fast	1,400	0	200
40 day fast	1,350	0	75

^{a} Modified from G. F. Cahill, Jr. and O. E. Owen, *Carbohydrate Metabolism and Its Disorders,* Academic Press, New York, 1968.

Reckoned as daily loss (Table 8.5), the available carbohydrate decreases rapidly, and after eight days the carbohydrate daily loss becomes negligible. Protein loss decreases progressively during the fast, but lipid loss is maintained over the entire period. The body adjusts to the lack of carbohydrate by drawing upon protein in a decreasing manner, and upon lipid to a major extent. Thus lipid may supply well over 90 percent and protein well under 10 percent of calories in a prolonged fast.

Since the body contains only 1,000 g of nitrogen, protein conservation is critical for survival. It has been estimated that loss of more than $\frac{1}{3}$ to $\frac{1}{2}$ of total nitrogen is not compatible with life. How does the body regulate this nitrogen excretion?

After prolonged starvation, nitrogen is excreted chiefly as ammonia (approximately $\frac{2}{3}$) by the kidney, with only a small proportion as urea (approximately $\frac{1}{4}$ to $\frac{1}{3}$). The excreted ammonia balances by neutralization the organic acids excreted (β-hydroxybutyric and acetoacetic) as well as the small quantity of the inorganic acids excreted such as phosphoric and sulfuric. Of considerable interest is the fact that the ratio of K^+ to nitrogen excreted (3 meq K^+/gram N) equals that present in the body. Na^+ loss is small and represents the extracellular fluid loss derived from tissue breakdown. It appears that the excretion of nitrogen as ammonia functions to maintain acid-base balance, thus preserving Na^+ and K^+ in order to maintain fluid volume.

Gluconeogenesis and ketogenesis, generally speaking, go together, being activated and inactivated in tandem. Starvation activates both, while administration of even a small amount of glucose decreases both. This probably represents the body's attempt to overcome the "sooty fuel" situation which results from burning ketone bodies by supplying carbohydrate and allowing a "clean fuel" combustion. The biochemical bases for the coordinated control of both through metabolite controls has been presented.

Ketone bodies are formed in the liver and utilized in the muscle. Gluconeogenesis takes place in the liver and in the kidney as well. After prolonged starvation, when gluconeogenesis from amino acids has failed, an extremely serious situation exists with regard to the brain. This organ usually utilizes glucose. It has recently become established that with prolonged starvation, the brain becomes progressively adapted to the utilization of ketone bodies, thus obviating the need for continued gluconeogenesis.

After prolonged starvation, glucose carbon is conserved by glycolytic recycling of glucose to pyruvate and lactate which are in turn reconverted to glucose, without oxidation. The same is true of glycerol carbon. At this time, oxidation is almost entirely that of lipid. Thus glucose is not used by muscle, but rather by those tissues, the blood cells, liver, kidney (medulla) which can recycle glucose carbon anaerobically. As mentioned already, brain progressively uses less and less glucose, and ketone bodies to a greater and greater extent. Protein is broken down decreasingly and the carbon and especially the nitrogen retained. Fatty acids are converted to ketone bodies and the ketone bodies are oxidized in muscle. Kidney (especially the cortex) oxidizes both fatty acids and ketone bodies.

Thus there is a realignment of organ (and cell) metabolic function during the stress of starvation. How this is accomplished is still debated, but in all likelihood there may be an altered enzyme synthesis with a new complement of catalysts, a tribute to the flexibility of the organism. If only man's thought processes could maintain the same degree of flexibility under changing stressful circumstances that his metabolic processes maintain, what a better world this would be!

In this chapter, we have described the control mechanisms of carbohydrate and lipid metabolism. Developing the concept of the four short-circuiting sites, the control of each site by metabolites as well as by enzyme interconversions has been discussed. This latter control in glycogen and in triglyceride metabolism appears to be related to hormone action. It specifically amplifies the signals of epinephrine, glucagon, and other hormones, acting with impressive speed. The former controls are exerted by end products of individual reactions or end products of metabolic sequences upon early sites usually before or following branching points. Several examples illustrate the *specific* and *absolute* nature of these metabolite controls (e.g., glucose-6-P, citrate, acetyl-S-CoA). Other examples detail the coordinated nature of the metabolite and substrate control (PFK). The metabolites include substrates and end products as well as nucleotides and energy carriers. The control by the latter substances will be further detailed in Chapter 10.

REFERENCES

Cahill, G. F. Jr., and O. E. Owen, "Some Observations on Carbohydrate Metabolism in Man," in *Carbohydrate Metabolism and its Disorders,* F. Dickens, P. T. Randle, and W. J. Whelan (eds.), Academic Press, N. Y., 1968.

Krebs, E. G., and D. A. Walsh, "Studies on the Mechanism of Action of Cyclic 3′,5′-

AMP in the Phosphorylase System," *Metabolic Regulation and Enzyme Action,* (A. Sols and S. Grisolia, eds.), Federation of European Biochemical Societies, **19,** 121 (1970).

Metabolic Roles of Citrate, T. W. Goodwin, ed., Academic Press Inc., New York, 1968.

Passonneau, J. V., and O. H. Lowry, "The Role of Phosphofructokinase in Metabolic Regulation," *Adv. in Enzyme Regulation,* **2,** George Weber, (ed.), Pergamon Press 265–274 (1964). A clear discussion of the regulation of PFK.

Piras, R., L. B. Rothman, and E. Cabib, "Regulation of Muscle Glycogen Synthetase by Metabolites; Differential Effects on the I and D Forms," *Biochemistry,* **7,** 56 (1968).

Stadtman, E. R., "Allosteric Regulation of Enzyme Activity," *Adv. in Enzymol.,* **28,** 41 (1966), Interscience Publishers.

Sutherland, E. W., G. A. Robison, and R. W. Butcher, "Some Aspects of the Biological Role of Adenosine 3',5'-Monophosphate (Cyclic AMP)," *Circulation,* **37,** 279–306 (1968).

Villar-Palasi, C., N. D. Goldberg, J. S. Bishop, F. Q. Nuttall, and J. Larner, "Hormonal Control of Glycogen Synthetase Interconversion," *Metabolic Regulation and Enzyme Action,* (A. Sols and S. Grisolia, eds.), Federation of European Biochemical Societies, **19,** 149, (1970).

INTEGRATION AND CONTROL OF PROTEIN AND NUCLEIC ACID METABOLISM

NINE

In the present chapter we will consider the control of the metabolism of the nitrogen-containing compounds. The types of controls which enter here are similar to those already discussed in Chapters 7 and 8. In addition, we will discuss the slower adaptive reactions by which the number of enzyme molecules is controlled (Section 7.8).

The control of nucleotide synthesis and amino acid synthesis and degradation will be treated first. Then, the patterns of altered protein synthesis as influenced by nutritional (substrate) and hormonal perturbations will be discussed. Some of the experimental approaches used to delineate the control sites in RNA and protein biosynthesis will be considered, since the exact chemical events are just starting to appear and, therefore, can only be discussed in preliminary terms. Lastly the control of protein synthesis in bacteria by 3'5'-cyclic adenylate will be discussed.

9.1 CONTROL OF NUCLEOTIDE METABOLISM

The reaction path of purine nucleotide metabolism with the sites of metabolic control is outlined in Figure 9.1. The initial reaction (I), two potential short-circuiting recycling sites (II and III), as well as the four reactions in which the nitrogenous bases are converted to nucleotides (IV-VII) are all sites of control. (See also Section 5.12.)

As already discussed (Chapters 5 and 7), the phosphoribosyl pyrophosphate amidotransferase reaction (I) is inhibited by the various purine nucleotide end products. Even though kinetic analysis indicated that the inhibition by purine nucleotides was competitive with substrate PRPP, it soon became evident that the mechanism was by way of the inhibitor binding at a site different from the substrate binding site. This assignment of an allosteric type of regulation was based on the following kind of observations: The sensitivity of the enzyme to inhibition by purine nucleotide varied greatly with a variety of experimental enzyme treatments including freezing, dialysis, storage at low temperature (4°), and Sephadex treatment, which did not

Figure 9.1 Pathways and control of purine nucleotide metabolism. Catalytic reactions ⟶; allosteric controls − − −→. I, II, III, sites of potential recycling; IV, V, VI, VII sites of incorporation of bases into nucleotides. All are subject to control. Other numbers refer to individual reactions. Modified from E. R. Stadtman, *Adv. Enz.*, **28**, 41 (1966).

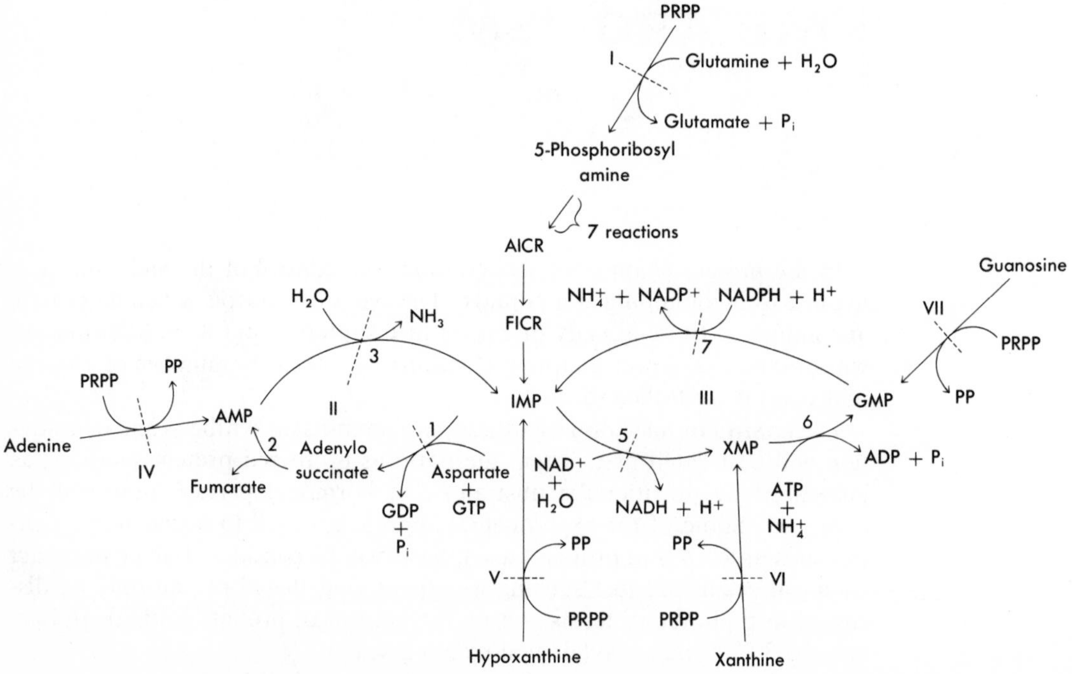

affect significantly the K_m of the enzyme for its substrates. Mixtures of *homologous* 6-hydroxy purine nucleotides (GMP + IMP) or 6-amino purine nucleotides (AMP + ADP) inhibited, but the inhibition observed was that of the most effective inhibitor present. However, with *heterologous* mixtures (6-amino + 6-hydroxy purine nucleotides AMP + GMP), the inhibition was *greater* than that calculated for a simple effect. This *cooperative inhibition* (Chapters 7 and 8) is consistent with two different allosteric binding sites, one for 6-amino nucleotides and the other for 6-hydroxy purine nucleotides.

The interconversions of GMP and IMP, and AMP and IMP are potential recycling sites (II and III). As such, they would lead to a wasteful hydrolysis of GTP, Eqs. (1) through (4), or ATP Eqs. (5) through (8).

$$\text{GTP}^{4-} + \text{aspartate}^{1-} + \text{IMP}^{2-} \longrightarrow \text{adenylosuccinate}^{4-} + \text{GDP}^{3-} + \text{P}_i^{2-} + 2\text{H}^+ \tag{1}$$

$$\text{adenylosuccinate}^{4-} \longrightarrow \text{AMP}^{2-} + \text{fumarate}^{2-} \tag{2}$$

$$\text{AMP}^{2-} + \text{H}_2\text{O} \longrightarrow \text{IMP}^{2-} + \text{NH}_3 \tag{3}$$

Sum $\quad \text{GTP}^{4-} + \text{aspartate}^{1-} \longrightarrow \text{GDP}^{3-} + \text{P}_i^{2-} + \text{fumarate}^{2-} + \text{NH}_3 + 2\text{H}^+ \tag{4}$

$$\text{IMP}^{2-} + \text{DPN}^+ + \text{H}_2\text{O} \longrightarrow \text{XMP}^{2-} + \text{DPNH} + \text{H}^+ \tag{5}$$

$$\text{XMP}^{2-} + \text{ATP}^{4-} + \text{NH}_4^+ \longrightarrow \text{GMP}^{2-} + \text{ADP}^{3-} + \text{P}_i^{2-} + 2\text{H}^+ \tag{6}$$

$$\text{GMP}^{2-} + \text{TPNH} + 2\text{H}^+ \longrightarrow \text{IMP}^{2-} + \text{TPN}^+ + \text{NH}_4^+ \tag{7}$$

Sum $\quad \text{ATP}^{4-} + \text{TPNH} + \text{DPN}^+ + \text{H}_2\text{O} \longrightarrow \text{DPNH} + \text{TPN}^+ + \text{ADP}^{3-} + \text{P}^{2-} + \text{H}^+ \tag{8}$

Again, specific end product regulation provides a sensitive control, turning key enzymes on and off to ensure metabolite flow in either direction. Thus, IMP dehydrogenase, Eq. (5), is inhibited by GMP, not by adenine nucleotides, while GMP dehydrogenase, Eq. (7), is inhibited by ATP, AMP, and IMP. Adenylosuccinate synthetase, Eq. (1), similarly is inhibited by ADP, and AMP deaminase, Eq. (3), is also regulated in typical allosteric fashion. The AMP concentration velocity relationship is sigmoidal, suggesting cooperative AMP binding, and ATP activates AMP binding by converting the sigmoidal to the hyperbolic Michaelis-Menten kinetics with decreased K_m for AMP.

All of the conversions of purine bases to purine nucleotides by reaction with PRPP (IV, V, VI, VII) (pyrophosphorylases) also appear to be subject to regulation. AMP pyrophosphorylase (IV) is inhibited by adenine nucleotides, IMP pyrophosphorylase (V) by guanine and inosine nucleotides, XMP pyrophosphorylase (VI) by guanine and inosine nucleotides, and GMP pyro-

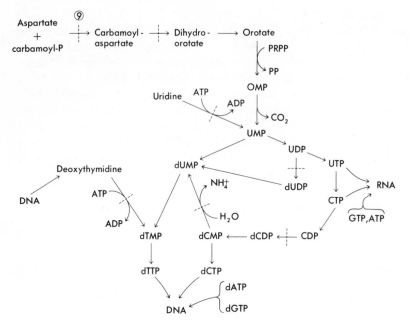

Figure 9.2   Pathways and control of pyrimidine nucleotide metabolism. Catalytic reactions ⟶; allosteric controls ---- 9 = aspartate transcarbamylase. Modified from E. R. Stadtman, *Adv. Enz.*, **28**, 41 (1966).

phosphorylase (VII) most effectively by guanine nucleotides. Thus, all are subject to end product inhibition.

Figure 9.2 presents the metabolism of pyrimidines and the sites of metabolic control. Aspartate transcarbamylase (ATCase) catalyzing reaction (9)

$$\text{aspartate}^{1-} + \text{carbamoyl-P}^{2-} \xrightarrow{\text{(ATCase)}} \text{carbamoyl aspartate}^{2-} + \text{P}_i^{2-} + \text{H}^+ \tag{9}$$

is subject to metabolic control and will be discussed.

The kinetics for the substrate aspartate are sigmoid (Figure 9.3, curve 1). This indicates that more than one aspartate molecule is bound and that binding of the first facilitates the binding of subsequent molecules. CTP is a specific end product inhibitor which is competitive with aspartate. With CTP, the sigmoid aspartate curve is shifted toward higher substrate concentrations (to the right), the K_m of the enzyme for aspartate is increased, $V_{\max}$ is unchanged, and the sigmoid character is still present (curve 2). ATP activates as well as reverses the CTP inhibition. With high ATP, the K_m of the enzyme for aspartate is decreased, $V_{\max}$ is unchanged, and the kinetics are altered from sigmoid to hyperbolic.

Even though CTP inhibition is competitive with aspartate, the two bind

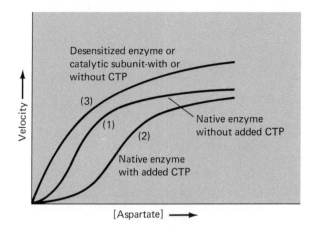

Figure 9.3

Control in native and loss of control in desensitized aspartate transcarbamylase. Curve 1: native enzyme without added CTP. Curve 2: native enzyme with added CTP. Note the inhibitory effect. Curve 3: desensitized enzyme with or without added CTP. Note loss of control in desensitized enzyme.

at separate sites on the enzyme. This is shown by the elegant experiment in which the enzyme is "desensitized" to inhibition by CTP but without loss of activity. A number of different treatments (including heating, incubation with urea or heavy metals) all done under specified conditions lead to such an altered enzyme-catalytically active, with hyperbolic aspartate kinetics, and not inhibited by CTP (curve 3).

Elegant physical chemical studies have demonstrated that procedures which desensitize, dissociate the native enzyme (molecular weight 310,000) into subunits of two kinds: regulatory (molecular weight 34,000, made up of two peptide chains, each 17,000) and catalytic (molecular weight 99,000, made up of three subunits, each 33,000). The intact molecule is composed of six regulatory peptide chains and six catalytic subunits. The regulatory subunit has no catalytic activity but binds CTP. The catalytic subunit is not inhibited by CTP and is catalytically active. This disaggregated enzyme is capable of being reaggregated under appropriate conditions and the original enzyme characteristics restored (see Wold, Chapter 3).

Another fascinating regulatory property is shown by the influence of substrate analogs (e.g., maleate). These molecules are themselves not utilized as substrates. When incubated with the enzyme at low concentrations, they increase enzyme activity but inhibit it at high concentrations (Figure 9.4). This *biphasic* action is explained by first binding of analogue to unoccupied substrate sites. This causes enhanced cooperativity (analogous to substrate activation), increasing enzyme affinity for true substrate with a resultant increase in enzyme activity. With higher concentrations of analog, the stimulating effect reaches a maximum and begins to be counteracted by the competitive inhibition of the analog acting against the substrate. This leads to inhibition of enzyme activity. This biphasic effect of the substrate analog is lost in the desensitized enzyme.

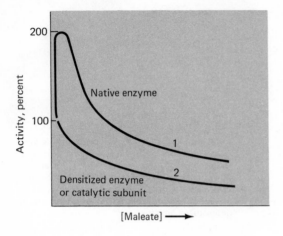

Figure 9.4

Effect of maleate on native and desensitized aspartate transcarbamylase. Curve 1: native enzyme; note the biphasic effect of increasing maleate. Curve 2: desensitized enzyme. Note loss of control by maleate. Substrate concentration is constant.

The physical separation of the catalytic and regulatory subunits represents one of the most important achievements in the study of regulatory enzymes.

9.2 CONTROL OF AMINO ACID METABOLISM

In Section 7.6 the four types of end product feedback inhibition in the biosynthesis of amino acids in bacterial systems was discussed. As shown in Table 9.1, this process of end product inhibition is general for many of the amino acids and is not restricted to bacteria but occurs in mammalian systems as well.

Two examples of enzymes catalyzing the metabolism of amino acids whose regulation have been well studied will be discussed. Both glutamate dehydrogenase and glutamine synthetase degrade or synthesize glutamate, which is located at the crossroad between amino acid metabolism and the TCA cycle and whose regulation is therefore of prime importance to the cell.

Glutamate dehydrogenase crystallized from liver has a high molecular weight (about 1,000,000) and can be dissociated into subunits under a variety of conditions. The state of aggregation is influenced markedly by amino acids, nucleotides, several hormones, and metal ions. Interestingly, dissociation into subunits is characterized by an increase in specificity of the enzyme for monocarboxylic acids as substrates (for example, alanine) with a decrease in activity for the dicarboxylic amino acids (for example glutamate).

The enzyme is made up of 3 to 4 identical monomers of molecular weight 300,000–350,000. These are themselves made up of identical subunits of molecular weight 50,000–55,000. There is a rapid equilibrium between polymers and monomers. At high protein concentrations, the enzyme is present as a polymer. *Combinations* of substances which favor dissociation include

TABLE 9.1   END PRODUCT INHIBITION IN AMINO ACID BIOSYNTHESIS[a]

Amino Acid	Organism or Tissue	Sensitive Reactions
Arginine	E. coli	Glutamate → N-acetyl glutamate
	Micrococcus glutamicus	N-Acetylglutamate → N-acetylglutamate-γ-semialdehyde
	E. coli	N-Acetylglutamate-γ-semialdehye → N-acetylornithine
	E. coli	Ornithine → citrulline
Cysteine	S. typhimurium	Serine → O-acetylserine
Cystine	Rat liver	Homocysteine → cystathionine
Histidine	S. typhimurium	ATP + PRPP → phosphoribosyl ATP
Isoleucine	E. coli	Threonine → α-ketobutyrate
Leucine	S. typhimurium	α-Ketoisovalerate + acetyl-S-CoA → β-carboxy-β-hydroxyisovalerate
Lysine	E. coli	Aspartate → β-aspartyl-P
Proline	E. coli	Glutamate → Δ^1-pyrroline-5-carboxylate
Serine	Rat liver	Phosphoserine → serine
Threonine	E. coli	Aspartate → β-aspartyl-P
	Rhodopseudomonas capsulatus	Aspartate-β-semialdehyde → homoserine
	E. coli	Homoserine → 4-phosphohomoserine
Tryptophan	E. coli	5-P-Shikimate → anthranilate
Valine	Aerobacter aerogenes	Pyruvate → acetolactate

[a]Modified from White, A., Handler, P., and E. L. Smith, *Principles of Biochemistry*, 4th edition, McGraw-Hill, New York, 1968.

DPNH and Zn^{2+}; DPNH and GTP (or GDP) with or without Zn^{2+}; DPN+ and GTP and Zn^{2+}; DPNH and steroid or diethylstilbesterol; DPNH and thyroxine or derivatives; DPNH and ATP. Various chelating agents such as orthophenanthroline or phenanthridine also favor dissociation. These changes are opposed by various metabolites including ADP, some amino acids, and organic mercurials such as methyl mercuric chloride. On the basis of considerable experimental work two types of monomer are proposed, one is enzymatically active (X) and the other, inactive (Y). Conversion of X to Y may result from a conformational change induced by the binding of effector substances cooperatively to X. The conversion may also result from a shift in the equilibrium brought on by the binding of effectors to Y.

Because of its key position in metabolism, it is of interest that mammalian glutamate dehydrogenase has a dual nucleotide specificity, acting with either DPN or TPN. The DPN-linked reaction is thought to function catabolically, while the TPN reaction is thought to function anabolically. ATP has no regulatory effect on TPNH oxidation, but it does inhibit DPNH oxidation. In addition, the regulatory effects on DPNH just discussed do not apply for

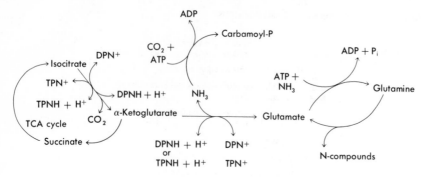

Figure 9.5   Glutamate dehydrogenase and tricarboxylic acid cycle interrelationships. Modified from E. R. Stadtman, *Adv. Enz.*, **28**, 41 (1966).

TPNH. These metabolic relationships are shown in Figure 9.5, which points out the similarity between the DPN-specific control of glutamate dehydrogenase and of the ICDH reaction discussed in Chapter 8.

Glutamine synthetase from *E. coli* has proved to be a fascinating example of regulation by covalent modification (Chapter 7). In this case, the enzyme is reversibly adenylated and deadenylated. The reaction catalyzed by glutamine synthetase is given in Eq. (10).

$$\text{glutamate}^{1-} + \text{NH}_4^+ + \text{ATP}^{4-} \longrightarrow \text{glutamine} + \text{ADP}^{3-} + \text{P}_i^{2-} + \text{H}^+ \tag{10}$$

It also catalyzes the transfer of the glutamyl group to hydroxylamine, Eq. (11).

$$\text{glutamine} + \text{NH}_2\text{OH} \longrightarrow \gamma\text{-glutamyl-NHOH} + \text{NH}_3 \tag{11}$$

If the cells are grown in the presence of NH_4^+, the activity of the enzyme is found to be very much decreased. The effect is quite specific for ammonia and is seen with bacteria related to *E. coli* but not with unrelated bacteria or with yeasts. As little as 10 minutes of treatment with ammonia causes a reduction of enzyme activity to about $\frac{1}{10}$ of control values.

Both types of enzyme activity, active and inactive, were purified to homogeneity. The molecular weight of both was found to be the same, 600,000. It was discovered that they differed in absorption spectrum and that the inactive enzyme contained bound AMP. It soon became apparent that the active enzyme became converted to the inactive form by covalent adenylation, the reaction catalyzed by a separate adenylating enzyme. A difference in metal specificity also distinguished the more active glutamine synthetase (GS) from the less active or adenylated form. The nonadenylated form utilized Mg^{2+}, while the adenylated form utilized Mn^{2+}. The adenylating enzyme,

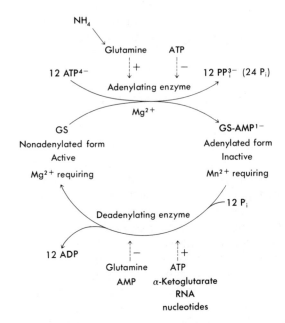

Figure 9.6

Regulation of glutamine synthetase by adenylation deadenylation. Catalytic reactions $\longrightarrow$; allosteric controls $---\rightarrow$. $+$ = positive; $-$ = negative. (See Figure 7.12). Modified from H. Holzer, *Adv. Enz.*, **32**, 297 (1969).

which used ATP as substrate, was affected positively by glutamine (Figure 9.6). NH_4^+ added to the culture medium was rapidly converted to glutamine, which acted as the intracellular effector, thus explaining the rapid inactivation by NH_4^+. ATP, itself a substrate, also affects the adenylating enzyme negatively (Figure 9.6).

The opposite conversion was catalyzed by a deadenylating enzyme utilizing P_i, with the release of ADP (Figure 9.6). The positive effectors of this reaction include ATP, α-ketoglutarate, and RNA. The negative effectors include glutamine and AMP. Thus, glutamine, the product, acts as end product inhibitor to inactivate GS by enhancing the adenylation as well as by decreasing the deadenylation. ATP, on the other hand, maintains the enzyme in its active form, as does α-ketoglutarate, thus favoring the synthesis of glutamine. AMP acts oppositely. GS is itself controlled by four known mechanisms, including *feedback inhibition, repression, cumulative feedback inhibition,* and enzyme-catalyzed *covalent modification.* The multiplicity of controls probably relates to the importance of this enzyme in metabolism.

9.3 CONTROL OF PROTEIN SYNTHESIS AND DEGRADATION

In Chapter 7 we discussed the control of the rate of protein synthesis in bacteria and showed that it is partially under genetic control and partially under control by the environment. Animal cells are considerably more complex than bacterial cells from the genetic point of view. It has been estimated, for example, that a mammalian cell may contain about 1,000 times as much genetic information as an *E. coli* cell. An *E. coli* chromosome can code for approximately 2000–4000 polypeptide chains, while a mammalian cell is potentially capable of synthesizing perhaps over a million proteins (assuming that the average size of the proteins is the same as in bacteria). Thus, there may be a difference of perhaps two to three orders of complexity between the two.

Because every animal cell (except the haploid mature sex cells, and certain specialized cells like the mature erythrocyte) contains the sum total of all the genetic information, most of which is never expressed, a highly efficient control of gene action and thus of protein synthesis must exist. It is now clear in higher animals that during major biologic shifts, such as embryonic development, birth, growth, and metamorphosis, marked changes in structure occur with changes in function. The complexity is further enhanced by the fact that these shifts are regulated by hormonal controls as well. These shifts are intimately associated with increases or decreases in the number of protein molecules. Altered enzyme activity, which is sufficient to control the less marked metabolic fluctuations, would not suffice to control these more marked biologic shifts. For example, consider that once an animal cell has become differentiated, its progeny always produces a unique set of proteins. By what means is the pattern of protein synthesis and its rate controlled in animal cells?

The pathway of DNA synthesis, RNA synthesis, amino acid activation and subsequent polymerization into protein has been discussed in Chapter 5 and in another volume of this series (Wold). It will be reviewed in outline form here. Recall that messenger RNA is first synthesized as directed by DNA template, Eq. (12) (transcription phase).

$$\text{nucleoside triphosphate XTP} \xrightarrow{\text{RNA polymerase}} (\text{XNP})_n + n\text{-PP}_i \tag{12}$$

where X = adenine, cytosine, uracil, guanine (ACUG). This reaction is inhibited by certain antibiotics including actinomycin D. The possibilities for the control of transcription are centered about the synthesis, degradation, and activity of mRNA. In effect, the number of molecules as well as their activity are, or could be, regulated. In bacterial systems the importance of the protein repressors, as well as the small inducers and corepressors, has been discussed. Are similar systems functional during the major biologic shifts? Do animal cells have repressors? Do the hormones act as or combine with the repressors? Are operators present?

Although the details of the degradation of mRNA are still under active investigation, it is already clear that the mRNA is very short-lived in bacteria (half-life of the order of minutes) as compared to animal cells (half-life of the order of hours or longer). This already suggests that the translation process may be an important site of control in animal cells.

$$\text{Amino-acyl-tRNA} \xrightarrow[\substack{\text{mRNA}\\ \text{GTP}\\ \text{Mg}^{2+}}]{\substack{\text{initiation and/or}\\ \text{transfer factors}\\ \text{ribosomes}}} \text{polypeptide} + \text{tRNA} \qquad (13)$$

Figure 5.22 (page 147) shows these reactions in diagrammatic form. Note the complexity of the process and the possibility of several potential sites of control. These include the rate of attachment of the ribosome to the mRNA. Ribosomes attach at only specific points on the mRNA, most likely the nucleotide sequences that code for the amino terminal of the polypeptide chain. What are the stereochemical factors that select this one point, and what are the factors that control the reading rate? ATP is required for amino acid activation, and GTP for peptide synthesis, possibly for frame shifting of growing polypeptide chains within the ribosome (Figure 5.22). The supply of these high energy phosphate compounds is another site of control. Yet another site is the number and activity of the tRNA molecules, which serve as adapters for polypeptide synthesis. Recently, for example, it has been shown that a number of different tRNA molecules are present which can serve as adapters for a single amino acid, some of which code for infrequent triplets in specific proteins. Thus, synthesis of certain proteins may be regulated by the availability of specific tRNA's. The supply of a prosthetic group, such as heme, may control the synthesis of its respective protein, globin, by end product inhibition. We know little about the enzymology of the polymerization or of the movement of the ribosomes along the mRNA. These are also potential sites of control.

Determination of Enzyme Turnover and Its Hormonal Control

In bacterial as well as in mammalian systems, protein synthesis can be experimentally demonstrated by increase in net mass. The conclusive experiment is one in which the incorporation of a radioactive amino acid is traced into a protein, usually an enzyme. The enzyme is first partially purified and then selectively precipitated by a specific antibody. Biosynthesis may then be determined by the radioactivity which has been incorporated into the enzyme, by the increased enzyme activity, as well as by protein-nitrogen precipitated by the antibody. Since this type of study will undoubtedly become more and more important, a typical case will be treated in detail.

Following a period of steroid (prednisolone) administration to rats, ^{14}C-leucine was injected. One hour later livers were removed, homogenized and the enzyme alanine aminotransferase extracted, partially purified, and precipitated with the specific antibody. There was about a five-fold increase in radioactivity incorporated into the enzyme of the steroid-treated as compared to the control rats (Table 9.2). The enzyme activity was correspondingly increased more than three-fold. Since the half-life of the enzyme was determined to be of the order of several days (as will be shown subsequently), these incorporation data (obtained after 1 hour) can be taken as good approximations of the relative rates of synthesis. This is true provided that there is not a large difference in the specific activity of ^{14}C-leucine in the respective control and hormone-treated precursor pools. To evaluate the possible effect of hormone administration on ^{14}C-leucine specific activities in the precursor pools, the radioactivity incorporated into total soluble protein of the liver was also determined (Table 9.2). There was only a small

TABLE 9.2 ^{14}C-LEUCINE INCORPORATION INTO LIVER ALANINE AMINOTRANSFERASE IN NORMAL AND STEROID-TREATED RATS[a]

Status	Enzyme Activity Units	C.P.M. Incorporated into Enzyme	C.P.M. Incorporated into Soluble Protein	Soluble Protein, mg.
Normal (N)	31.4	21.0	14,200	8.3
Prednisolone (P)	108.0	99.0	18,500	8.5
P/N	3.44	4.71	1.3	1.0

[a] Modified from H. S. Segal, Y. S. Kim, and S. Hopper, *Adv. Enz. Reg.*, **3**, 29 (1965), Pergamon Press, New York.

increase with steroid administration, not sufficient to account for the large increase in radioactivity incorporated into the specific enzyme. The increase in radioactivity in the enzyme can, therefore, be taken as a direct measure of increased rate of synthesis. It may, therefore, be concluded that hormone administration increased enzyme synthesis.

Kinetic analysis of the hormonal control of enzyme synthesis and degradation allows quantitative estimation of the separate rates. Let $d(E)/dt$ be the rate of enzyme increase; then it follows that

$$\frac{d(E)}{dt} = k_1 - k_2(E) \tag{14}$$

where k_1 is defined as the rate constant for enzyme synthesis and k_2 is defined as the rate constant for enzyme breakdown. It is assumed that the rate of enzyme synthesis is independent of enzyme concentration and that the rate of breakdown is first order in enzyme concentration.

Integration of Eq. (14) gives Eq. (15)

$$\ln \frac{[(k_1/k_2) - (E)]}{[(k_1/k_2) - (E_{init})]} = -k_2 t \tag{15}$$

where (E_{init}) is the initial enzyme concentration. When the new steady state is reached, $d(E)/dt = 0$. Therefore, from Eq. (14), $k_1/k_2 = (E_{final})$. Substituting in (15), we obtain

$$\ln \frac{[(E_{\text{final}}) - (E)]}{[(E_{\text{final}}) - (E_{\text{init}})]} = -k_2 t \tag{16}$$

When the enzyme activity is half-way to the new level, then we have

$$(E) = \frac{(E_{\text{final}}) + (E_{\text{init}})}{2} \tag{17}$$

Substituting in Eq. (16), we obtain

$$\ln \tfrac{1}{2} = -k_2 t_{\frac{1}{2}} \quad \text{or} \quad t_{\frac{1}{2}} = \frac{0.693}{k_2} \tag{18}$$

Therefore, the time at which one half of the new steady-state level is reached is inversely proportional to the rate constant for enzyme breakdown.

Figure 9.7 shows the time course of alanine aminotransferase (AAT) increase with steroid administration and the decrease following steroid removal. With hormone administration the new steady-state level is achieved in about five days. After discontinuing the hormone, the enzyme level returns to the normal steady-state level with a slower fall-off rate than the rate of rise. To calculate the two half-lives (control and hormone-stimulated), the equations

Figure 9.7   Time course of alanine aminotransferase after steroid administration and withdrawal. Modified from H. L. Segal, Y. S. Kim and S. Hopper, *Adv. Enz. Reg.,* **3,** 29 (1965).

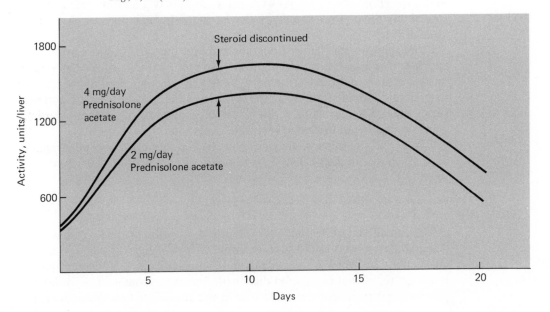

TABLE 9.3A   ENZYME LEVEL AS A FUNCTION OF TIME [a]

Normal	Steroid-treated
$\dfrac{d(E)}{dt} = k_1 - k_2 (E)$	$\dfrac{d(E)}{dt} = k_1^1 - k_2^1 (E)$
at the steady state $k_1 = k_2 (E_0)$	$k_1^1 = k_2^1 (E_0^1)$
at any time t $\ln [(E) - (E_0)] = [\ln (E_0^1) - (E_0)] - k_2 t$	$\ln [(E_0^1) - (E)] = \ln [(E_0^1) - (E_0)] - k_2^1 t$

TABLE 9.3B   CALCULATED RATES OF SYNTHESIS OF ALANINE AMINOTRANSFERASE IN NORMAL AND STEROID-TREATED RAT LIVER [a]

	(E_0) units/g liver	k_2 $(days^{-1})$	Calculated k_1 (units/g liver) $x(days^{-1})$	(mg/g liver) $x(days^{-1})$
Normal (N)	31	0.2	6.3	0.02
Prednisolone (P)	108	0.6	65.4	0.22

[a] Tables 9.3A and 9.3B modified from H. S. Segal, Y. S. Kim, and S. Hopper, *Adv. Enz. Reg.*, **3**, 29 (1965), Pergamon Press, New York.

of Table 9.3 were used. Plots of $\ln [(E) - (E_0)]$ versus t (days) and $\ln [E'_0) - (E)]$ versus t (days) were made. k_2, the degradation rate constant, was about three times larger in the hormone-treated than in the control animals.

From the rate constant for degradation and the steady-state levels of the enzyme, it is possible to calculate the rates of synthesis of the enzyme in normal and steroid-treated animals (Table 9.3). k_1 increased about ten-fold with steroid administration. Thus, hormone administration led to increased steady state AAT levels as a result of increased rates of synthesis partially compensated by an increased rate of degradation.

The $T_{1/2}$ for a number of enzymes have been determined in similar manner and are shown in Table 9.4. A wide range of values from hours to days is seen.

Influence of Nutritional State on Enzyme Turnover

The nutritional state has been shown to control protein synthesis and degradation. A well established example is that of liver arginase. The specific activity of liver arginase of rats fed diets made up of 70 percent protein is 1.5–2.5 times that of rats fed diets with 8 percent protein. This is due to a greater number of arginase molecules in the animals fed on the high protein

TABLE 9.4   HALF-LIFE (T$_{1/2}$) VALUES FOR ENZYMES

Enzyme	Organ	T$_{1/2}$
Δ-Aminolevulinate synthetase	Liver	60–74 min
Tyrosine aminotransferase	Liver	1½–2 hours
Tryptophan pyrrolase	Liver	2–4 hours
Threonine dehydrase	Liver	3 hours
Catalase	Liver	24–30 hours
Alanine aminotransferase	Liver	84 hours
Arginase	Liver	4–5 days
Aldolase	Muscle	20 days

diet as determined by the technique of immunologically precipitable protein.

If the animals on the 8 percent protein diets are starved, and if the animals on the 70 percent protein diets are switched to 8 percent protein diets, and the separate rates of synthesis and degradation estimated as described, the following may be observed (Figure 9.8). During starvation, there is a net increase of total arginase (left upper bars) which occurs in the absence of enzyme degradation (left lower bars). The stability of arginase under these conditions may be contrasted to that of other liver proteins which are in a state of breakdown. After change from a high to low protein diet, there is a marked decrease in total arginase (right-upper bars) which results from altered rates of both synthesis and degradation (right lower bars). During the first three days, there is a decreased rate of synthesis and an increased rate of breakdown. During the second period, synthesis stops, while breakdown is still going on. In the last period, the new steady state is achieved characteristic of the new diet. From this experiment it can be appreciated that diet alters both the rate of enzyme synthesis and degradation.

Control by Substrate of Enzyme Synthesis

Protein enzyme synthesis is also *controlled* by substrate. An important example is the regulation of tryptophan pyrrolase in liver by tryptophan itself. If tryptophan is administered to an adrenalectomized rat, an increase in tryptophan pyrrolase activity is observed. An increase is also observed with steroid administration. When steroid and tryptophan are given together, the increases in enzyme activity are generally additive, suggesting that two different mechanisms are involved. The finding that the steroid effect is inhibited by actinomycin D while the tryptophan action is not is also in keeping with this conclusion.

Recent experiments with purified tryptophan pyrrolase demonstrated that in order for the enzyme to be fully active, it must be preincubated with

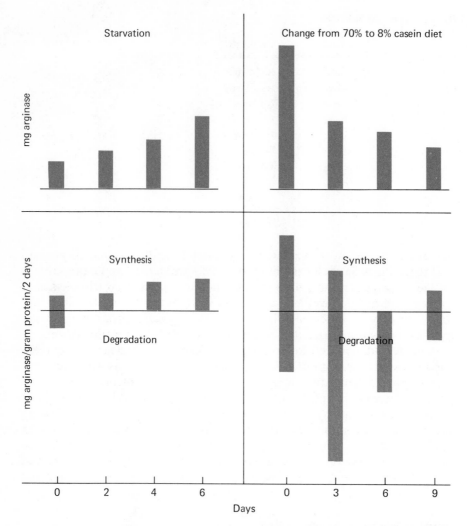

Figure 9.8   Arginase turnover in liver with fasting and diet change. Upper bars total amount of enzyme; lower bars rate of enzyme synthesis and degradation. Bar height above line = synthesis; below line = degradation. Modified from R. T. Schimke, R. Ganschow, D. Doyle, and I. M. Arias, *Fed. Proc.,* **27,** 1223 (1968).

hematin (a cofactor), a reducing agent, and tryptophan itself. An activity assay was accordingly developed using these additives together with a preincubation period to determine "total" enzyme activity. The enzyme was also assayed under "ordinary" conditions without preincubation with cofactor and activators to determine "active" enzyme. In Table 9.5, the enzyme

TABLE 9.5 TRYPTOPHAN PYRROLASE ACTIVITY FOLLOWING STEROID AND SUBSTRATE ADMINISTRATION[a]

Induction by	Enzyme Assay (units/g liver)		
	Nonactivation Conditions	Activation Conditions	Ratio
	(1)	(2)	(1)/(2)
Hydrocortisone	6.4	16.0	0.40
Tryptophan	24.8	34.0	0.73

[a] Modified from W. E. Knox, *Adv. Enz. Reg.*, **4**, 287 (1966), Pergamon Press, New York.

activities assayed as just described in livers of animals treated with steroid and with tryptophan are compared. A marked difference is observed. After tryptophan activation, the enzyme is already more fully activated than after steroid treatment. From these and other results, the following sequence of events was deduced. First, the apoenzyme is biosynthesized, Eq. (19), **a.**

$$\text{precursors} \xrightarrow{\text{Steroid}} \underset{\substack{\text{(inactive)} \\ \mathbf{a}}}{\text{apoenzyme}} \xrightarrow[\text{hematin}]{\text{L-tryptophan}} \underset{\substack{\text{(inactive)} \\ \mathbf{b}}}{\text{oxidized holoenzyme}} \xrightarrow[\substack{+ \\ \text{ascorbate} \\ \mathbf{c}}]{\text{L-tryptophan}} \underset{\text{(active)}}{\text{reduced holoenzyme}} \qquad (19)$$

This protein is inactive as a catalyst. The apoenzyme is, therefore, conjugated with hematin, **b,** its prosthetic group, to form the oxidized form of the holoenzyme, which is also catalytically inactive. This is reduced, **c,** with ascorbate to the active form of the holoenzyme. There are, thus, two inactive forms of the enzyme and one active form. Steroids promote the biosynthesis of the apoenzyme, and this step is inhibited by actinomycin D. Tryptophan promotes the conversion of the two inactive forms to the active form of the enzyme in vitro as well as in vivo. Thus, the *double assay procedure* (with and without activation) was a key point in working out the difference in mechanism of action of tryptophan and steroid in promoting increased tryptophan pyrrolase levels in liver. This combined mechanism of regulation by promotion of biosynthesis by steroid and promotion of conversion of inactive to active enzyme by substrate is a fascinating example of dual regulation.

Substrates have also been shown to act by decreasing enzyme degradation.

Change in Enzyme Patterns

Control of protein enzyme levels is readily observed during major biological shifts such as those listed in Table 9.6. One of the fascinating aspects of

**TABLE 9.6   BIOLOGICAL SHIFTS ASSOCIATED WITH CONTROL OF
PROTEIN ENZYME LEVEL**

Embryological development

Metamorphosis
  Insect
  Amphibian

Neonatal development

Growth and Development
  Puberty

Dietary perturbations
  Starvation
  Obesity

Environmental alterations
  Drugs
  Chemical agents

these studies is the manner in which *patterns* of metabolism are altered by emphasizing or deemphasizing whole *groups* of enzymes. Studies of the mechanisms of control during these major shifts have and will continue to yield rich rewards in terms of understanding biology at the chemical level.

9.4   APPROACHES USED TO STUDY THE MECHANISM OF ACTION OF HORMONES TO CONTROL PROTEIN BIOSYNTHESIS AT THE CHEMICAL LEVEL

As indicated by the reactions of protein biosynthesis, the potentialities for control exist at all possible sites, that is, transcription of DNA into RNA, amino acid activation, and the translation of RNA into the polypeptide sequence. Although no complete mechanism of hormonal control of protein biosynthesis has been worked out, a number of valuable approaches have appeared and will be discussed.

A number of hormones act to regulate protein synthesis in tissues. This is readily shown either in vivo or in vitro by the stimulation of the incorporation of labeled amino acids into mixed total proteins. A number of such observations with a variety of hormones are listed in Table 9.7A. Furthermore, hormones control the synthesis and/or degradation of a number of specific proteins and enzymes which are also listed in Table 9.7B. Note the wide variety of mammalian, insect, and plant hormones studied.

Of special importance in mammals are the glucocorticoids, insulin, glucagon, and the androgens and estrogens, and thyroid hormones. Each of these hormones controls protein enzyme synthesis or degradation. Note specially those cases where *groups of enzymes* are controlled. Groups such as those catalyzing reactions in gluconeogenesis are of considerable interest

TABLE 9.7A   HORMONAL STIMULATION OF PROTEIN SYNTHESIS IN VIVO AND IN VITRO[a]

Hormone	Species	In Vivo	In Vitro
Growth hormone	Rat, man	Liver, kidney, heart spleen, adrenal	Liver slices, cell-free system, adrenal quarters
ACTH	Rat	Adrenal	Adrenal quarters, cell-free system
TSH	Chicken, rat	Thyroid	Thyroid slices
Thyroxine, triiodothyronine	Rat, man	Liver, kidney, heart	Liver mitochondria, liver microsomes or ribosomes
	Frog, tadpole		Liver slices
Testosterone	Rat, mouse, guinea pig	Seminal vesicle, prostate, kidney	Slices, homogenates, muscle minces, cell-free preparations from seminal vesicle, prostate, kidney, muscle
Estrogen	Rat, hen	Rat uterus, hen oviduct	Slices, homogenates, cell-free preparations of rat uterus and hen oviduct
Cortisone	Rat	Liver	Liver microsomes
Insulin	Rat	Liver, diaphragm, skeletal muscle	Diaphragm, liver slices, cell-free preparations from liver and heart.

TABLE 9.7B   ENZYME OR PROTEIN

Hormone	Specific Protein Synthesized
Thyroxin triiodothyronine	Cytochrome C, isocitrate dehydrogenase, respiratory components and membranes
Testosterone	
Estrogen	Phosphovitin
Cortisone	Tryphophan pyrrolase, transaminase(s), gluconeogenic enzymes
Insulin	Glucokinase, pyruvate kinase, malic enzyme.

[a] From J. R. Tata, *Prog. in Nucleic Acid Res. and Molec. Biol.*, **5**, 191 (1966).

because the altered enzyme activities could be related directly to the altered metabolism. Under these conditions, in vivo functions for the enzymes could, therefore, be assigned.

Inhibitors

A number of inhibitors of protein synthesis have been widely used (Table 9.8). As can be seen, the inhibitors are divided into four groups and act at all sites in the process. Because of its structure, actinomycin D combines with guanine bases and thus inhibits DNA-dependent RNA synthesis, Eq. (12). Its action, measured by the inhibition of incorporation of orotate into nucleic acid, can lead to essentially complete inhibition of RNA synthesis.

TABLE 9.8   INHIBITORS OF PROTEIN SYNTHESIS

Group 1: Inhibitors of nucleoside (deoxynucleoside) triphosphate synthesis

a. Azaserine	Inhibits reactions using NH_2 from glutamine
b. Aminopterin and Amethopterin	Inhibit synthesis of tetrahydrofolic acid (coenzyme in the synthesis of nucleotides)
c. Sulfonamides	Inhibit p-aminobenzoic acid competitively
d. 5-Fluorodeoxyuridine	Inhibits (competitively) thymidine biosynthesis (specific inhibitor of DNA synthesis)

Group 2: Inhibitors of DNA-synthesis (replication)

a. Mitomycin C Phleomycin	Causes fragmentation of DNA (cross-link formation?)

Group 3: Inhibitors of RNA-synthesis

a. Actinomycin D Chromomycin A3	Complexes with G in DNA to block transcription (Not clear why replication is not affected)
b. Chloramphenicol Cycloheximide	Blocks synthesis of rRNA and functional ribosomes

Group 4: Inhibitors of protein synthesis

a. Tetracyclines (Terramycin, Aureomycin) and Streptomycin	Bond to ribosomes and give faulty(?) reading of mRNA
b. 5-Methyl tryptophan	Competes with try for tRNA try
c. Puromycin Tenuagonic acid	Blocks growth of polypeptide chain Blocks release of finished product from ribosomes

Puromycin acts at translation [see Eq. (13)] by inhibiting the elongation of peptides. Its action is determined by measuring the incorporation of labeled amino acids into proteins. With inhibitor present in sufficient concentration, the incorporation may be reduced *almost* completely.

Conclusions derived from inhibiting effects *alone* are usually not justified because inhibitors may and usually do have several actions. One of the clearest examples is puromycin which, in addition to its action on protein synthesis, acts separately as a competitive inhibitor of 3′,5′-cyclic adenylate in its hydrolysis by phosphodiesterase and probably at other cyclic adenylate sites as well. Conclusions derived from studies of inhibitions of hormone effects can also be confusing when they relate to hormones that have multiple effects, because it has not been established whether multiple effects derive from a single action of the hormone or from multiple actions. In the case of insulin, for example, the stimulation of transport of sugars, amino acids, or glycogen synthesis in muscle is not inhibited by actinomycin D or puromycin, but the stimulation of RNA and protein synthesis in muscle is inhibited. On the other hand, all of the actions of some hormones (sex hormones, thyroid) appear to be inhibited by the inhibitors of RNA and protein synthesis. Finally, the action of inhibitors is markedly dependent on experimental conditions, thus leading to conflicting reports. Among the most important are timing of the experiment and the dose of inhibitor used. Excessive inhibitor doses may lead to nonspecific toxic effects. With low

TABLE 9.9   A HORMONE CLASSIFICATION IN TERMS OF TIME OF ONSET OF ACTION AND GENERAL TYPE(S) OF EFFECTS

Hormone	Time of Onset of Action	General Type of Hormone Effects
Epinephrine and catecholamines	Seconds–minutes	Metabolic
Glucagon	Seconds–minutes	Metabolic and growth
Insulin	Minutes–hours	Metabolic and growth
ACTH	Minutes–hours	Metabolic and growth
Cortisone	Minutes–hours	Metabolic and growth
Testosterone	Hours–days	Growth
Estrogen	Hours–days	Growth
Growth hormone	Hours–days	Growth
TSH	Hours–days	Growth
Ecdysone	?	Growth
Thyroid hormones	Days	Growth

doses, the effect may not be observed. It is useful to remember that *dose-response curves give a great deal more information than single-dose experiments.*

RNA Synthesis

RNA synthesis is known to be stimulated by every hormone which stimulates growth as well as by several hormones which are "metabolic" hormones. Table 9.9 is a "rough" classification of hormones in terms of time of action and type of effects produced. In most cases, the stimulation of RNA synthesis precedes the stimulation of protein synthesis in the cytoplasm. This is particularly well illustrated in the case of the very slowly acting thyroid hormone. Following a single injection of triiodothyronine into a thyroidectomized rat, the sequence of events in liver is shown in Figure 9.9. The early stimulation of nuclear RNA synthesis precedes the increased activity of the nuclear RNA polymerase enzyme activity (Mg^{2+} stimulated) as well as the ribosomal RNA synthesis and microsomal protein synthesis. Hormones accelerate the synthesis of all types of RNA.

By another approach, it has proved possible to detect hormonal control of nuclear "messenger-like" RNA. RNA is extracted from nuclei and assayed for its biological template activity using an *E. coli* ribosomal "indicator system" catalyzing the conversion of labeled amino acids into proteins. In this way, it was demonstrated that RNA from nuclei of castrate rats had decreased template activity compared with RNA from normal rats. Testosterone administration reversed this effect. This appears to be some of the clearest evidence for the hormonal control of the synthesis of specific types of RNA.

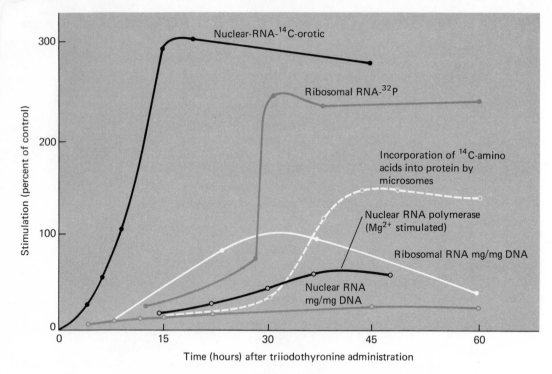

Figure 9.9   Biochemical signposts of triiodothyronine action in rat liver. Note the early
effects observed on the incorporation of ^{14}C-orotate into nuclear RNA and
the somewhat later effects on ribosomal RNA synthesis, microsomal protein
synthesis, and nuclear RNA polymerase activity. From J. R. Tata, Hormones and the Synthesis and Utilization of Ribonucleic Acids, *Progress in
Nucleic Acid Research and Molecular Biology,* **5,** 191 (1966).

RNA Polymerase

The activity of the DNA-dependent RNA polymerase enzyme in nuclei
has been assayed following hormonal perturbation. The mammalian enzyme has not as yet been resolved free of endogenous DNA. Accordingly,
the enzymology is "dirty" in the sense that assays measure the activity of the
enzyme and the endogenous DNA template together. The polymerase is
dependent on the four nucleoside triphosphates as substrate and is inhibited
by actinomycin D. It is of considerable interest that the activity of the enzyme is increased after hormone treatment (Figure 9.10). From this experiment alone, it is impossible to say whether this means that the template
DNA is increased or whether the enzyme activity itself is increased.

Figure 9.10

Effects of hormone administration on nuclear RNA polymerase activity.
Administration of growth hormone, triiodothyronine, and testosterone all
cause an increase in enzyme activity. Note the differences observed between
Mg^{2+} and Mn^{2+} + ammonium sulfate additions, suggesting that there may
possibly be two different enzymes or two forms of the enzyme. From J. R.
Tata, Hormones and the Synthesis and Utilization of Ribonucleic Acids,
Progress in Nucleic Acid Research and Molecular Biology, **5,** 191 (1966).

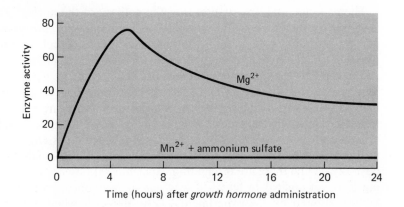

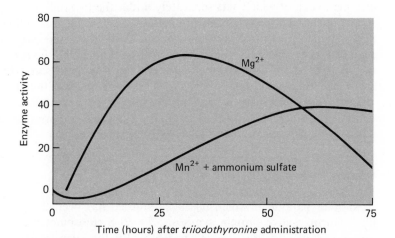

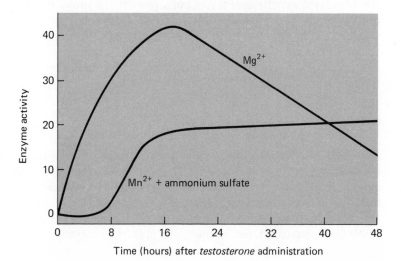

The experimental observation that the activity of the nuclear polymerase is markedly increased in the presence of high salt concentrations (e.g., 10 percent saturated ammonium sulfate) is also of considerable interest. In the presence of the increased ionic strength, the enzyme is altered such that it acquires a Mn^{2+} requirement in place of Mg^{2+}, which is the metal normally required in the absence of salt. The RNA synthesized in the presence of high salt and Mn^{2+} differs in base composition and nearest-neighbor base frequency from that synthesized with Mg^{2+} in the absence of salt. In the presence of high salt and Mn^{2+}, the RNA is more "messenger-like", while in the presence of Mg^{2+} alone, the RNA is more "ribosomal-like" in composition. While these are fascinating experimental observations, their meaning is as yet unclear in terms of whether there is one enzyme whose specificity is altered by the experimental conditions, or whether there are two enzymes, each of which acts separately under the two different conditions.

The hormonal perturbations are equally fascinating, but difficult to interpret. The effect of three hormones on the two polymerase enzyme activities is shown in Figure 9.10. It can be seen that, kinetically, the *earliest* effect is on the Mg^{2+}-requiring enzyme activity assayed without salt, which synthesizes the "ribosomal-type" of RNA. This suggests that the stimulation of ribosomal RNA synthesis may be an important early event in hormone action. The significance of this enzymatic "marker" of hormone action must await further purification and study of the enzyme itself.

Polysome Profiles

Another parameter which has been studied has been the polysome profiles. During active protein synthesis, 70–80 S ribosomes are "aggregated" into polysomes by the messenger RNA. By the sucrose density gradient centrifugation experiment, it has been possible to show that the proportion of total ribosomes recovered as polysomes is depressed after hormone gland ablation. After injection of the appropriate hormone, normal levels of polysomes are restored. This is in keeping with hormone-stimulated nuclear messenger RNA synthesis, and the increased template activity of nuclear RNA.

Effects of Added Synthetic Polynucleotides

Further experimental efforts have been directed at simplifying the protein-synthesizing portion of the process itself. 80-S ribosomes prepared from mammalian tissues are stimulated by synthetic polyribonucleotides much like 70-S *E. coli* ribosomes are stimulated. Using tRNA charged with ^{14}C-amino acids, it has been possible to study the messenger RNA content of ribosomes prepared from hormonally perturbed animals. This is done by measuring protein synthesis with endogenous messenger RNA, and then adding excess polyribonucleotide to fully stimulate the system (a "plus-minus assay" in effect). In such an experiment the activity of prostatic ribosomes without polynucleotide was shown to be markedly reduced after orchiectomy and restored in activity following testosterone administration. The maximum synthetic capacity of the system as expressed by the activity with added polynucleotide was not affected by the hormonal perturbations. This indicates that the enzyme itself was not altered, but that there was an altered messenger RNA content of the ribosomes as a result of the hormonal perturbations. Much more work is required to carefully study this situation, including experiments with a number of different hormones to decide whether this pattern is indeed a general one or limited to the particular case studied.

It would appear from the work done thus far that evidence has been brought forward which indicates that hormones act to control the messenger RNA content, and thus may be thought of to somehow control transcription. Since mammalian messenger RNA is considered to be relatively long-lived compared with its bacterial counterpart, it is thought possible that control of translation may also be present. Evidence to prove this idea will be most eagerly sought for in the future.

9.5 THE CONTROL OF ADAPTIVE ENZYME SYNTHESIS IN BACTERIA BY 3'5' CYCLIC ADENYLATE

The actions of 3'5' cyclic adenylate to control adaptive enzyme synthesis in bacteria have been elegantly studied recently with considerable success. In a phylogenetic survey study, it was originally discovered that *E. coli* contained cyclic adenylate, and that glucose added in the growth medium decreased the concentration of the cyclic nucleotide. It had been known for some time that glucose repressed some enzyme synthesis in bacteria. From these two pieces of information it was deduced that the repression by glucose might be due to a decrease in the level of cyclic adenylate. To test this hypothesis, cyclic adenylate was added to an *E. coli* culture in which the synthesis of β-galactosidase was repressed by glucose. As is shown in Figure 9.11, where β-galactosidase activity (units/ml) is plotted against growth rate (measured by absorbance at 560 nm), after the addition of glucose, there is a "transient repression" which lasts 20–30 minutes during which time there is almost a complete cessation of β-galactosidase synthesis. This is followed by a renewal of β-galactosidase synthesis, but at a decreased rate. Cyclic adenylate addition overcomes both types of repression and restores the rate to normal. It is now known that the synthesis of a number of enzymes in *E. coli* and in other bacteria as well is stimulated by cyclic adenylate (Table 9.10).

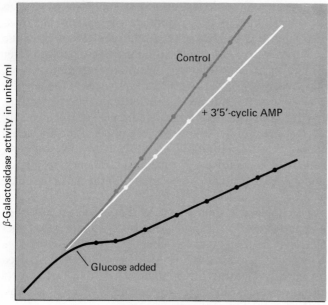

Absorbance at 560 nm.

Figure 9.11

E. coli was grown on a minimal medium supplemented with thiamine (5 µg/ml) and glycerol (0.5 percent). At the start of the experiment isopropyl thiogalactoside (IPTG), the inducer, was added. Ten minutes later the culture was divided into three parts. They are represented on the graph as follows: the control group, in color; glucose added (0.01M), in black; glucose (0.01M) plus 3'5' cyclic adenylate (5×10^{-3} M) added, in white. From I. Pastan and R. Perlman, *Science,* **169,** 339 (1970).

TABLE 9.10   CYCLIC AMP STIMULATION OF ENZYME SYNTHESIS[a]

Bacterial organism	Enzyme
Escherichia coli	β-galactosidase
	lac permease
	galactokinase
	glycerol kinase
	α-glycerol-P-permease
	L-arabinose permease
	fructose phosphotransferase
	tryptophanase
	D-serine deaminase
	thymidine phosphorylase
Salmonella typhimurium	galactokinase
Aerobacter aerogenes	β-galactosidase

[a] From I. Pastan and R. Perlman, *Science,* **169,** 339 (1970).

Since added cyclic adenylate overcame the glucose repression, cyclic adenylate concentrations were measured in bacteria repressed by glucose. Using sensitive analytical methods which we need not detail here, it was found that concentrations were decreased to approximately $\frac{1}{10}$ those of control. Addition of other repressive compounds also lowered cyclic adenylate concentrations, and the decreased levels were qualitatively correlated with the severity of the repression.

To further examine this hypothesis, cyclic adenylate deficient mutants were isolated by a procedure which involved selection from a single plate of colonies which could not ferment lactose and galactose. Such a mutant strain was found to contain undetectable cyclic adenylate and was markedly deficient in adenyl cyclase activity, the enzyme forming cyclic adenylate from ATP. When an inducing agent was added (isopropyl thiogalactoside, IPTG), the mutant made only 5 per cent of the β-galactosidase as the parent strain. Added cyclic adenylate increased synthesis toward normal. In fact, added cyclic adenylate corrected a number of other metabolic defects in the organism as well, including restoring tryptophanase and D-serine deaminase activities.

To study the reasons for the effectiveness of cyclic adenylate, the question was asked "Does cyclic adenylate affect transcription or translation?"

When the *amount and the rate* of lac mRNA synthesis was studied by selective hybridization techniques, it was shown that added cyclic adenylate increased the *amount and the rate* of lac mRNA synthesis. Conversely in glucose-repressed cells, a decreased *amount and rate* of lac mRNA synthesis was noted. Added cyclic adenylate increased the *amount and rate* of lac mRNA synthesis in glucose-repressed cultures. These elegant experiments which correlate the rate of mRNA synthesis, the amount of mRNA and the rate of enzyme synthesis, demonstrate that cyclic adenylate acts to control transcription.

Does the cyclic nucleotide therefore control transcription by increasing the frequency of initiation of mRNA synthesis, or does it increase the rate of the subsequent polymerization? Some evidence, in favor of the former, is provided by an experiment with the inhibitor rifampicin, which specifically inhibits RNA initiation and not polymerization. Rifampicin inhibits the cyclic adenylate stimulation.

This conclusion agrees well with the work carried out with regulator gene mutants. β-galactosidase synthesis in i$^-$ and o$^-$ gene mutants was repressed normally by glucose and responded normally to cyclic adenylate. Promotor (p$^-$) mutants however, had an altered response to cyclic adenylate. One mutant in which most of the p and part of the i gene were deleted was completely unresponsive to cyclic AMP. Another mutant had a decreased sensitivity to cyclic adenylate. There is also evidence that (p$^-$) mutants are resistant to glucose repression.

Thus, the point of action of cyclic adenylate in transcription has been elegantly delineated by these experiments. Whether it acts on the enzyme, or on the DNA is not known at present. Figure 9.12 shows schematically the control by cyclic adenylate of transcription of the lac operon in *E. coli*.

There is also evidence that cyclic adenylate acts to control translation. When cyclic adenylate was added after messenger RNA synthesis was

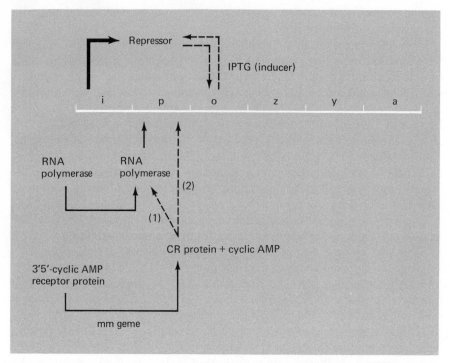

Figure 9.12   3'5' Cyclic AMP Control of Transcription of lac Operon. See Figure 7.13. i, P, and O are regulator, promotor, and operator genes respectively while Z, Y, and a genes code for β-galactosidase, galactose permease and transacetylase respectively. Genes for the RNA polymerase and 3'5' cyclic AMP receptor protein (-CR) are also shown. Note the two possible sites of action of 3'5'cyclic AMP when combined with its receptor protein, the polymerase (1) and the DNA of the P gene (2). From I. Pastan and R. Perlman, *Science,* **169,** 339 (1970).

stopped by actinomycin D or proflavin, it was found that tryptophanase synthesis was stimulated. Since there was no detectable effect on the rate of tryptophanase mRNA breakdown, nor on the rate of conversion of precursor to active enzyme, it would appear that the rate of polypeptide chain elongation was increased..

Thus, studies with bacteria have demonstrated that the cyclic nucleotide acts to control transcription and probably also translation as well.

In this chapter we have described the control of purine and pyrimidine nucleotide and amino acid metabolism and the control of protein biosynthesis. Some of the sites of control by hormones and by major biological shifts such as neonatal development are known. The mechanisms of control are still to be determined. The site of action of cyclic AMP to promote enzyme synthesis in *E. coli* was shown to be localized at the promotor or p gene in transcription. There is also probably control of translation as well.

REFERENCES

Bitensky, M. W., Yielding, K. L., and Tomkins, G. M., *J. Biol. Chem.,* **240,** 663 (1965).

Burch, H. B., "Substrates of Carbohydrate Metabolism and their Relation to Enzyme Levels in Liver from Rats of Various Ages," *Adv. Enz. Reg.,* **3,** 185 (1965), Pergamon Press.

Holzer, H., "Regulation of Enzymes by Enzyme-Catalyzed Chemical Modification." *Adv. Enz.,* **32,** 297 (1969), Interscience Publishers.

Knox, W. E. "The Regulation of Tryptophan Pyrrolase Activity by Tryptophan," *Adv. Enz. Reg.,* **4,** 287 (1966), Pergamon Press.

Pastan, I. and R. L. Perlman, *Science,* **169,** 339 (1970).

Schimke, R. T., Ganschow, R., Doyle, D., and I. M. Arias, *Fed. Proc.,* **27,** 1223 (1968).

Segal, H. L., Kim, Y. S., and S. Hopper, "Glucocorticoid Control of Rat Liver Glutamic-Alanine Transaminase Biosynthesis," *Adv. Enz. Reg.,* **3,** 29 (1965), Pergamon Press.

Stadtman, E. R., "Allosteric Regulation of Enzyme Activity," *Adv. Enz.,* **28,** 41 (1966), Interscience Publishers.

Tata, J. R., "Hormones and the Synthesis and Utilization of Ribonucleic Acids," *Progress in Nucleic Acid Research and Molecular Biology,* **5,** 191 (1966).

William-Ashman, H. G., Liao, S., Hancock, R. L., Jurkowitz, L., and D. A. Silverman, *Rec. Prog. Horm. Res.,* **20,** 247 (1964).

INTEGRATION
AND CONTROL OF
ENERGY METABOLISM

TEN

In this chapter, we will discuss the control of energy metabolism. We will see how important a role specific inhibitors played in elucidating the control of respiration, phosphorylation, and ion transport. The development of the concept of the requirement of a supramolecular organization for biochemical function will be introduced. A human genetic block will also be considered from the point of view of its influence on our ideas of the control of energy metabolism. Finally, by way of bringing the control of all of metabolism together, the control through the *energy charge* concept of the adenylate system will be discussed. Here, it can be appreciated how control operates throughout all of metabolism to gear energy production and energy utilization to meet cellular requirements.

10.1 SUBSTRATE CONTROLS, INHIBITORS, AND CROSSOVER POINTS

Stripped down to its essential form, the chain of respiratory carriers, as already discussed (Chapter 3), for mitochondrial transport of electrons consists of the following Eq. (1).

$$\text{DPN} \longrightarrow \text{FP} \longrightarrow \text{cyt b} \longrightarrow \text{cyt c} \longrightarrow \text{cyt a} \longrightarrow O_2 \tag{1}$$

From thermodynamic considerations, it was shown previously that the three energy-conserving phosphorylation steps occurred at DPN $\longrightarrow$ FP, cyt b $\longrightarrow$ cyt c, cyt a $\longrightarrow$ O_2.

The regulation of respiration could conceivably arise through control at one or more of three loci, (1) O_2 supply, (2) substrate supply, or (3) the ATP-synthesizing mechanism itself. As a result of many different types of experiments, it is clear that control at (3), the ATP-synthesizing mechanism, is of greatest significance.

One of the earliest experiments demonstrating this control was done with rat liver mitochondria oxidizing pyruvate. By adding glucose and a purified yeast hexokinase preparation it was possible to demonstrate a marked stimulation of respiration. This "ATP-trapping system" converted the terminal P of ATP formed during respiration into the more stable glucose-6-P. ADP was formed as nucleotide product which, by acting as phosphate acceptor, itself stimulated respiration.

Control by ADP and P_i

With the polarographic method, it was possible to *continuously* monitor O_2 uptake. Using this technique, the effect of ADP exhaustion and readdition could be demonstrated *directly* (Figure 10.1). When P_i was added to mitochondria oxidizing glutamate as substrate, respiration was slow, 8 mμ atoms of oxygen $\times$ min^{-1}. On adding ADP (0.2 μM), the rate immediately increased ten-fold to 80 mμ atoms of oxygen $\times$ min^{-1}, and then leveled off at a

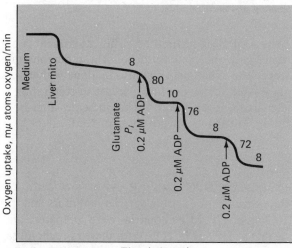

Figure 10.1

Effect of ADP and P_i in control of respiration. Numbers correspond to rates of oxygen uptake measured polarigraphically in mμ atoms of O_2 per minute. Control rate = 8. On adding glutamate, P_i, and ADP note 10 fold increase in rate to 80. Note the repeated effect of ADP addition. From L. Ernster and R. Luft, *Adv. in Metabolic Disorders, Vol. I*, R. Levine and R. Luft, editors, p. 95, Academic Press, Inc., New York, 1964.

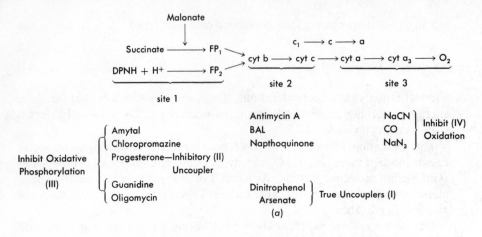

Types of Respiratory Inhibitors & Uncoupling Agents

    I. *True Uncouplers*
       Eliminate phosphorylation and either not affect or stimulate respiration rate.
       (a) Dinitrophenol
       (b) Arsenate
    II. *Inhibitory Uncouplers*
       Depress respiration rate but inhibit phosphorylation even more.
       (a) Progesterone
    III. *Inhibitors of Oxidative Phosphorylation*
       Inhibit respiration only when coupled to phosphorylation.
       (a) Guanidine   (c) Amytal
       (b) Oligomycin (d) Chlorpromazine
    IV. *Inhibitors of Oxidation*
       Inhibit respiration either uncoupled or coupled.
       (a) NaCN
       (b) CO
       (c) NaN_3

(b)

Figure 10.2 (a) The simplified respiratory pathway and the sites of action of inhibitors.
(b) Four classes of respiratory inhibitors and uncoupling agents.

new slower rate of 10 when the ADP became limiting. This experiment could be repeated a number of times with the same mitochondria to demonstrate the reversibility of the process. The experiment can also be done with excess ADP and limiting P_i. Upon P_i addition, a marked increase in respiration is again observed but not so marked as with ADP. This indicates that both ADP and P_i control respiration, but P_i less effectively than ADP.

Inhibitors and Crossover Points

The three sites of phosphorylation, DPN $\longrightarrow$ FP, cyt b $\longrightarrow$ cyt c, cyt a $\longrightarrow$ O_2, have been directly demonstrated using specific inhibitors and the crossover point concept (Chapter 7). Mitochondria were prepared and treated to make them permeable to DPNH + H$^+$. With these mitochondria, it was shown that for each oxygen atom used, about three $\frown$ P bonds were formed. This is designated as a P/O ratio of 3. If a reducing agent such as ascorbate was used to generate reduced cytochrome c, or if chemically reduced cytochrome c was used with permeable mitochondria, it was shown that when cytochrome c was reoxidized a P/O ratio approaching 1 was obtained. The fact that the coupled phosphorylation in this reaction was sensitive to inhibition by dinitrophenol was taken as evidence that it was truly oxidative phosphorylation. This localized one of the three phosphorylation sites to cyt c $\longrightarrow$ O_2 (Figure 10.2, site 3). With succinate as substrate, which bypassed the DPN site and fed electrons directly into a different FP, a P/O ratio approaching 2 was obtained. Since the FP $\longrightarrow$ cyt b potential difference was too small to account for an ATP energy-conservation step (see Chapter 3), this then localized the second site to cyt b $\longrightarrow$ cyt c (Figure 10.2, site 2). The DPNH $\longrightarrow$ FP site was separately shown by an interesting experiment. With DPNH + H^+ as substrate, the oxidation was localized to FP by using ferricyanide as electron acceptor (from FP) and antimycin A, an antibiotic respiratory inhibitor, to inhibit oxidation via the cytochromes. Under these conditions, a P/O ratio approaching 1 was obtained (Figure 10.2, site 1).

Since the various components of the respiratory chain have distinctive absorptions which differ in the oxidized and reduced states, it is possible to follow *dynamically* the changes in oxidation-reduction states when inhibitors are added or conditions are otherwise changed. For example, when antimycin A is added to metabolizing mitochondria, there is an oxidation of cytochromes a and c, while cytochrome b and DPN become reduced. This is illustrated diagrammatically in Figure 10.3 (curve 1). This crossover point between cytochromes b and c marks the point at which antimycin A has acted to inhibit respiration.

Similar studies were made to detect respiratory crossover points when phosphorylation was limited by ADP exhaustion in mitochondria carrying out both respiration and phosphorylation—so-called "tightly-coupled" mitochondria. When respiration was decreased because of a lack of ADP, a crossover point was detected between reduced cytochrome c and oxidized cytochrome a (Figure 10.3, curve 2). If ADP were added, the normal state was restored, indicating that the process was completely reversible. Thus, one site of phosphorylation (cyt c $\longrightarrow$ O_2, site 3) was independently identified. If 0.1 M azide was added to the ADP-depleted mitochondria, the crossover point shifted "downstream"; cytochrome b was reduced and cytochrome c was oxidized (Figure 10.3, curve 3). This marked the second phosphorylation site (site 2). In similar manner, the third site was identified when cyanide was added to mitochondria in the ADP-depleted site. Under these conditions, the crossover point was shifted further downstream; DPN was reduced and FP was oxidized (Figure 10.3, curve 4). Thus, by this type of experiment, the three phosphorylation sites were identified. Similar studies identified the specific sites of action of a number of respiratory inhibitors. These are indicated in Figure 10.2. As mentioned, the flavoproteins which accept electrons from succinate and DPNH are different ones and are indi-

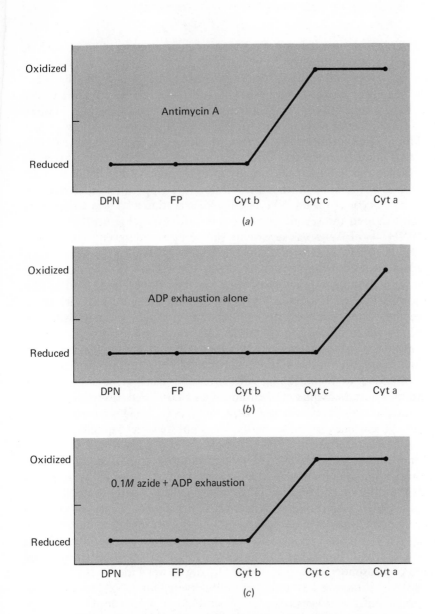

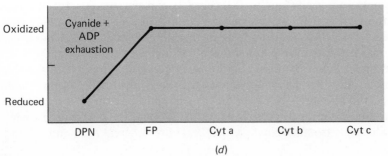

(a)

(b)

(c)

(d)

cated in the figure as FP_1 and FP_2, respectively. The two components of cytochrome a are also shown, cytochrome a the electron acceptor, and cytochrome a_3 the component which activates oxygen.

10.2   UNCOUPLING OF RESPIRATION AND PHOSPHORYLATION

Much of our knowledge of respiratory phosphorylation and its control comes from what has been termed the *phenomenon of uncoupling*. This implies that mitochondria, which becomes uncoupled, are able to respire but lack the control of respiration by P_i and ADP. Note that this situation is analogous to the case of an enzyme (e.g., ATCase, Section 9.1), which has been "desensitized" such that it is catalytically active but has lost the control of catalysis. In the latter case, the separation of catalytic and control subunits has been accomplished.

The control characteristics of a mitochondrial respiratory system are shown in Figure 10.4 in diagrammatic form. The product of the three phosphorylation sites, an *hypothetical* high-energy intermediate, is designated $\smallsmile$ I. $\smallsmile$ I is then converted to the *hypothetical* transfer compound X $\smallsmile$ I. The control by ADP and (to a lesser extent) by P_i is shown in the graph at the left, where increased ADP and P_i concentration leads to increased respiration rate. This occurs *with* increased ATP formation. On the right, control by uncoupling agents is shown. Increased uncoupler (e.g., dinitrophenol) concentration or (Ca^{2+}) leads to increased respiration rate but *without* ATP formation.

Two stages of uncoupling have been experimentally distinguished (Figure 10.5). In the control tightly-coupled system, addition of ADP + P_i leads to increased respiration with a high P/O ratio. With a relatively low concentration of an uncoupling agent (e.g., 10^{-5} *M* dinitrophenol), a reasonable phosphorylation occurs with reasonable efficiency (P/O ratio) *even in the face of a more or less complete loss of respiratory control by* P_i *and ADP* (*loosely coupled*). With a higher concentration (e.g., 10^{-4} *M* dinitrophenol), there is a complete loss of both phosphorylation and respiratory control (*complete uncoupling*).

Many studies have shown that whenever uncoupling occurs there can be demonstrated an enhanced enzymatic hydrolysis of ATP to ADP + P_i (ATPase activity). Much evidence indicates that this ATPase activity constitutes the respiratory phosphorylation pathway acting in the reverse direction. It would appear, then, that the uncoupling agents do not inactivate this enzymatic pathway but somehow disconnect it from respiration.

Figure 10.3

Schematic representation of crossover points in oxidative phosphorylation. (*a*) effect of antimycin A; (*b*) effect of ADP exhaustion alone; (*c*) effect of 0.1 M azide + ADP exhaustion; (*d*) effect of cyanide + ADP exhaustion. Note the shift of the crossover point "downstream."

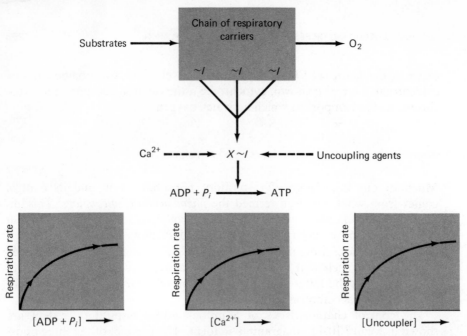

Figure 10.4   Schematic representation of respiratory control in mitochondria. The control by ADP + P_i, Ca^{2+}, and uncouplers to increase respiration is shown. $\sim$I is a hypothetical high energy intermediate; X $\sim$ I, a hypothetical high energy transfer compound. From B. Chance, Control of Energy Metabolism, *Colloquium of the Johnson Research Found,* Edited B. Chance, R. W. Estabrook, and J. R. Williamson, Academic Press, Inc., New York, 1965.

Figure 10.5   Loosely coupled and uncoupled oxidative phosphorylation. Experiment 1: tightly coupled, without dinitrophenol; experiment 2: loosely coupled with 10^{-5} M dinitrophenol; experiment 3: uncoupled with 10^{-4} M dinitrophenol. From G. F. Azzone, O. Eeg-Olofsson, L. Ernster, R. Luft and G. Szaboleski, *Exptl. Cell Res.,* **22,** 415 (1961).

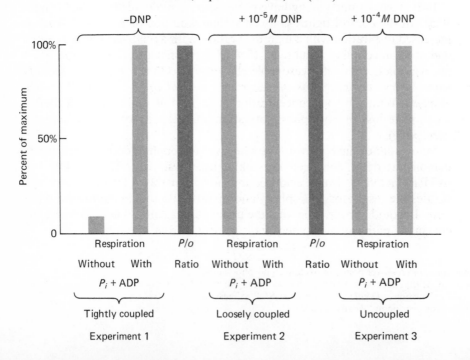

Interestingly, fractionation studies of the ATPase activity have shown that it can be separated into two major fractions, one of which (termed F_1) is a protein of molecular weight 280,000 and has the enzymatic activity *but is no longer sensitive to uncoupling agents*. The other fraction (F_0), a complex lipo-protein, is itself enzymatically inactive so far as ATP hydrolysis is concerned. When F_0 is added back to F_1, the sensitivity to uncoupling agents is restored. Clearly, the analogy to the separation of catalytic and control subunits in the case of ATCase is strong. In Figure 10.2, uncoupling agents have been classified into four types. Type I, the true uncoupler, acts to eliminate the phosphorylation either without affecting or even stimulating respiration. Type II inhibits respiration as well as phosphorylation; Type III inhibits respiration only when it is coupled to phosphorylation; Type IV inhibits respiration alone under any circumstances.

10.3 ATPase AND ION TRANSPORT

Throughout this book, we have constantly emphasized those reactions in which there is a net gain or loss in charge. The respiratory phosphorylation of ADP to ATP is an example of such a reaction in which formally a proton is taken up, Eq. (2).

$$H^+ + ADP^{3-} + P_i^{2-} \longrightarrow ATP^{4-} + H_2O \tag{2}$$

In the opposite direction, when ATP is hydrolyzed, a proton is produced. Experimentally, if the reaction is run in a bicarbonate buffer, the proton liberation can be followed by CO_2 gas production.

In mitochondria, marked proton (as well as other ionic) translocations take place. These ionic shifts (K^+, Ca^{2+}, etc.) are closely coupled to ATP hydrolysis or ATPase action. The fact that this transport function of mitochondria is inhibited by uncoupling agents indicates its close relationship to respiratory phosphorylation. For example, let us consider the effect of added Ca^{2+} on mitochondrial respiration. Shown in Figure 10.6 is a simultaneous trace of several different respiratory and structural mitochondrial parameters. Addition of Ca^{2+} leads to an initial burst of respiration (oxygen rate) (curve *a*), which subsequently returns to the control rate. Simultaneously, cytochrome c becomes more oxidized (curve *b*), as does reduced pyridine nucleotide (curve *c*). Accompanying these changes of increased electron flow, there are changes in mitochondrial structure, as evidenced by the increased light scattering (curve *d*). As shown in the figure, the same cycle of events is also brought on by ADP addition or by the addition of the uncoupling agent, dicoumarol (see also Figure 10.4). Ca^{2+} is transported into and accumulates in the mitochondrion under these conditions. We would like at this point to emphasize the significance of reactions in which protons are produced or liberated by linking such reactions to this ion transport function.

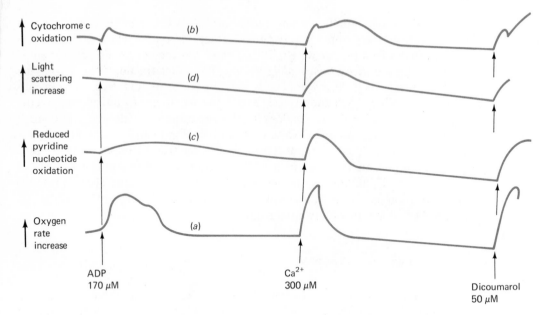

Figure 10.6   Effect of ADP, Ca^{2+}, and dicoumarol on several parameters of respiration and mitochondrial function, cytochrome c oxidation (*b*), light scattering (*d*), reduced pyridine nucleotide oxidation (*c*), and oxygen consumption (*a*). At the points indicated by the arrows ADP (170 μm) or Ca^{2+} (300 μm) or dicoumarol (50 μm) were added to the respiring mitochondria. Note the similarity of effects. Modified from B. Chance, *Control of Energy Metab.*, Academic Press, Inc., New York, 1965.

Let us consider a series of reactions consisting first of the familiar hydrolysis of ATP to ADP and P_i in which a proton is produced.

$$ATP^{4-} + H_2O \longrightarrow ADP^{3-} + P_i^{2-} + H^+ \tag{3}$$

Recalling that H_2O is a reactant (the O of which is incorporated into P_i), we may ask, "What is the formal stoichiometry if we consider the ionization of water?" See Eq. (4). Summing Eqs. (4) and (3), we obtain Eq. (5), which states

$$H^+ + OH^- \longrightarrow H_2O \tag{4}$$

$$ATP^{4-} + OH^{1-} \longrightarrow ADP^{3-} + P_i^{2-} \tag{5}$$

that the stoichiometry can be equally well satisfied by reacting ATP with

OH^-. Let us now look into the sequence and introduce an oxidation-reduction reaction between an oxidized charged element OR^- and a proton, Eq. (6),

$$OR^- + H^+ \longrightarrow OH^- + R^+ \tag{6}$$

$$R:\ddot{O}:+ H^+ \qquad H:\ddot{O}:^- + R^+$$

from which we obtain by metathesis $OH^- + R^+$. Summing Eqs. (5) and (6), we obtain Eq. (7). This states that

$$ATP^{4-} + OR^- + H^+ \longrightarrow ADP^{3-} + P_i^{2-} + R^+ \tag{7}$$

ATP hydrolysis can be coupled to a conversion of H^+ together with OR^-, an anionic oxygen-containing moiety, to R^+, a cationic deoxygenated moiety. Note that R has been oxidized in terms of electrons (charge) but deoxygenated in terms of oxygen. If now we consider that ROH can ionize, we have Eq. (8),

$$ROH \rightleftharpoons H^+ + {}^-OR \tag{8}$$

Summing Eqs. (7) and (8), we obtain Eq. (9),

$$ATP^{4-} + ROH \longrightarrow ADP^{3-} + P_i^{2-} + R^+ \tag{9}$$

which states that the splitting of ATP can be coupled to the deoxygenative conversion of ROH into R^+ with the loss of its oxygen into P_i. ROH can either ionize into OR^- which contains oxygen, or be converted into R^+ which does not. R^+ is, thus, the analogue of H^+ when water reacts.

Suppose that we now consider that ROH can react reversibly with a second ionizable function HX to form the new compound RX. This is shown in the reverse direction in reaction (10).

$$R-X + H_2O \rightleftharpoons HX + ROH \tag{10}$$

If we add Eqs. (10) and (9), we obtain Eq. (11).

$$ATP^{4-} + R-X + H_2O \longrightarrow ADP^{3-} + P_i^{2-} + R^+ + HX \tag{11}$$

Now, if we add the fact that HX can ionize, Eq. (12),

$$HX \rightleftharpoons H^+ + X^- \tag{12}$$

and sum Eqs. (12) and (11), we obtain Eq. (13).

$$ATP^{4-} + R-X + H_2O \longrightarrow ADP^{3-} + P_i^{2-} + H^+ + R^+ + X^- \tag{13}$$

This final equation tells us that in the overall sense, the splitting of ATP (with H_2O) can be coupled to the *ionization* of R—X into R^+ and X^-.

It is now possible to reconstruct a model of the mitochondria such that this system is used to translocate protons (Figure 10.7). A key feature of this model is that it depends in an *absolute* sense on a supramolecular organization of the enzyme systems involved. *This is a new concept in metabolism.* The model is divided into a central membrane portion, an inner phase 1, and an outer phase 2. The total ATPase is made up of the three sections labeled A, B, and C. Separately, section A contains the R—X hydrolase (10), section C, the R—X synthetase (13), and section B contains an R—X moving function or translocase. When these three functions are coupled to ATP synthesis (direction of arrows), protons are fed into the system in phase 2 (outside), water is formed and fed back out into phase 2, while inside in phase 1, ATP is synthesized and protons accumulate. In this model, the stoichiometry is two protons per ATP synthesized. In the reverse direction, when ATP is hydrolyzed, protons would accumulate outside, in phase 2. Both the coupling reactions of RX synthesis and breakdown and the translocation in space of the coupling system take place in the membrane. Note that the F_1 protein, the ATPase insensitive to uncoupling agents, can be thought of as the R—X synthetase contained in section C. F_0, the coupling factor, would represent the rest of the system. When the system is intact, an uncoupling agent such as oligomycin would block by inhibiting the reactions of A and B. When F_1 (section C) was separated, the ATPase action would be present because H_2O would substitute for R—X. Although this is an hypothetical model, it explains a great deal of experimental detail. Furthermore, it allows us to see how proton (or in fact, other ion transport) can be coupled to ATP synthesis or hydrolysis. A central feature is that ATP hydrolysis (13) may be coupled to drive ionizations which then permit ion transport to occur. In other words, ATP may be said to be used to "pump" ions. Of great importance in the future will be the elucidation of the nature of R—X and the mechanism of its translocation.

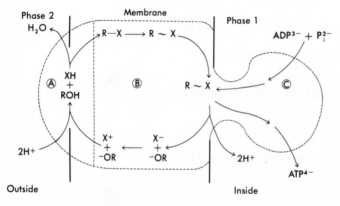

Figure 10.7

The Mitchell Model of oxidative phosphorylation. From P. Mitchell, Translocation through Natural Membranes, *Adv. Enzymol.*, **29**, 33 (1967).

10.4   ANTIBIOTIC-STIMULATED ION TRANSPORT

It has recently been discovered that a number of antibiotics and *Streptomyces* metabolites as well as certain synthetic macrocyclic compounds act to induce ion transport into and out of mitochondria, red blood cells, and other systems. A great deal of interest has been focused on these substances because they produce striking effects selectively on the transport of K^+ and not Na^+. This is of considerable importance since it offers a new approach to investigate the fact that the capacity of biological membranes to discriminate between Na^+ and K^+ underlies a number of important physiological processes, including excitation and conduction of excitable tissues, secretion of intestinal fluids, and reabsorption of fluid from the kidney proximal tubules.

The two opposing actions of two antibiotics, valinomycin and nigericin, are shown in Figure 10.8. Addition of valinomycin to mitochondria results in an uptake of K^+, a counter movement of H^+, and a decrease in light scattering due to water uptake and mitochondrial swelling. The opposite set of changes are seen when nigericin is added, that is, a K^+ output, H^+ uptake, and increase in light scatter.

The schematic structure of valinomycin, a cyclic polypeptide, is shown in Figure 10.9, which also shows the structure of monensin, an analog related to nigericin. As indicated, valinomycin is a closed cyclic polypeptide, while monensin is a linear molecule containing a carboxyl function which, when ionized, cyclizes by hydrogen bonding. Both valinomycin and monensin enclose cations, as does alamethacin, a third type and also cyclic. Alamethacin contains a carboxyl group but the carboxylate is not involved in the cyclization. In the nigericin-monensin class, the cation-complexing function re-

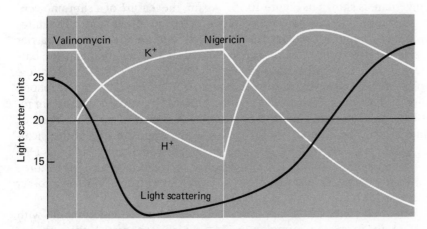

Figure 10.8   The influence of antibiotics nigericin and valinomycin on mitochondrial ion transport swelling. Note the opposite effects of the two antibiotics. From B. Pressman, *Fed. Proc.*, **27**, 1283 (1968).

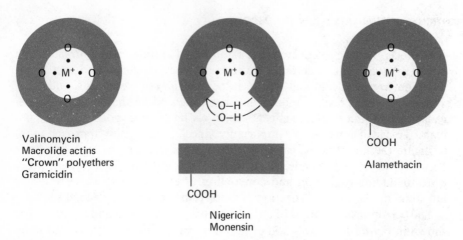

Valinomycin
Macrolide actins
"Crown" polyethers
Gramicidin

Nigericin
Monensin

Alamethacin

Figure 10.9   Diagrammatic structures of three antibiotic classes represented by valinomycin, nigericin, and alamethicin. With nigericin, the ionized active form
as well as the unionized inactive forms are shown. From B. Pressman, *Fed.
Proc.*, **27**, 1283 (1968).

quires the presence of a carboxylate ion rather than the carboxyl group. As
shown in Figure 10.9, the presence of an unionized carboxyl group leads to
an acyclic configuration which does not complex. For structural reasons,
these substances are able to specifically complex K^+. The remarkable ability
to discriminate between ions is apparently an inherent property of the macro-
lides themselves, which are sort of giant detergents with hydrophilic interiors
and hydrophobic exteriors.

A model devised to explain the action of the two antibiotics, valinomycin
and nigericin, is shown in Figure 10.10. Again, the feature of a supramolecular organization is apparent (see also W.old for further discussion). The mitochondrial ion pump is considered to be linked with an adjoining ion barrier
region of the membrane. Valinomycin (V) enters the membrane at the barrier region and reacts with the hydrated metal ion ($M^+ \cdot H_2O$) to form the
complex M^+V^*, which diffuses to the pump containing its own ionophore,
labelled I. The ion is transferred to I forming M^+I^*, while valinomycin re-
verts back to its ground state V and is free to diffuse back to the barrier for
another cycle. The complex M^+I^* moves to the opposite side of the membrane where it reacts with an interphase element which converts I^* to I^0, a
state which has little affinity for M^+, which is then discharged. I^0 is restored
to I by an energizing element from $\sim$ P available from ATP or another
source, and I is ready to recycle another time.

Nigericin (N) acts in the opposite vectorial sense. It can combine with
$M^+ \cdot H_2O$ to form the complex N^-M^+ which can travel through the
barrier to the ion pump. However, it is unable to release the ion to the
ionophore, since the latter is presumably unable to supply the proton required to convert nigericin from its carboxylate to its carboxyl form (a con-

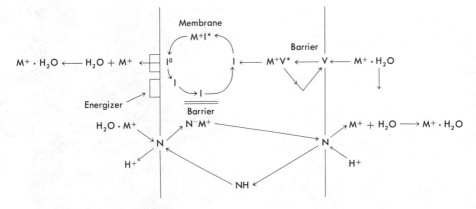

Figure 10.10   Model of valinomycin and nigericin in ion transport. V = valinomycin at
ground state; V* = same activated; M⁺ = metal ion; I = membrane ionophore at ground state; I* = membrane ionophore at activated state combined with M⁺; I⁰ = same uncombined with M⁺; N = nigericin; N⁻ =
ionized form; NH = unionized form. From B. Pressman, *Fed. Proc.,* **27,**
1283 (1968).

formation unable to complex). When the proton is supplied, the nigericin can
tranverse the membrane to discharge the ion and establish the transmembrane
equilibrium,

$$\frac{[M^+]\ \text{internal}}{[M^+]\ \text{external}} = \frac{[H^+]\ \text{internal}}{[H^+]\ \text{external}}$$

10.5   GENETIC BLOCK

A report has appeared of a case of increased metabolic rate in a patient
without hyperthyroidism in which the mitochondria were present in a
"loosely-coupled" state.

The patient, a woman in her 30's, had a basal metabolic rate 200 percent
above normal. She had suffered with the disease since childhood. The
hypermetabolism could not be ascribed to hyperthyroidism since measures
which depress thyroid function had no effect.

Mitochondria were isolated from a biopsy of muscle and compared with
control muscle mitochondria similarly obtained. Respiration was measured
with and without a phosphate acceptor.

In Figure 10.11, polarographic measurements are shown. In the normal
mitochondria (Experiment 1), on ADP addition, the normal increase in
respiration is observed. Oligomycin inhibits the respiration. In the patient's
mitochondria (Experiment 2), there is a marked respiration which is little influenced by P_i or ADP and which is not inhibited by oligomycin. ATPase
was also determined in the absence and presence of the uncoupling agent
dinitrophenol, DNP. The ATPase activity, which was low was stimulated by

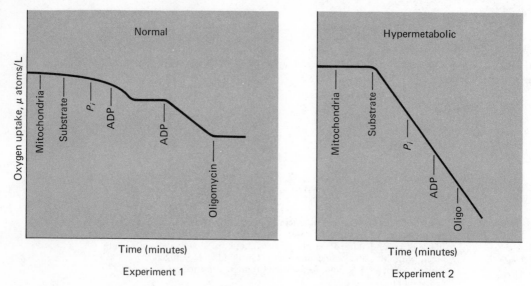

Figure 10.11 Respiratory control in mitochondria from a control patient and from a patient with a hypermetabolic disease. Control = experiment 1; patient = experiment 2. Note the lack of an effect of added ADP or P_i on respiration and the failure of oligomycin to inhibit in experiment 2 as compared with experiment 1. From L. Ernster and R. Luft, *Adv. Metab. Diseases,* **1,** 95 (1964).

DNP in the case of the control mitochondria. The ATPase of the patient's mitochondria was already elevated without added DNP and not much further increased by added DNP.

Although the final mechanism is not known, there is every reason to believe that some defect in the coupling mechanism is present. Clearly, future investigations of this disease with fractionation experiments of the ATPase itself would be expected to yield important information in the basic mechanism of the coupling itself (as well as on ion transport) in this condition of altered mitochondrial function.

10.6 INTEGRATED CONTROL OF METABOLISM BY ENERGY CHARGE

As we have already seen, in addition to other key metabolites, the adenylate compounds control key reactions in carbohydrate, lipid, and nitrogen metabolism. It would seem reasonable that ATP forming and utilizing systems would respond to the energy balance in the cell in terms of all the adenylate compounds rather than to any single adenylate compound. In the cell, the total adenylate pool (AMP + ADP + ATP) is essentially constant over short time periods (see Table 6.4). The amount of energy stored can, therefore, be considered to be proportional to the number of anhydride phosphate bonds per adenosine. This number would vary from 0 to 2. In many ways this system resembles an electrochemical storage cell in its ability to accept, store, and supply energy as anhydride phosphate. In order to provide a more convenient scale, varying from 0 to 1, a new system termed *energy charge* was defined, which is equal to *one half the phosphate anhydride bonds per adenosine*. Since the total anhydride phosphates would, in terms of concentrations, be equal to 2ATP + ADP, the energy charge could be equal to (ATP + $\frac{1}{2}$ ADP)(ATP + ADP + AMP).

The adenylate system can be described in an overall way by Eq. (14).

$$AMP + 2P_i \rightleftharpoons ATP + 2H_2O \tag{14}$$

This represents the sum of two equations, (15) and (16).

$$2ADP + 2P_i \rightleftharpoons 2ATP + 2H_2O \tag{15}$$

$$ATP + AMP \rightleftharpoons 2ADP \tag{16}$$

Equation (16) is the reaction catalyzed by adenylate kinase and Eq. (15) represents ATP resynthesis or utilization by any process. Free energy of hydrolyses and energy charge differ since only ATP and ADP contribute to free energy of hydrolysis, but ATP, ADP, and AMP contribute to energy charge. The relationship between energy charge and relative concentrations of the adenylate compounds under these conditions is given in Figure 10.12.

Figure 10.12   Relationship between the energy charge and concentrations of the adenylate compounds. From D. E. Atkinson, *Biochemistry*, **7**, 4030 (1968).

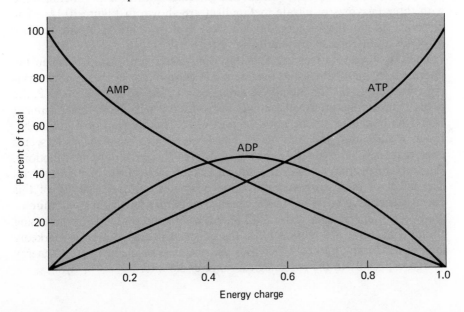

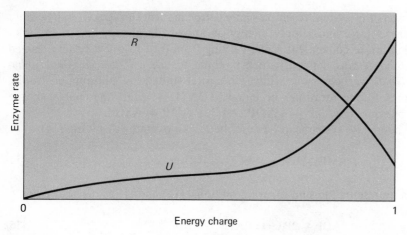

Figure 10.13   Idealized effect of energy charge on the enzymatic rate of an energy utilizing
enzyme (U) and an energy regenerating enzyme (R). From D. E. Atkinson,
Biochemistry, **7**, 4030 (1968).

Processes that utilize ATP shift the system to the left, those that form ATP
shift it toward the right.

The response of an idealized energy-regenerating and energy-utilizing
system to control by energy charge is shown in Figure 10.13.

For an *energy-regenerating* system (R), the activity would be high at low
charge and then fall off steeply at high charge. The opposite would be true
for an *energy-utilizing* system (U). The activity would be low at low charge
and then increase rapidly at high charge. Examples of experimental data
with three enzymes of citrate metabolism are shown in Figure 10.14. PFK
responds as a typical energy-regenerating system while ATP citrate lyase
responds as a typical energy-utilizing system.

There is a very interesting and important interrelationship between the
intermediary metabolites and the adenylate compounds in energy-regenerating and energy-utilizing metabolic sequences. In the generation of ATP, the
pools of metabolic intermediates would be diminished. Their replenishment
would be linked to regeneration of the ATP. This overlap of function between metabolites and adenylates has been termed *amphibolic*. It seems
clear that there must be overlapping control of these overlapping functions.
This type of overlap of control is shown in the case of PFK in Figure 10.14.
The effect of increasing energy charge is to decrease the activity of this
energy-generating enzyme. In the absence of citrate under these conditions,
the effect of energy charge is small (curve *a*). In the presence of increasing
citrate concentrations (curves *b*, *c*), the effect of energy charge is markedly
increased. Citrate markedly increases the steepness of the response to energy
charge, especially in the *physiological range of 0.8 to 0.9*.

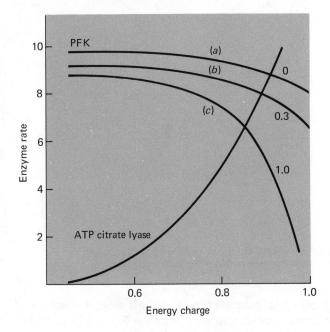

Figure 10.14

Control by energy charge and citrate and example of an amphibolic effect. Note the R nature of the response to energy charge in the absence of citrate (curve *a*) and the increased sensitivity in the presence of increased citrate (curves *b* and *c*). Note the U nature of the response of the ATP citrate lyase. L. Shen, L. Fall, G. M. Walton and D. E. Atkinson, *Biochemistry,* **7,** 4041 (1968).

The effect of energy charge on several enzymes of polysaccharide carbohydrate, TCA cycle, amino acid, and nucleotide metabolism have been investigated. In all instances, the control is in keeping with the enzyme's function (Table 10.1). In Figure 10.15, the control by ATP, as energy charge, is shown to regulate all of metabolism. The control is either negative in the energy-producing reactions of polysaccharide breakdown, glycolysis, or the TCA cycle, or positive in the energy-requiring reactions of amino acid syn-

TABLE 10.1   EFFECT OF ENERGY CHARGE ON ENZYMES

Enzyme	Area	Type	Function
Phosphorylase *b* kinase	Polysaccharide	R	Glycogenolysis
PFK	Carbohydrate	R	Glycolysis
Pyruvate dehydrogenase	Preceding TCA cycle	R	Oxidation
Citrate synthase	TCA cycle	R	Oxidation
Isocitrate dehydrogenase	TCA cycle	R	Oxidation
ATP citrate lyase	Citrate metabolism	U	Acetyl-S-CoA production
Aspartokinase-lysine sensitive (*E. coli*)	Lysine synthesis	U	Amino acid synthesis
PR-ATP synthase (*E. coli*)	Histidine biosynthesis	U	Amino acid synthesis
PRPP synthase (*E. coli*)	Nucleotide biosynthesis	U	Nucleotide synthesis

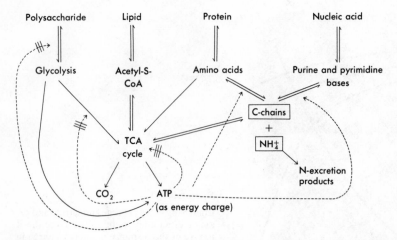

Figure 10.15   Generalized model of control by energy charge of metabolism including polymer-monomer rate conversions. Note the predictions present in this model.

thesis and purine or pyrimidine base syntheses. In this way, it can be appreciated how the entire metabolism can be regulated. From Figure 10.15, it can be predicted that new control sites will be discovered, especially in the areas of polymer biosynthesis and breakdown. Furthermore, it is anticipated that control mechanisms probably exist which utilize the redox potential of oxidized and reduced cofactors to control reactions in metabolic sequences.

In this chapter, we have derived the controls associated with the energy metabolism. We have shown how energy metabolism is regulated by its own substrate, ADP and P_i, and how it may be coupled or uncoupled from respiration. The relationship to ion transport in terms of models involving supramolecular organization of enzymatic systems was discussed. The importance of H^+-forming and utilizing reactions was also elaborated. Finally, the universality of the adenylate compounds as controlling agents in terms of the energy charge was discussed.

REFERENCES

Atkinson, D. E., "Citrate and the Citrate Cycle in the Regulation of Energy Metabolism," *Metabolic Roles of Citrate* (T. W. Goodwin, ed.) Academic Press, Inc., New York, 1968.

Atkinson, D. E., "The energy charge of the adenylate pool as a regulatory parameter; Interaction with feedback modifiers," *Biochem.,* **7** 4030 (1968).

Chance, B., *Control of Energy Metabolism* (B. Chance, R. W. Estabrook and J. R. Williamson, eds.), A. Colloquium of the Johnson Research Found., Academic Press, Inc., New York 1965.

Ernster L., and R. Luft, "Mitochondrial Respiratory Control: Biochemical, Physiological, and Pathological Aspects," *Advances in Metabolic Disorders* (R. Levine and R. Luft, eds.), Vol. I, Academic Press, Inc., New York, 1964.

Klungsøyr, L., Hageman, J. H., Fall, L., and D. E. Atkinson, "Interaction between energy charge and product feedback in the regulation of biosynthetic enzymes," *Biochem.,* **7** 4035 (1968).

Mitchell, P., "Translocation through natural membranes," *Adv. Enzymol.,* **29,** 33 (1967).

Pressman, B., Physiology Society Symposium on Biological and Artificial Membranes, *Fed. Proc.,* **27,** 1283 (1968).

Shen, L. C., Fall, L., Walton G. M., and D. E. Atkinson, "Interaction between energy charge and metabolite modulation in the regulation of enzymes of amphibolic sequences; phosphofructokinase and pyruvate dehydrogenase," *Biochem.* **7,** 4041 (1968).

Membranes of Mitochondria and Chloroplasts, (E. Racker, ed.), Van Nostrand Reinhold Co., New York, 1970.

Villar-Palasi, C., and S. H. Wei, Phosphorylase *b* to *a* Conversion by Non-Activated Phosphorylase *b* kinase. An *in vitro* Model of the Mechanism of Phosphorylase *a* Increase with Muscle Contraction, *Proc. Natl. Acad. Sci.,* **67,** 345 (1970).

GLOSSARY

Allosteric activator. An allosteric effector which enhances enzyme activity (Figure 7.1, curve 3+, 4++).

Allosteric effector. Any small molecule, including substrate, which modifies enzyme activity by binding at sites other than the catalytically active site.

Allosteric enzyme or protein. Regulatory enzymes or proteins which bind allosteric effectors.

Allosteric inhibitor. An allosteric effector which decreases enzyme activity (Figure 7.1, curve 5−).

Amphibolic. The overlap in function between metabolic intermediates and adenylate compounds in an energy-generating system.

Concerted feedback inhibition. Two or more end products are required simultaneously to obtain inhibition of an early reaction.

Cooperative feedback inhibition. Each end product of a branched metabolic pathway inhibits partially, but two or more end products together inhibit more than the sum of the individual inhibitions.

Corepressor. A small molecule capable of combining with the repressor to form an active complex which combines with the operator and prevents mRNA synthesis.

Cumulative product inhibition. The inhibition of each product of a branched pathway is separate and independent.

Cytosol. The soluble portion of the cytoplasm after all particles are removed.

Desensitization. The loss of the allosteric responsiveness with the retention of enzymatic activity.

Enzyme multiplicity. More than one enzyme catalyzing the same reaction.

Feedback inhibition. Inhibition of the first or an early enzyme of a pathway by the metabolic end product.

Flux. Metabolic flow or velocity in vivo. Flux equals Ak_a where A is tissue substrate concentration and k_a equals V_{max}/K_m. Therefore flux equals AV_{max}/K_m.

Hill coefficient. The numerical value of the slope of the Hill plot. It signifies the number of allosteric effector molecules bound to the enzyme.

Hill plot. A plot of $\log [v/V_{max} - v]$ versus $\log [S]$.

Hyperbolic kinetics. Ordinary, first order, Michaelis-Menten kinetic plot of initial velocity against substrate concentration (Figure 7.1, curve 2–0).

Inducer. A small molecule capable of combining with the repressor to form an inactive complex which cannot combine with the operator, and therefore, permits mRNA synthesis.

Induction. The de novo synthesis of an enzyme from amino acids dictated by a structural gene and requiring the presence of a small molecule, the **Inducer.**

Initiator gene (i). One of the regulator genes. It codes for the repressor protein which binds to the DNA at the operator (o) gene.

K_i, inhibitor constant. The equilibrium (dissociation) constant of the reaction $E + I = EI$.

K_m, Michaelis constant. This substrate concentration at which $v = V/2$.

K_s, substrate constant. The equilibrium (dissociation) constant of the reaction $E + S = ES$.

Lysosome. Large cytoplasmic particles containing many hydrolytic enzymes with acid pH optima which are presumably concerned with intracellular digestive processes.

Mitochondria. Large cytoplasmic particles in which terminal oxidation and oxidative phosphorylation take place.

Negative crossover point. In the same linear sequence (see **Positive crossover point**) if there is a decreased metabolic flux at a particular step, say C ⟶ D, then the steady state levels of C will increase and those of D will decrease. This change may also be noted in substrates behind (B+) or ahead (E−) of the negative crossover point.

Operator gene. One of the regulator genes. It is the gene required to initiate the transcription of the entire operon and is located on the chromosome at the start of the operon.

Operon. A cluster of structural genes on a chromosome dictating and regulating the synthesis of the enzymes of a metabolic pathway.

Phenomenon of uncoupling. In general, the phenomenon which occurs when mitochondria have the ability to respire but lack the ability to respond to added ADP and P_i (partial) or lack the ability to synthesize ATP (complete).

Positive crossover point. Given the linear reaction sequence A $\xrightarrow{1}$ B $\xrightarrow{2}$ C $\xrightarrow{3}$ D $\xrightarrow{4}$ E, catalyzed by the respective enzymes 1, 2, 3, and 4, and having no feedback control. If metabolic flux is increased at a particular step, say B ⟶ C, then the steady state levels of B will decrease and those of C will increase. This change may be also noted in substrates behind (A−) or ahead (D+) of the positive crossover point.

Promotor gene (p). One of the regulator genes. It is thought to be the site on the DNA at which RNA polymerase attaches and catalyzes the synthesis of mRNA.

Regulator gene. A gene not necessarily located on the same chromosome as the operon which controls its rate of enzyme synthesis.

Repression. The prevention of the formation of an enzyme as dictated by a structural gene in the presence of a small molecule, the **Corepressor.**

Repressor. The product of a regulatory gene (i), most likely a protein, capable of combining with an inducer to form an inactive complex, or with a corepressor to form an active complex. The active form of the repressor combines with an operator to prevent mRNA formation.

Ribosome. Small cytoplasmic particles made up of RNA and protein which are the site of protein synthesis.

S. Sedimentation coefficient given in Svedberg units, describing the velocity attained per unit of applied force by a particle moving through a liquid medium. See also the volume in this series by Van Holde.

Sigmoid or cooperative kinetics. Sigmoid or S shaped kinetic plot of initial velocity against substrate concentration, indicating that at least two molecules of substrate interact with the enzyme and that the reaction is of a higher order than one. "Cooperative" refers to the fact that the binding of the first molecule somehow affects the binding of the second.

Substrate(s). The reactant(s) in an enzymatic reaction which is converted to product.

Turnover number. Number of moles of substrate converted to product per mole of enzyme per minute.

v, **velocity.** The observed velocity of the enzyme reaction.

V_{max}, **maximum velocity.** The maximum value of *v*, corresponding to saturation of the enzyme with substrate as given by the Michaelis equation.

APPENDIX

TABLE A.1 SOME BIOCHEMICALLY IMPORTANT ISOTOPES

Isotope	Radiation	$T_{1/2}$
$_{1}H^{2}$	—	—
$_{1}H^{3}$	β^{-}	12.46 yr
$_{6}C^{14}$	β^{-}	5,700 yr
$_{7}N^{15}$	—	—
$_{8}O^{18}$		
$_{9}F^{18}$	β^{+}	112 min
$_{11}Na^{22}$	β^{+}, γ	2.6 yr
$_{11}Na^{24}$	$\beta^{-\prime}, \gamma$	15.06 hr
$_{15}P^{32}$	β^{-}	14.3 days
$_{15}P^{33}$	β^{-}	25.4 days
$_{16}S^{35}$	β^{-}	87.1 days
$_{17}Cl^{36}$	$\beta^{-}, \beta^{+},$ K capture	4.4×10^{5} yr
$_{17}Cl^{38}$	$\beta^{-\prime}, \gamma$	37.3 min
$_{19}K^{42}$	β^{-}, γ	12.4 hr
$_{20}Ca^{45}$	β^{-}	152 days
$_{25}Mn^{52}$	$\beta^{+}, \gamma,$ K	6.0 days
$_{25}Mn^{54}$	K, γ	310 days
$_{26}Fe^{55}$	K, γ	4 yr
$_{26}Fe^{59}$	β^{-}, γ	45.1 days
$_{27}Co^{56}$	$\beta^{+}, \gamma,$ K	72 days
$_{27}Co^{58}$	$\beta^{+}, \gamma,$ K	72 days
$_{29}Cu^{61}$	$\beta^{+}, \gamma,$ K	3.3 hr
$_{29}Cu^{64}$	$\beta^{-}, \gamma,$ K, β^{+}	12.8 hr
$_{30}Zn^{65}$	$\beta^{+}, \gamma,$ K	250 days
$_{53}I^{131}$	β^{-}, γ	8.1 days

TABLE A.2   GENETIC METABOLIC DISEASES IN MAN

Diseases of Carbohydrate Metabolism

  Diabetes mellitus
  Familial lactic acidosis
  Fructose intolerance
  Fructosuria
  Glycogen storage
    Glucose-6-phosphatase(I)
    α-Glucosidase(II)
    Debranching enzyme system(III)
    Branching enzyme(IV)
    Muscle phosphorylase(V)
      (McArdle's disease)
    Liver phosphorylase(VI)
    Phosphorylase kinase
    Phosphorylase kinase kinase
      (protein kinase)
    Phosphofructokinase
  Aglycogenosis (glycogen synthase)
  Hyperoxaluria
  Pentosuria
  Renal Glycosuria

Diseases of Lipid Metabolism

  Familial hyperlipoproteinemia
  α,β-Lipoproteinemia
  Lipoidosis cerebroside
  Lipoidosis ganglioside
  Lipoidosis glycolipid
  Lipoidosis sphingomyelin
  Lipoidosis sulfatide
  Tangier disease

Diseases of Steroid Metabolism

  Adrenogenital syndromes

Diseases of Amino Acid Metabolism

  Albinism
  Alcaptonuria
  Arginino succinaciduria
  Ataxia telangiectasia
  Blue diaper syndrome
  Branched chain ketoaciduria
  Citrullinemia
  Cystathioninuria
  Cystinuria
  Dopa-uria
  Familial dysautonomia
  Formiminotransferase deficiency
  Goiter
  Hartnup disease
  Histidinemia
  Homocystinuria
  3-Hydroxykynureninuria
  Hydroxyprolinemia
  Hyperammonemia
  Hyperglycinemia
  Hyperglycinemia with hyperoxaluria
  Hyperlysinemia
  Hypersarcosinemia
  Hyperserotoninemia
  Hypervalinemia
  Hypoglycemia—leucine induced

  Imidazole amino aciduria
  Indolylacroyl glycinuria
  Joseph's syndrome
  Methionine malabsorption
  Oculo-cerebro-renal syndrome
  Osteopathy, peptiduria, and
    mental retardation
  Phenylketonuria
  Prolinemia
  Pyridoxine dependency
  Tryptophanuria
  Tyrosinemia

Diseases of Purine and Pyrimidine Metabolism

  Gout
  Hyperuricemia
  Orotic aciduria
  Xanthinuria
  Hemochromatosis
  Wilson's disease

Diseases of Porphyrin and Heme Metabolism

  Hyperbilirubinemia
  Porphyrias

Diseases of Connective Tissue Muscle or Bone

  Central core disease and
    nemalinemyopathy
  Hurler's syndrome
  Hypophosphatasia
  Muscular dystrophies
  Periodic paralysis
  Pseudohypoparathyroidism and
    pseudo-pseudohypoparathyroidism
  Systemic amyloidoses

Diseases of Blood and Blood-forming Tissues

  Hemophilia and diseases of clotting
  Elliptocytosis
  Glucose-6-phosphate dehydrogenase
    deficiency
  Hemoglobinopathies and thallassemia
  Hemolytic anemia
  Hereditary spherocytosis
  Methemoglobinemia
  Pyruvate kinase deficiency

Diseases of Epithelial Transport

  Cystic fibrosis
  Fanconi syndrome
  Renal tubular acidosis
  Vitamin D-resistant rickets with
    hypophosphatemia
  Vasopressin-resistant diabetes insipidus

Diseases of Circulating Enzymes or Plasma Proteins

  Acatalasia
  Agammaglobulinemia
  Pseudocholinesterase deficiency

Modified from *Metabolism,* P. L. Altman and D. S. Dittmer (eds.), Federation of American Societies for Experimental Biology, (1968).

TABLE A.3   COENZYMES AND COFACTORS

Name	Structure	Vitamin	Function
Diphosphopyridine nucleotide (DPN) or Nicotinamide adenine dinucleotide (NAD)	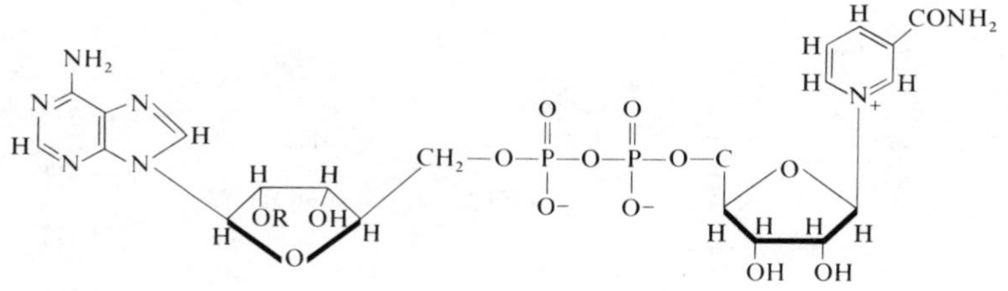	Nicotinic acid	Hydrogen carrier
Triphosphopyridine nucleotide (TPN) or Nicotinamide adenine dinucleotide phosphate (NADP)	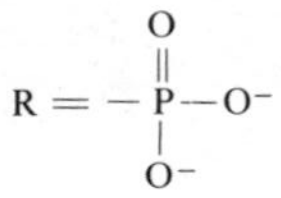	Nicotinic acid	Hydrogen carrier
Lipoic Acid-dithiooctanoate			Hydrogen and acyl carrier
Flavin adenine dinucleotide (FAD)	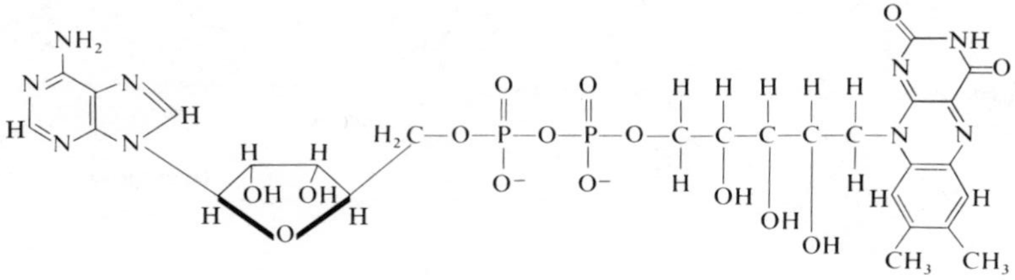	Riboflavin	Hydrogen carrier

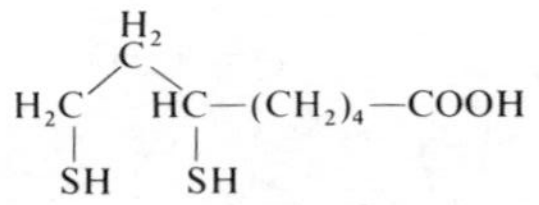

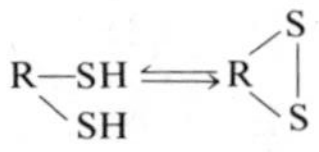

277

TABLE A.3   COENZYMES AND COFACTORS (continued)

Name	Structure	Vitamin	Function
Flavin mononucleotide (FMN)	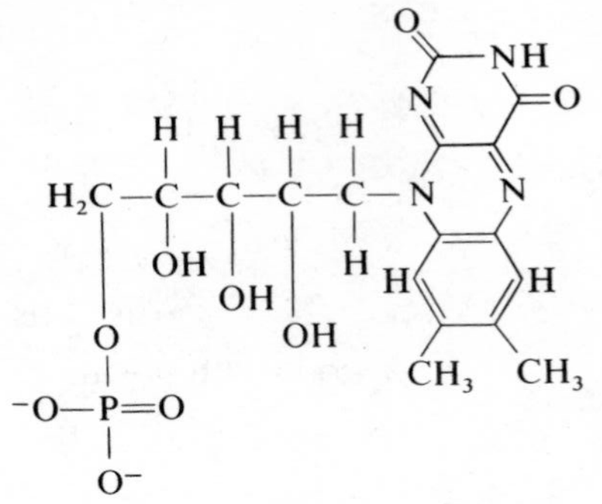	Riboflavin	Hydrogen carrier
Glutathione (GSH) (γ-glutamyl-cysteinyl-glycine)	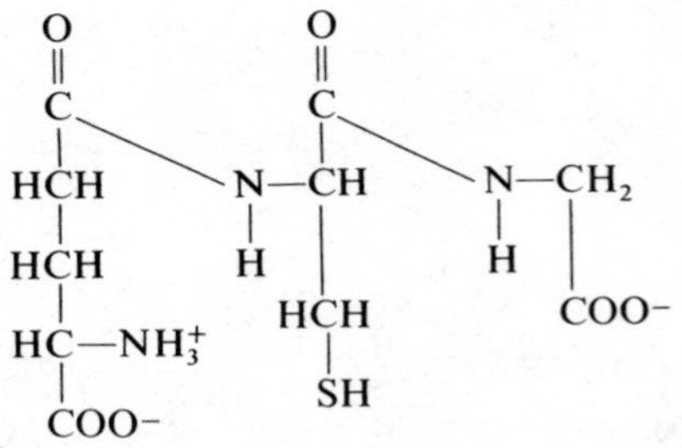		Hydrogen carrier

$$2 \, RSH \rightleftharpoons R-S-S-R$$

Hydrogen carrier

Vitamin C

Ascorbic acid

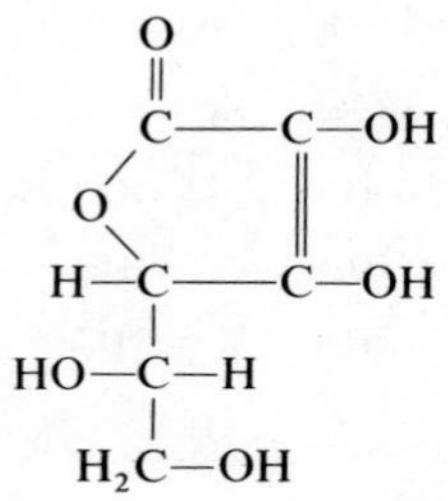

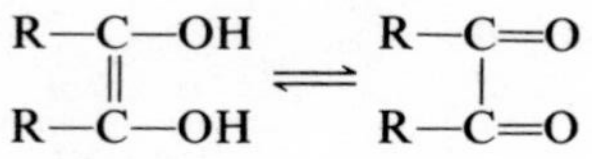

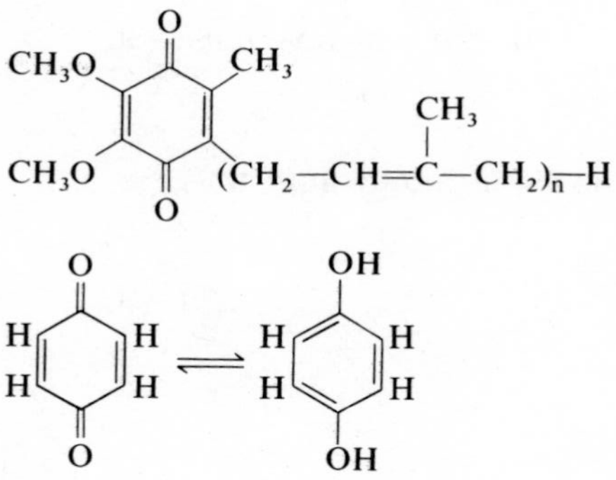

Hydrogen carrier

Ubiquinone

TABLE A.3 COENZYMES AND COFACTORS (continued)

Name	Structure	Vitamin	Function
Vitamin K	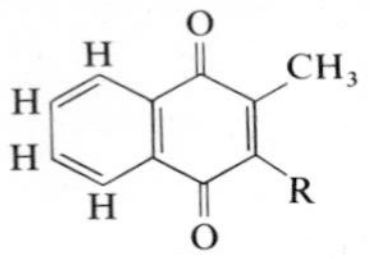 menadione $R = H$ K_1 $R = -CH_2-CH=C-CH_2-(CH_2-CH_2-CH-CH_2)_3-H$ K_2 $R = -(CH_2-CH=C-CH_2)_n-H$	Vitamin K	Hydrogen carrier
Cytochrome c	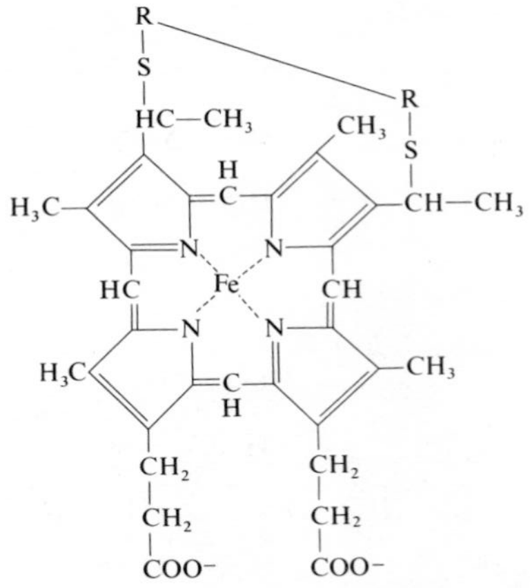 $Fe^{2+} \rightleftharpoons Fe^{3+}$ $R\!\!-\!\!\!-R$ = protein		Electron carrier

Thiamine pyrophosphate (TPP)

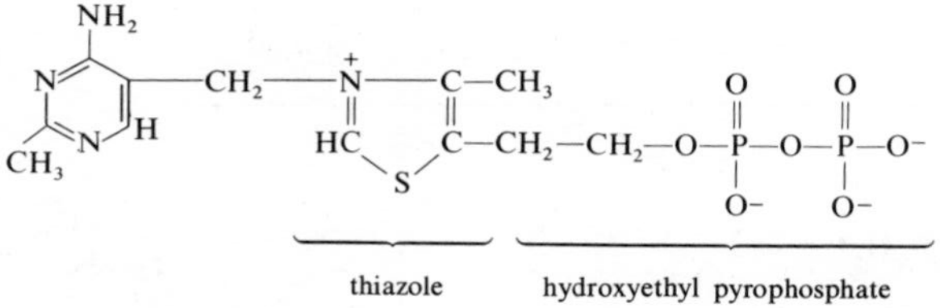

thiazole

hydroxyethyl pyrophosphate

Thiamine   C-1 carrier

Hydroxyethyl thiamine pyrophosphate (HETPP)

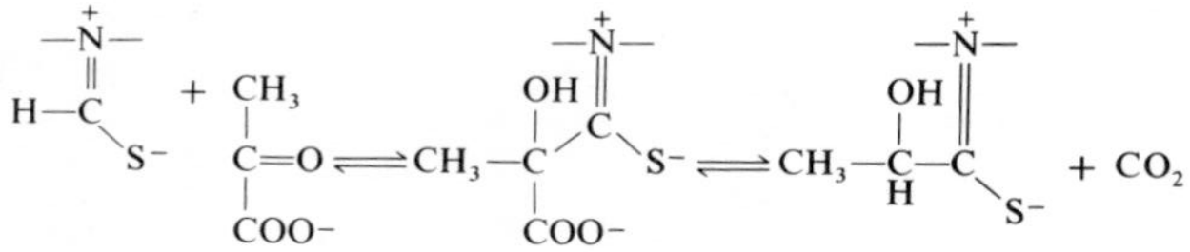

$+ CO_2$

Coenzyme A (CoA) (acetylation coenzyme)

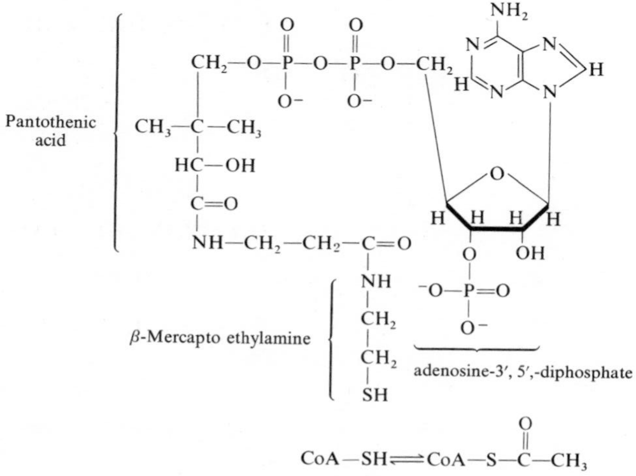

Pantothenic acid

β-Mercapto ethylamine

adenosine-3',5'-diphosphate

Pantothenic acid   Acyl carrier

$CoA\!-\!SH \rightleftharpoons CoA\!-\!S\!-\!C\!-\!CH_3$

TABLE A.3 COENZYMES AND COFACTORS (continued)

Name	Structure	Vitamin	Function
Biotin	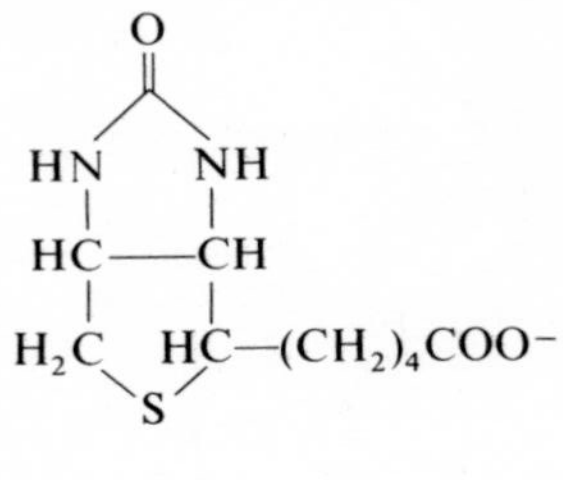	Biotin	C-1 carrier (CO_2)
N-Carboxybiotin	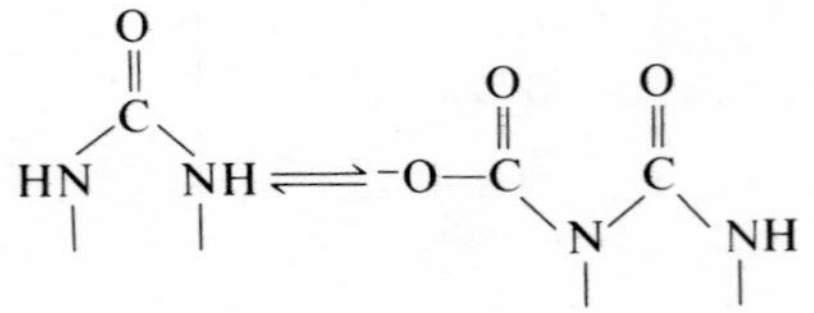		
Tetrahydrofolic acid (THFA)	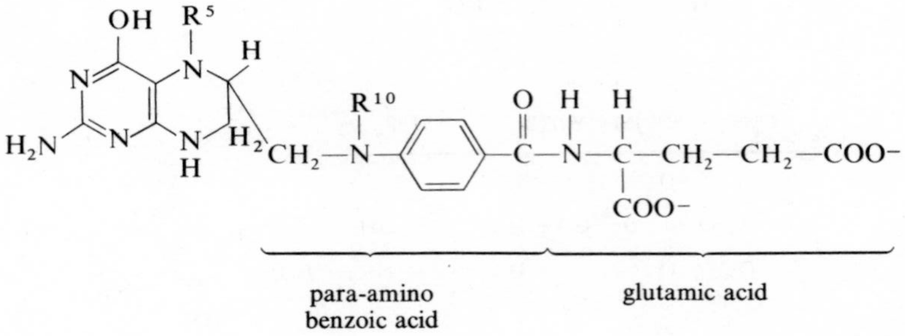	Folic acid	C-1 carrier methyl hydroxymethyl formyl formimino

	R^5	R^{10}
THFA	—H	—H
5-formyl-THFA	—CHO	—H
10-formyl-THFA	—H	—CHO
5,-10-methenyl-THFA	5 $\overset{+}{N}$=CH—N 10	
5,-10-methylene-THFA	5 N—CH₂—N 10	
5-hydroxymethyl-THFA	—CH₂OH	—H
5-formimino-THFA	—CH=NH	—H

S-Adenosyl methionine

or

active methione

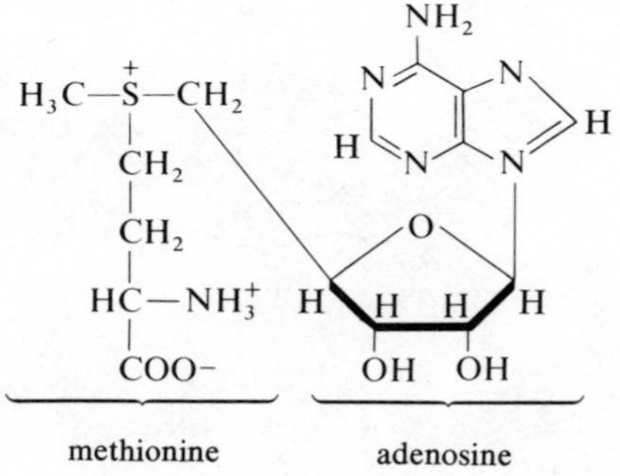

methionine

adenosine

C-1 methyl carrier

TABLE A.3 COENZYMES AND COFACTORS (continued)

Name	Structure	Vitamin	Function
Vitamin B$_{12}$	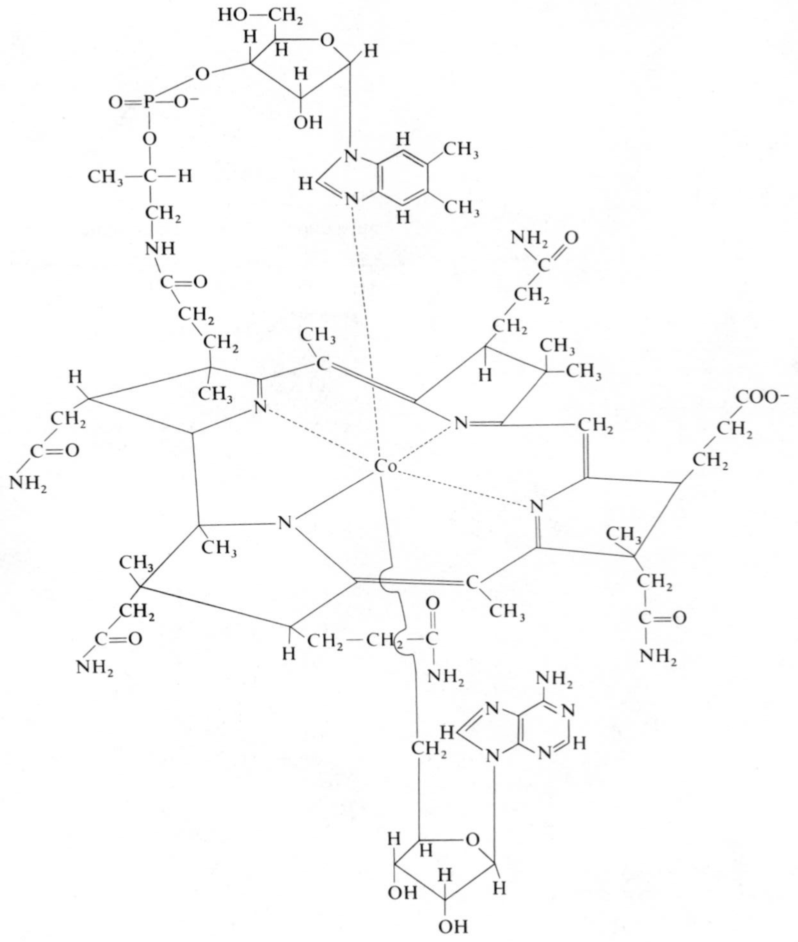 *(chemical structure of vitamin B$_{12}$)*	Vitamin B$_{12}$	C-1 carrier

Pyridoxal phosphate (PLP)

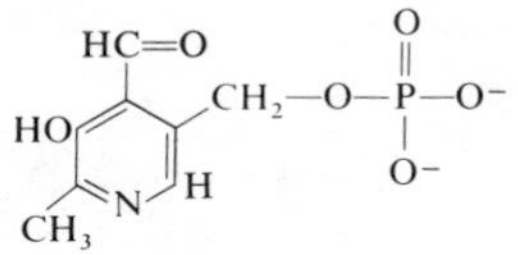

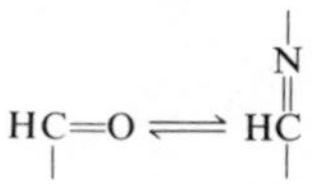

Pyridoxine

Coenzyme for
transamination,
deamination,
decarboxylation,
racemization,
dehydration

**Nucleotides and
nucleotide pyrophosphates**

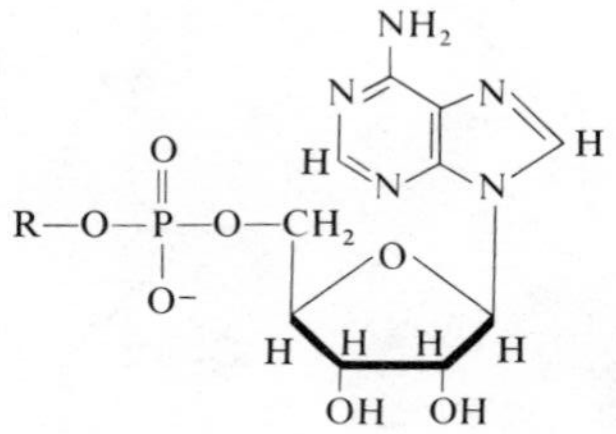

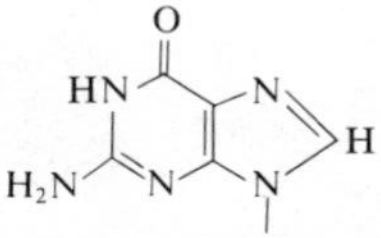

R = H   adenylic acid (AMP)

R = ⁻O—P—O⁻   adenosine diphosphate (ADP)

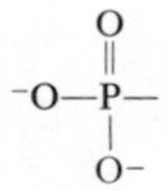

R = ⁻O—P—O—P—O⁻   adenosine triphosphate (ATP)

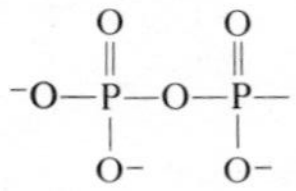

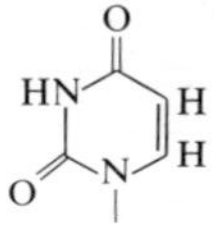

guanylic acid (GMP)
guanosine diphosphate (GDP)
guanosine triphosphate (GTP)

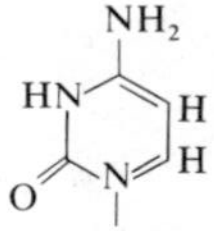

cytidylic acid (CMP)
cytidine diphosphate (CDP)
cytidine triphosphate (CTP)

uridylic acid (UMP)
uridine diphosphate (UDP)
uridine triphosphate (UTP)

Phosphate
carriers

Name	Structure	Vitamin	Function
3′,5′-Cyclic adenylic acid	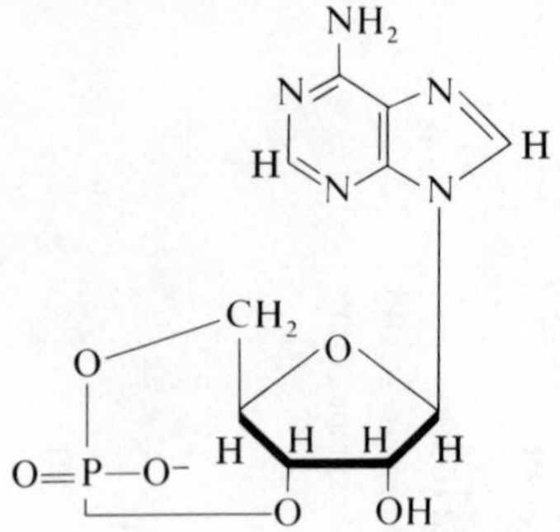		Control agent in phosphorylations
3′,5′-Cyclic guanylic acid	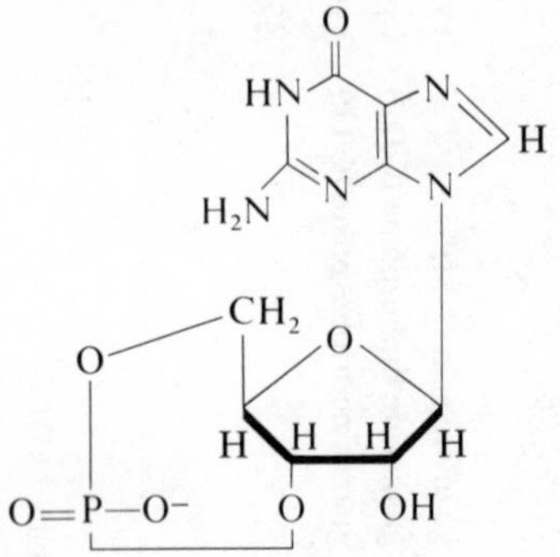		
Glucose-1,6-diphosphate	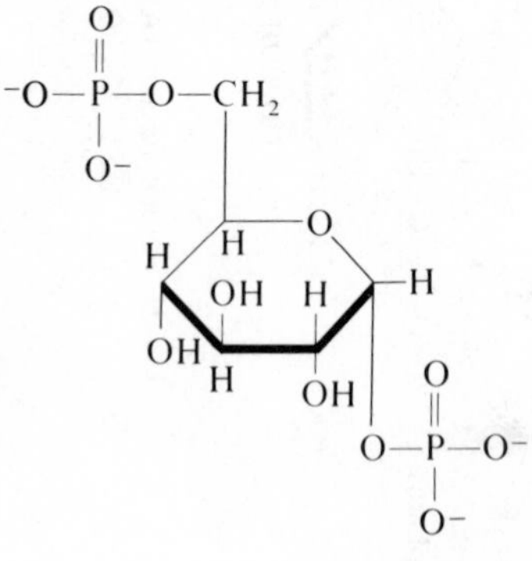		Cofactor in phosphate transfer reactions

Name	Structure	Vitamin	Function
Ribose-1,5-diphosphate	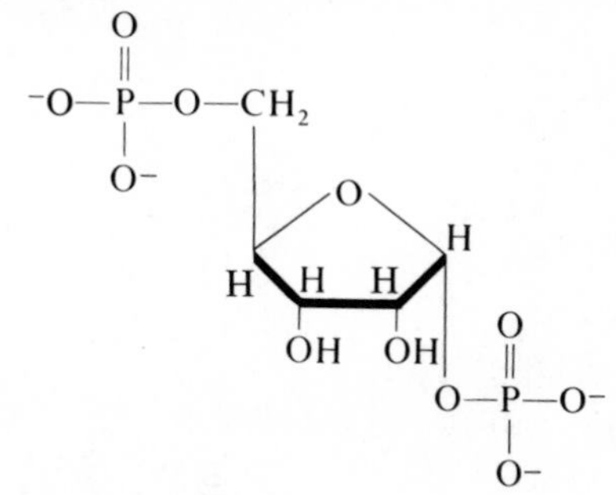		Cofactor in phosphate transfer reactions
2,3-Diphosphoglyceric acid	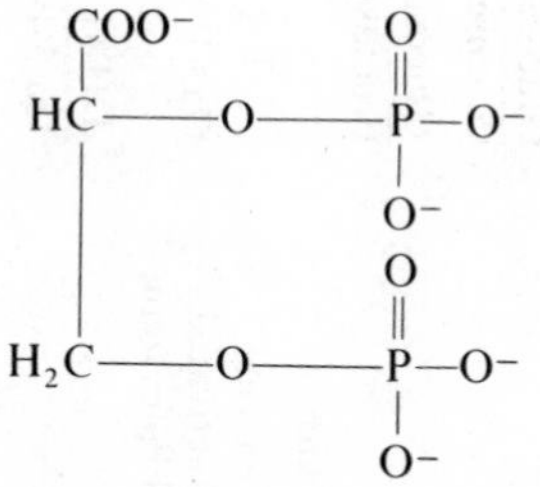		Cofactor in phosphate transfer reactions

Ribose-1,5-diphosphate

$$\begin{array}{c} O \\ \parallel \\ {}^-O-P-O-CH_2 \\ \mid \\ O^- \end{array}$$

furanose ring with H, H H, OH OH, O-P(=O)(O⁻)-O⁻

2,3-Diphosphoglyceric acid

$$\begin{array}{c} COO^- \\ HC-O-P(=O)(O^-)-O^- \\ \mid \\ H_2C-O-P(=O)(O^-)-O^- \end{array}$$

TABLE A.4 PROPERTIES OF THE ENZYMES AND REACTIONS OF GLYCOLYSIS, GLUCONEOGENESIS, GLYCOGENESIS, LIPID HYDROLYSIS, β-OXIDATION, AND FATTY ACID SYNTHESIS

Enzyme	Molecular Weight	Coenzyme or Activators	Inhibitors	Equilibrium Constant (approx.) pH 7.4	ΔG° (cal mole^{-1})
Phosphorylase b	~200,000	AMP, Pyridoxal phosphate	ATP	$\dfrac{P_i}{\text{Glucose-1-P}} = 5$	-970
Phosphorylase a	~400,000	Pyridoxal phosphate			
Phosphoglucomutase	60,000	Glucose-1,6-P$_2$, Mg^{2+}	Glucose-6-P	$\dfrac{\text{Glucose-6-P}}{\text{Glucose-1-P}} = 17$	$-1{,}680$
Phosphoglucose isomerase	48,000			$\dfrac{\text{Glucose-6-P}}{\text{Fructose-6-P}} = 2.3$	
Phosphofructokinase	360,000	Mg^{2+}, ADP, AMP, P$_i$	ATP, citrate		
Aldolase	150,000	Yeast enzyme reactivated by Zn^{2+}, Co^{2+}, Fe^{2+}, Cu^{2+}	Yeast enzyme is inactivated by PP$_i$, cysteine	$\dfrac{\text{F-1, 6-P}_2}{\text{Ga3-P} \times \text{DHAP}} = 10^4$	
Phosphotriose isomerase				$\dfrac{\text{DHAP}}{\text{Ga-3-P}} = 25$	
Triose phosphate dehydrogenase	140,000	DPN$^+$	Iodoacetate	$\dfrac{\text{Ga-3-P} \times \text{DPN}^+ \times \text{P}_i}{\text{1,3-diPglyc} \times \text{DPNH}} = 1$	$-1{,}420$
Phosphoglycerate kinase		Mg^{2+}		$\dfrac{\text{3-P-glyc} \times \text{ATP}}{\text{1,3-diPglyc} \times \text{ADP}} = 3{,}000$	
Phosphoglycero-mutase	60,000	Mg^{2+}, 2,3-diphosphoglycerate		$\dfrac{\text{3-PGA}}{\text{2-PGA}} = 10$	
Enolase	87,000	Mg^{2+}, Mn^{2+}	F$^-$, PP$_i$, Ca^{2+}	$\dfrac{\text{2-PGA}}{\text{PEP}} = 0.22$	

Enzyme	Molecular weight	Cofactors / activators	Inhibitors	Equilibrium constant	ΔG
Pyruvate kinase	230,000	Mg^{2+}, K^+, fructose-1,6-P_2	Ca^{2+}		
Lactate dehydrogenase	140,000	DPN^+	Oxamate	$\dfrac{\text{Lactate} \times DPN^+}{\text{Pyr} \times DPNH} = 3 \times 10^5$	
Hexokinase glucokinase	96,000	Mg^{2+}	Glucose 6-P	$\dfrac{\text{Glucose-6-P} \times ADP}{\text{Glucose} \times ATP} = 630$	
Glycerolphosphate dehydrogenase	78,000	DPN^+	Dihydroxy-acetone-P fructose-1,6-P_2	$\dfrac{\text{Dihydroxyacetone-P} \times H^+ \times DPNH}{\text{L-Glycerol-3-P} \times DPN^+} = 1 \times 10^{-12}$ M	
Alcohol dehydrogenase	84,000	DPN^+	Ethanol DPN^+ acetaldehyde DPNH	$\dfrac{\text{Acetaldehyde} \times DPNH \times H^+}{\text{Ethanol} \times DPN^+} = 8 \times 10^{-12}$ M	
Pyruvate carboxylase	650,000	Biotin, acetyl-S-CoA Mg^{2+}	Oxalate 5' AMP 3' AMP CTP, d CTP GTP, UTP, ITP TTP, CDP, CMP		−5000 cal
Phosphoenolpyruvate carboxykinase	73,300	Acetyl-S-CoA, Mg^{2+}	HCO_3^-; GDP GMP	$\dfrac{IDP \times PEP \times CO_2}{ITP \times \text{oxaloacetate}} = 0.372$ M	
Fructose-1,6-di-phosphatase		Mg^{2+}, ATP	F^-, AMP	Hydrolysis favored	

TABLE A.4 PROPERTIES OF THE ENZYMES AND REACTIONS OF GLYCOLYSIS, GLUCONEOGENESIS, GLYCOGENESIS, LIPID HYDROLYSIS, β-OXIDATION, AND FATTY ACID SYNTHESIS (continued)

Enzyme	Molecular Weight	Coenzyme or Activators	Inhibitors	Equilibrium Constant (approx.) pH 7.4	$\Delta G°$ (cal mole^{-1})
Glucose-6-phosphatase	350,000	Mg^{2+}	Citrate	Hydrolysis favored	
UTP uridyl transferase or ADP adenyl transferase		Mg^{2+}		$\dfrac{PP_i \times UDPG}{UTP \times glucose\text{-}1\text{-}P} = 0.3$	
Glycogen synthase	~260,000 (D form)	Glucose 6-P	UDP, UMP, ATP, ADP, AMP	Synthesis favored	−3,200
Phospholipase A	30,000–35,000			Hydrolysis favored	
Phospholipase C	100,000	Ca^{2+}		Hydrolysis favored	
Phospholipase D		Dodecylsulfate phosphatidic acid Triphosphoinositide monoacetyl-P	Cetyltrimethyl-ammonium bromide	Hydrolysis favored	
Lipase	40,000–200,000	Bile salts Fatty acids		Hydrolysis favored	
Phosphatidate phosphatase			Mg^{2+}		
Thiokinase	30,000–60,000	Flavin		$\dfrac{AMP \times PP_i \times acyl\text{-}S\text{-}CoA}{ATP \times fatty\ acid \times CoA} = 1.5$	
Acyl-S-CoA dehydrogenase	220,000		Crotonoyl-S-CoA	$\dfrac{Crotonoyl\text{-}S\text{-}CoA \times reduced\ pyocyanine}{Butyryl\text{-}S\text{-}CoA \times pyocyanine} = 0.22$	
Enoylhydratase	210,000			$\dfrac{Crotonoyl\text{-}S\text{-}CoA \times H_2O}{L(+)\text{-}3\text{-}Hydroxybutyryl\text{-}S\text{-}CoA} = 16.2$	
3-Hydroxy acyl-S-CoA dehydrogenase		DPN		$\dfrac{3\text{-}Oxyacyl\text{-}S\text{-}CoA \times DPNH \times H^+}{L(+)\text{-}Hydroxyacyl\text{-}S\text{-}CoA \times DPN^+} =$ (3-hydroxybutyryl-S-CoA) 6.3×10^{-10} M (3-hydroxyhexanoyl-S-CoA) 2.5×10^{-11} M	

Enzyme	Turnover number	Cofactors/activators	Inhibitors/substrates	Equilibrium
Acetyl-S-CoA acetyl-transferase				$\dfrac{CoA \times acetoacetyl\text{-}S\text{-}CoA}{(Acetyl\text{-}S\text{-}CoA)^2} = 2 \times 10^{-5}$ M
Acetyl-S-CoA carboxylase	540,000–1,800,000	Citrate Isocitrate	Fatty acyl-S-CoA esters	Essentially irreversible
Acetoacetyl-S-CoA reductase		TPN		Essentially irreversible
Enoyl-S-CoA hydratase	210,000			$\dfrac{Crotonoyl\text{-}S\text{-}CoA \times H_2O}{L(+)\text{-}3\text{-}Hydroxybutyryl\text{-}S\text{-}CoA} = 16.2$
Pyruvate decarboxylase	175,000–1,000,000	Thiamine		Essentially irreversible
Citrate synthase	86,000		Fluoroacetyl-S-CoA Fatty acyl-S-CoA	$\dfrac{Acetyl\text{-}S\text{-}CoA \times H_2O \times oxaloacetate}{Citrate \times CoA} = 1.2 \times 10^{-4}$ M
Citrate (isocitrate) hydrolyase		Iron	Fluorocitrate	Citrate 90.9% cis-Aconitate 2.9% Isocitrate 6.2%
Isocitrate dehydrogenase	300,000–400,000	DPN AMP (yeast or *A. niger*) ADP (heart)	ATP, DPNH (heart)	
Isocitrate dehydrogenase	61,000	TPN	Isocitrate	$\dfrac{2\text{-}Ketoglut \times CO_2 \times TPNH}{threo\text{-}D\text{-}s\text{-}isocit \times TPN^+} = 7.7 \times 10^{-1}$ M
Succinate dehydrogenase	200,000	Iron Flavin	Fumarate Malonate	
Fumarate hydratase (fumarase)	194,000		Adipate Succinate Glutarate Malonate d-Tartrate Mesaconate d-Malate Citrate trans-Aconitate and others	$\dfrac{Fumarate}{L\text{-}Malate} = 0.23$
Malate dehydrogenase	52,000–148,000	DPN	Oxaloacetate Dicarboxylic Hydroxy acids	$\dfrac{Oxaloacetate \times DPNH \times H^+}{L\text{-}Malate \times DPN^+} = 6.4 \times 10^{-13}$ M

TABLE A.5 ENDOCRINE GLANDS AND THEIR HORMONE SECRETIONS

Gland	Hormone	Action
Adrenal cortex	Steroids Aldosterone Corticosterone Cortisol	H_2O and salt metabolism; gluconeogenesis and other metabolic controls; inflammation and immunity; hypersensitivity; circulatory maintenance
Adrenal medulla	Epinephrine and Norepinephrine	Control of metabolism, blood vessel tone, respiration
Gastrointestinal tract	Gastrin Secretin Pancreozymin Cholecystokinin	HCl secretion Pancreatic juice secretion Pancreatic enzyme secretion Gall bladder contraction
Corpus luteum	Steroids Progesterone Relaxin	Uterine preparation for ovum; pregnancy maintenance; breast development Relaxation of pelvis in preparation for delivery
Ovary	Steroids Estrone and Estradiol	Normal menstruation and secondary sexual development
Testis	Steroid Testosterone	Normal sexual function and secondary sexual development
Seminal vesicle	Prostaglandins	Regulate metabolism and blood vessel tone
Pancreas	Insulin Glucagon	Synthesis and storage of carbohydrate, lipid and protein Glycogenolysis and lipolysis
Parathyroid	Parathormone (PTH)	Ca^{2+} and P metabolism—blood levels of Ca^{2+} ↑
Anterior pituitary (adenohypophysis)	Prolactin (lactogenic hormone) Adrenocorticotrophin (ACTH) Thyrotrophin (TSH) Somatotrophin (growth hormone) Luteinizing hormone (LH or ICSH) Follicle stimulating hormone (FSH)	Breast development and milk secretion; development of corpus luteum Adrenal cortical steroid production; lipolysis Thyroid hormone production; lipolysis Growth; control of metabolism Luteinization; progesterone production development of interstitial cells in testis; androgen production Follicle development in ovaries and ovulation, stimulates development of seminiferous tubules in testis
Posterior pituitary (neurohypophysis)	Oxytocin Vasopressin	Uterine contraction; milk ejection H_2O reabsorption in kidney tubules; blood vessel contraction
Intermediate lobe of pituitary	Melanocyte stimulating hormone (MSH)	Pigment spread
Pineal	Melatonin (5-hydroxytryptophol) Adrenoglomerulotropin	Pigment aggregation Aldosterone secretion
Thymus	Thymosin	Stimulation of lymph cell development
Thyroid	Thyroxin (T_4) Triiodothyronine (T_3) Calcitonin	Control of metabolic rate and oxygen consumption Ca^{2+} and P metabolism, blood levels of Ca^{2+} ↓
Placenta	Chorionic Gonadotrophin	Similar to pituitary Gonadotrophins

TABLE A.6   REGULATORY METABOLITES—MACRO AND MICRO

Macro ($\sim 10^{-3} - 10^{-5}\ M$)	Micro ($\sim 10^{-5} - 10^{-8}\ M$)
Glucose-6-P	3',5'-cyclic AMP
Fructose-1,6-diphosphate	3',5'-cyclic GMP
1,3-Diphosphoglycerate	Prostaglandins
Citrate	
Acetyl-S-CoA	
AMP, ATP, ADP	
GTP, UDP, and other nucleotides	
DPN+, DPNH + H+	
Fatty acids	
Fatty acyl-S-CoA	
Amino acids	

INDEX